LOVE IN THE AGE OF AUTISM

LOVE IN THE AGE OF AUTISM

NAVIGATING A JOYFUL
AND ROMANTIC MARRIAGE
IN THE FACE OF ADVERSITY

GAYLE DELONG,
JONATHAN ROSE, AND
JENNIFER ROSE

FHB | FIRST HILL BOOKS

FIRST HILL BOOKS
An imprint of Wimbledon Publishing Company
www.anthempress.com

This edition first published in UK and USA 2025
by FIRST HILL BOOKS
75–76 Blackfriars Road, London SE1 8HA, UK
or PO Box 9779, London SW19 7ZG, UK
and
244 Madison Ave #116, New York, NY 10016, USA

British Library Cataloguing-in-Publication Data
A catalogue record for this book is available from the British Library.

Library of Congress Cataloging-in-Publication Data: 2025931127
A catalog record for this book has been requested.

ISBN-13: 978-1-83999-431-9 (Pbk)
ISBN-10: 1-83999-431-2 (Pbk)

Cover Credit: Jonathan Rose

Clockwise from upper right: Gayle, Flora, Jennifer, and Jonathan

This title is also available as an e-book.

CONTENTS

PREFACE

Gayle DeLong was an outspoken "Warrior Mom"—a label that she wore as a badge of great pride. She fought relentlessly to lift the burdens of autism from her two daughters, Jennifer and Flora, and from the ever-growing population of autistic and vaccine-injured individuals throughout the world. By profession, she taught international business and finance, but she adapted her formidable statistical skills to tackle vaccine-safety issues, which (she decided) were more important than analyzing bank mergers. She was absolutely fearless and impervious to personal attacks. Her work was halted only by death: she lost her battle with breast cancer in early 2022.

She was also the most wonderful thing that ever happened to me, her surviving husband. I could never look into her bright, sparkling eyes without feeling absolutely happy. Doing the most mundane domestic chores with her—Gayle called it "playing house"—somehow filled me with spiritual joy. She was beautifully romantic, though she preferred the word "mushy." To our neighbors we were known as the couple who always held hands on our evening walks, as if that was something unusual, though it seemed perfectly natural to us.

This, then, is a story with three interwoven themes—love, autism, and cancer—and how the first helped our family endure the other two. It reproduces (with some editing) a diary that Gayle kept during her final two years, 2020 and 2021, fully intended for publication. She titled it "Musings," and she typically typed entries into her computer first thing in the morning. She left me free to read it, but I did not do so until she was on her deathbed. Then I (a professional historian) realized it was a powerful and revealing documentary, reflecting what Gayle and thousands of autism moms like her were thinking and experiencing. It was also a journal of the plague years, chronicling the devastating impact of the Covid lockdowns on special needs families, as the services they desperately needed were shut down. I promised Gayle that

I would see the manuscript through to publication. Shortly after her death, I discovered nine pocket diaries that she had kept from 2007 to 2013, recording the effects of treatments on Jennifer (who will receive the royalties for this volume) and Flora, and these are also incorporated into this book.

Love in the Age of Autism is radically unlike anything offered by the mainstream media. It is an unflinchingly honest account of what autism can do to the young people it afflicts and their family members. If you cannot deal with the realities of autism and prefer the complacent feel-good fantasies of *The Good Doctor*, read no further. Emotionally fragile autistic individuals may find this book too disturbing. Among other issues, it frankly confronts a taboo subject. Domestic violence perpetrated by autistic young people is shockingly common. Drs. Stephen Kanne and Micah Mazurek of the Thompson Center for Autism and Neurodevelopmental Disorders at the University of Missouri investigated 1,380 children with Autism Spectrum Disorder and "found that 56% were engaging in aggressive behaviors towards caregivers, while a smaller number (32%) engaged in these behaviors towards non-caregivers. Similarly, 68% of the children had previously behaved aggressively towards caregivers and 49% towards non-caregivers. These are extremely high rates, especially when compared with those for people who have intellectual disability (ID) but not autism. Aggressive behavior has been documented in only 7–11% of these individuals."[1] Gayle DeLong offers a detailed case study written by a victim of such violence.

But this is, first of all, a love story, and it begins on that supremely happy note.

---

1 https://www.iancommunity.org/cs/simons_simplex_community/aggression_and_asd.

TOGETHERNESS

It pays to advertise.

We met through a personal ad. It was 1994, the predigital era, so I inserted a miniautobiography in a paper-and-ink newsletter called "Academic Companions." In response Gayle had to type out a letter and mail it. With a stamp. I never saved the ad, and I only remember describing myself as "unmaterialistic, uncool, unhip, unattached" and "lackadaisically Jewish." But I did save her letter, and later had it framed and hung in our bedroom:

September 26, 1994

Dear Professor,

Your ad in the "Academic Companions" list is amusing and refreshing. You seem to be content.

I'm a Ph.D. student in international business and finance. I hope to finish in about two years and then to teach. Finding the right pursuit in life took time—I'm 36—but I'd rather take time and find something fulfilling. I'm from a small town in Pennsylvania [Lancaster], but I enjoy the adventure that New York offers.

I'd like to meet you; if you feel the same, please call […].

She was studying at NYU, so we arranged to meet at a sushi joint on LaGuardia Place. Here is what she recollected on our 25th anniversary: "He made me feel comfortable in his life from the very first moment we met. At the Japanese restaurant in the Village near NYU. 'Gayle!' he greeted me, as though we had known each other for a thousand years." And I suppose, in a sense, we had.

New York City in the 1990s now looks like a lost lovers' paradise. The cultural opportunities for dating were limitless, nothing was locked down, and the subway to Gayle's bachelorette pad in Brooklyn was safe. I could take her out to

1

a Lebanese restaurant and walk over to the Brooklyn promenade, the perfect spot to make a pass (successful). Looking out at the Lower Manhattan skyline, Gayle asked me what word it brought to mind. "Home," I said. As a country girl from Lancaster, she said it reminded her of another four-letter word. She never adjusted to the incessant street clamor of New York, which for me was my mother's heartbeat.

On one of our first dates I took her to see the film *Vanya on 42nd Street*. Chekhov tore my heart out, but she could not comprehend why members of the same family would work so hard at making each other miserable. (She hadn't yet met my family.) We then walked over to a Soho gallery exhibition of Roy Lichtenstein, the pop artist who spoofed comic book panels. I was embarrassed when the paintings turned out to be female nudes, but Gayle relished it all. She cheerfully admitted that she loved the images in *Penthouse* magazine. She had lived for a while in Denmark, and I still have her anthology of Danish erotica (what better way to learn the language?). When I first visited her apartment, I noticed a huge portrait of Albert Einstein on her kitchen wall, and I correctly deduced that she had the hots for smart Jewish guys. And when I gobbled up her hors d'oeuvres, she concluded that all my appetites were healthy. Not long after our first date, in a solidly American spirit of individual initiative, she invited herself up to my East Village apartment for dinner and postprandial sex.

Afterward she had some misgivings. Perhaps things had moved too far, too fast. As a doctoral student she was about to prepare for comprehensive examinations, a rite of passage that demanded months of intensive study. I realized that she valued her personal autonomy, and admired her for that. So I prudently suggested that we dial the relationship down a notch. We could continue to see each other as friends while putting sex on hold. I would stand ready to resume amorous relations whenever she was ready, but I would leave it to her to give the green light.

That gave us a chance to know each other better, and what we learned we liked. Gayle was stunned to discover that her penultimate boyfriend and I had attended the same college (Princeton) at the same time (Class of 1974). But whereas he never ceased to brag about his Ivy Leaguery, my attitude toward Princeton was Don't Ask, Don't Tell. Gayle was no less shocked when I suggested we catch a matinee at the theater the following Sunday. "I'd love to," she assured me, "but you do know what's happening next Sunday?" I had no idea, and I feared I had forgotten something terribly important. She finally had to tell me that it was the SuperBowl, and I had to admit that I didn't even know which teams were playing. If she hadn't been preoccupied with her comps, she might have proposed to me on the spot. We did see Jackie Mason's one-man Broadway show, where he performed the kind of ethnic humor that is today illegal. But 1995 was a more tolerant and enlightened era. And Gayle was warming up to me, as she recalled in one of her last diary entries:

> I was thinking about the moment I fell in love with him. We were waiting for Jackie Mason to come on stage & Jonathan described an event as a "bacchanal" just like in a little-known Don McLean song. I thought, "Woah. This guy is smart & fun & he seems to like me." He smelled good, too. Fresh & clean.

Once her comps were behind her, Gayle was ready to serve notice that she wanted full-throttle sex. It was a bitterly cold Valentine's Day. We had dined at a dreadful Chinese restaurant and walked back to the subway. But before she could put in her request, I saw her shivering on the platform and I blurted out, "You must be frigid."

Quite the contrary. Once, on the way to her apartment, I picked up an alternative weekly that ran a sex advice column, where a young woman wrote that she had six orgasms a night. Let's just say that we were not impressed. After making love Gayle was never shy about asking for seconds (or thirds).

Then one afternoon, as function of normal wear and tear, my condom broke. I was embarrassed and apologetic, but she said—and I'm never going to forget these words—"I could think of worse things than to be impregnated by you."

Wow. You didn't often hear that from New York single women, but it made me realize that Gayle was ready to build something permanent and marvelous with me. I immediately began plotting to propose to her. Step one: Cancel all dating services. Step two: Invite her to the family Passover seder, where she could check out my relatives (and their quirks). Step three: Find a cozy little bed and breakfast in New Hope, Pennsylvania. We dined at a romantic restaurant, where nervousness made me devour several dinner rolls, though it was the last day of Passover. "There's only so much I can do for my religion," I explained. Then I got down on my knee and proposed. Gayle understandably guarded her independence, and asked for time to think it over. The next day we were browsing a used bookstore, when I grabbed her hand and whispered, "I love holding your hand." "I almost agreed to marry you at that moment," she later recalled, "but it took yet another two days. So sorry."

Significantly, the theme song that Gayle chose for our wedding was Cole Porter's "Don't Fence Me In." We were both confirmed individualists, which may explain why we took so long to find marriage partners. (I was 42, she was almost 37.) Individualists can be picky, but they recognize each other, and they can be passionately loyal. As long as you respected Gayle's right to think for herself, she would stand by you and love you no matter what.

Before I met her, Gayle had worked for the General Accounting Office in Washington, where she learned to loathe bureaucracy. In this poem she wrote in 1991 we see Gayle the incorrigible maverick, who always distrusted authority, bucked the system, and insisted on doing things her way. It was a remarkable anticipation of how she would later fight autism and cancer:

The Replaceable Poem

Work at the government numbs creative brains.
It makes normal humans ask, "Am I insane?"

How can institutions a mind so thoroughly trash,
And destroy hearty souls with a mighty crash?

The hierarchy divides, brings animosity:
BOSS versus STAFF. Result? Mediocrity.

The treatment is shabby, respect is unknown.
Each person is a unit, each body a clone.

Forget about humor: Smiles must be fought.
You see, if you laugh, you're not a robot.

And they cheer themselves for hirings diverse.
Yet original thoughts are to them a curse.

You are different, new ideas from you flow.
You test assumptions, disrupt the status quo.

At first they berate you—perhaps out of fear?—
Then finally ignore you: Be thankful, my dear.

To those who are new—it's a simple case!—
Fit in or perish: you're easy to replace.

Gayle was living proof of the principle that a girl who enjoys a loving relationship with her father will become a woman who enjoys loving relationships with men. George DeLong was a poor Pennsylvania farm boy who enlisted in the Navy and fought at Pearl Harbor. He was on board the USS *Oklahoma* when it was torpedoed and capsized. He survived in an air pocket for 36 hours before a hole was cut in the hull and he was rescued. Most of the sailors on the *Oklahoma* never made it out alive. From that point on he relished every day of life as an unexpected bonus. Each morning he would ask, "What great and wonderful things are going to happen today?" He improved his mind belowdecks by reading Baruch Spinoza, a philosopher so freethinking that he was excommunicated by the scandalized Amsterdam Jewish community. That independence of mind and irrepressible optimism he conveyed to his daughter, with whom he spent long hours conversing in divey bars, as any devoted father should. A Democratic politician in Republican Lancaster County, he never won elective office. He was a flag-waving liberal, an endangered species today. He loved the country that had given him so much opportunity (including attending college on the GI Bill) and he wanted others to have the chances he had. In the 1960s his family was harassed for hosting an African exchange student, and he was involved in the National Conference of Christians and Jews, an organization that fought anti-Semitism. He also had liberal ideas about sex: I found on his bookshelf a paperback of Eustace Chesser's *Love without Fear: How to Achieve Sex Happiness in Marriage*, a pre-Kinsey guide to marital fulfillment. All that contributed to making Gayle the marvelous woman I knew.

Our daughter Jennifer arrived less than a year (but more than nine months) after the wedding. I was in the delivery room, and (a bit squeamishly) I cut her umbilical cord. I emailed our friends and family: "Jonathan Rose was seen last night in a Greenwich Village hotspot with his arms around two dynamite chicks. The scene was the maternity ward at St. Vincent's Hospital. Daughter Jennifer, a leggy redhead, arrived fashionably late. Mother Gayle is beaming [...]."

As I walked home to our apartment very early that morning, I was approached by an engaging young man who persuaded me that he knew my mother. Having established that opening, he explained that he needed thirty dollars because his car had run out of gas. The rational half of my brain was fully aware that this was a scam, but the other half told me: *What does it matter? I'm a father.* And I gave him the thirty bucks. We didn't have much money then, but it was a trivial price to pay for a newborn child. "That's the most romantic thing I've ever heard," Gayle said when I told her, "and if you ever do that again, I'll divorce you."

Gayle was still wobbly from childbirth when (two weeks later) we celebrated our first anniversary at the Oak Room at the Algonquin Hotel. There I began a tradition that would continue throughout our marriage: I got down on my knee and proposed to her all over again. (A waiter asked if I had lost something under the table.)

On weekends we took Jennifer in her stroller to East Village bruncheries, where waitresses with fifteen earrings would coo over her, and she would offer her bottle to derelicts in the street. Academic couples usually find it difficult to locate jobs near to each other, but Gayle landed a post at Baruch College, the business school of the City University of New York, practically on our doorstep and just one hour from my college (Drew University). Baruch had always served the children of immigrants, including my father back in the 1930s, and he was immensely proud that his daughter-in-law was teaching at his alma mater.

Gayle was adamant that there would be no Offspring Number 2 until we moved to the suburbs, even if that meant commuting into the city. So we found a house in Morristown, near my job. For the first time in my life, there was no subway station nearby, and I couldn't call the super if something needed fixing. I quickly learned to love suburban domestic tranquility, and marveled at the delightful normality of it all. We had a kitchen picture window looking out on a leafy backyard with a rivulet marking our property line. A K-2 school was directly across the street. A short walk brought us to the police station, where the chief was Andy Griffith. Gayle asked him about the crime rate. "What's crime?" he smirked. We connected with neighborhood parents, and we took the girls to visit their various cousins. It had taken Gayle and me a long time to settle down, and now we finally felt that we were on track. Every night, after we put the girls to bed, Gayle would propose a well-earned and immensely enjoyed reward: "A drink and a screw?"

But adversity is the real test of a marriage, and in our New Jersey Eden we were about to be confronted with a disorder we had scarcely heard of. In Manhattan there had been a few warning signs, which we ignored. We sent Jennifer to a daycare where she got along splendidly with everyone, including the other white kid, but the staff advised us that she was spacing out at intervals. We brushed that aside as insignificant. In Morristown we found a new pediatrician who suspected autism, but we were incredulous. Jennifer was a very huggy child, and we had bought into the stereotype that autistic children don't want to be touched. However, Gayle's sister noticed that Jenny was not developing speech on schedule. Shortly after the arrival of her younger sister, Flora, we had Jennifer tested by a neurologist, and he confirmed the autism diagnosis. When we returned to our car, we broke down and sobbed. Was our brief shining moment of normal life over? Would we ever be able to take our girls to a restaurant?

At first Flora seemed perfectly normal and healthy, with bright smiles and good eye contact. We kept a very close eye on her to see if autism would repeat itself. Very gradually, it did. Every year we had a holiday family picture taken, so we have hard photographic evidence of the change. By increments, Flora's eyes became ever more remote and wandered from the camera. On her fifth birthday she received her second MMR shot, and I distinctly noticed "She's regressing," but Gayle couldn't stand to hear it, and we did not immediately associate the two events.

We felt utterly helpless as our children descended ever deeper into autism. There was no prescribed treatment except for Applied Behavior Analysis, a kind of Pavlovian conditioning which only bored our girls and accomplished nothing. As the father of the family, I felt it was my responsibility to keep my cool when everyone else was losing theirs, but one day in April 2005 I broke down in front of my own father. "Are Jenny and Flora ever going to be able to hold a job, live independently, get married, raise children?" I wailed (uncharacteristically).

My dad, startled but eager to help, referred me to the *New York Times Book Review*, which had favorably treated a new and relevant book: David Kirby's *Evidence of Harm*. We ordered a copy, and when I went to Washington on academic business, I read it on the Metroliner. As soon as I arrived at the hotel I phoned Gayle and said decisively, "It's the mercury."

For that was Kirby's theory. A steady rise in the incidence of autism, coinciding with a large increase (after 1986) in the number of mandated childhood vaccinations, inevitably raised the question of whether the two were connected. A great many autism parents said that their children had regressed into autism shortly after receiving shots, but most doctors dismissed these reports as coincidental and anecdotal. In November 2002 the *New York Times Magazine* put forward a "Not-So-Crackpot Autism Theory," suggesting that the cause might be thimerosal, a mercury-based preservative used in several vaccines.[1] That hypothesis was worked out at length in *Evidence of Harm*, which was sympathetically discussed by Polly Morrice in the April 17, 2005 *New York Times Book Review*, under the arresting headline "What Caused the Autism Epidemic?" Kirby and

---

1 Arthur Allen, "The Not-So-Crackpot Autism Theory," *New York Times Magazine*, November 10, 2002, 66–69.

Morrice stopped short of explicitly endorsing the thimerosal hypothesis, but they clearly considered it a compelling theory worth investigating, and both suggested that parents might be better equipped to treat autism than doctors. The Centers for Disease Control (CDC) had funded a study that seemed to exonerate thimerosal, but Morrice saw a possible "smoking gun" in a statistical analysis performed by SafeMinds (an autism parents group), which "contended that the government analyses of such data were flawed in a way that obscured or eliminated the original findings of statistically significant risks." Morrice also highlighted the example of Lyn and Tommy Redwood, who "struggled to obtain a diagnosis for their son Will, who at 17 months started to lose his language and withdraw socially. When Will turned 4, his latest 'expert' doctor ran out of options: 'Why don't you just take him fishing?'" The Redwoods took charge of their son's treatment, resorting to chelation (which can remove mercury from the body), and Will showed remarkable improvement. "If one certain conclusion can be drawn from 'Evidence of Harm,'" Morrice concluded, "it's that Will's parents made the right decision about going fishing."[2]

If this theory was correct, then autism had been caused (inadvertently) by doctors and public health experts, who never find it easy to acknowledge iatrogenic diseases. Even more explosively, Morrice noted that UK doctor Andrew Wakefield (then little known in America) had "argued that autism was an immune-system disorder brought on by live measles virus in the MMR vaccine." That in fact is a common misreading of Wakefield's notorious 1998 *Lancet* article, in which he and his coauthors had only suggested an autism-MMR link as a hypothesis, admittedly unproven but worth further investigation. However, the MMR contained no thimerosal, raising the possibility that the fault might not lie solely in an additive (which could easily be removed from vaccines) but also in the vaccine itself. And if *that* theory was correct, then the whole medical paradigm of vaccination was in jeopardy.

Two months after the Morrice review, on June 25, the *Times* sharply reversed course, a move that involved some linguistic maneuvering. The April review had been subtitled "the battle between the medical establishment and parents," but nobody likes establishments, so the June article (on the front page) respun the story with the headline "On Autism's Cause, It's Parents vs. Research," suggesting that parents did no research. The article cited (dismissively) a few studies supporting a connection between thimerosal and autism,

2 Polly Morrice, "What Caused the Autism Epidemic?" *New York Times Book Review*, April 17, 2005, F20.

but for the most part it relied on assurances from government agencies, "prestigious" medical organizations, and "experts." The *Times* reported that "hundreds of doctors list their names on a Web site endorsing chelation to treat autism, even though experts say that no evidence supports its use with that disorder." But that statement raised troubling questions in the minds of thoughtful readers. These "experts" were unnamed, so how could we verify their expertise? If hundreds of doctors reported positive results from chelation, why did they not count as experts? Is "expert" a linguistic badge that journalists award to favored individuals to give them an artificial air of authority? Certainly the article never applied that label to parents, who were portrayed as emotional, irrational, submerged in "scientific illiteracy," "desperate," and even potentially violent. The *Times* reported that the CDC had called on the FBI to protect them from autism parents, and had instructed its employees "how to respond if pies are thrown in their faces." No pies or bombs were thrown (parents of handicapped children can rarely find time to hatch assassination plots), yet public health officials did face a real threat. As one of them said, "That's really scary for us because if science doesn't count, how do we make decisions?"[3]

Parents were not rejecting science, but they were staking a claim to being scientific themselves—and that, for the "experts," was scarier still. The "Parents vs. Research" slogan therefore aimed to reestablish the authority of medical authorities, which had drastically eroded with the rise of alternative medicine; to assert that the words of doctors and laypeople would no longer carry equal weight; and to affirm that "science" was the exclusive property of professionals, where parents must not trespass. But the parents radically rejected all of this exclusionary language. As one angry letter to the editor responded, "These children *are* the evidence, and their parents *are* the experts."[4]

These parents were ahead of their time, the vanguard of a "citizen scientist" movement which is now increasingly accepted as a partner in medical research (as illustrated by Amy Dockser Marcus in *We the Scientists: How a Daring Team of Parents and Doctors Forged a New Path for Medicine*). The gross mismanagement of the Covid pandemic by public health "experts" has glaringly revealed the failings of top-down bureaucratized corporate-driven medicine and given impetus to a new treatment model where parents and patients collaborate with physicians. The PubMed database now enables laypeople

---

3 Gardiner Harris and Anahad O'Connor, "On Autism's Cause, Its Parents vs. Research," *New York Times,* June 25, 2005, A1.
4 Belinda Aggarwal, Letter to the Editor, *New York Times,* July 1, 2005, A16.

to thoroughly research the scientific literature on any medical subject, to the point where, on a particular topic, they may be more "expert" than their doctors. Gayle made exhaustive use of PubMed when she dealt with autism and (later) cancer. "Democracy requires a very deep level of citizens constantly trying to understand one another's problems," explains Prof. Philip Kitcher of Columbia University. "So does science." And on this front, advancing human knowledge, Gayle was a pioneer.

(That said, nothing in this book should be taken as a recommendation for any kind of medical treatment. We are simply offering a historical record of the treatments we used for our girls. And while we were convinced that adverse reactions to vaccination could cause autism, we never ruled out other possible contributing causes, such as toxins in the general environment.)

We had already begun chelation for both girls, under the supervision of Dr. Stuart Freedenfeld of Stockton Family Practice. Starting at the end of 2007 and continuing through summer 2013, Gayle recorded our daughters' responses to treatment in a series of pocket diaries. These are not just medical documents: they are a record of the hopes and disappointments of autism parents.

Flora had good days and bad days. We naturally took the good days as signs that the treatments might be working. She seemed to comprehend details about *Charlotte's Web* ("Something's clicking [...]) [12/29/07]. We were amused by tricks of language while she was seated on the toilet: (Me: "You're not doing anything." Flora: "I am doing anything.") [12/30/07]. And when Flora simply smiled at Gayle when she picked her up at school, her mom was elated ("Oh, bliss!") [1/2/08]. One teacher was "thrilled about Flora's progress—complete & prompt answers, better eye contact, talking back." [1/10/08]. Before she saw Dr. Freedenfeld, Flora would cry through the night in bed. It turned out that, like many autistic individuals, she was suffering from gastrointestinal distress. After a change in diet, she slept so soundly that for a moment her mother thought she had died.

At first Jennifer seemed the more difficult of the two: "Jenny had altercation in Italian class. Disappointed in grade. I wonder how much teachers aren't telling me/us. Did I mention I hate autism?" But already her language skills were clearly improving. In 2006 she began her brilliant literary career by producing *The Backpack News*, a personal newsletter which she distributed at school. (She was distantly related to I. F. Stone, a controversial journalist who also published his own newsletter.) And in early 2008, on one of our family evening walks, she looked up and spontaneously asked, "What's that? Where are the stars?" [1/11/08]. A few days later "Flora seems to be slipping," but "Jenny [was] engaging in conversation. Different topics" [1/15/08]. These included the 2008 presidential race, where our family supported Obama in the primaries [1/27/08]. "I loathe Clinton and her CDC," Gayle wrote [1/31/08]. "We're finally getting to know the real Jenny—a really nice kid!" [2/4/08]. But in fact there were two Jennys, and one was still prone to fearsome melt-downs. "This past week was hell as was last week. Daily reports of Jenny's misbehavior. UNTIL […] Jonathan & I spoke to principal et al. Let them know we know Jenny's civil rights" [3/14/08]. On the other hand, Jenny was a "GREAT hostess" when her cousins visited [4/26/08]. "Jenny talking about so many different topics these days, asking questions pertaining to the conversation. FABULOUS!" [5/11/08].

Now Flora seemed stalled, obsessing over old calendars ("We have a long way to go.") [2/1/08]. Like some of the intellectually handicapped, when she was given a date in the remote past, she immediately knew the day of the week, but acquiring useful skills was another question entirely. Dr. Freedenfeld was "pessimistic about Flora," Gayle wrote. "I'm not ready to give up. There are some flickers […]" [4/8/08]. "Flora isn't responding to Prednisone. Damn. Damn. Damn" [4/18/08]. "Flora so out of it. I really wanted to have a conversation with her for my 50th birthday. It would take a miracle for that to happen" [5/6/08]. In the long run, there would be momentary ups and downs, but no net progress. We would seize on the good days, only to realize during the bad days that we had been grasping at straws, and then we would once again look for any positive signs. For both of us, and Gayle especially, this meant the constant stress of hopes raised and hopes dashed in an endless cycle. "Yesterday hated my life. Today I love my life. Go figure" [4/24/08]. Even more concisely, Gayle expressed what every autism parent feels: "Hope, anger, despair, then hope again" [7/28/08].

In June 2008, Gayle visited her mother in Lancaster. "She showed Jenny a picture of me giving Mayor Coe a 'Pearl Harbor' pearl in 1965. I was a year younger than Flora. She looks so much like me. I lost it. Mom held me as I bawled. I promised Mom I'm not giving up yet. I promise Flora, I will never give up" [6/29/08]. And the cycle of elation and heartbreak continued. "VERY slow w/homework. A VERY SICK LITTLE GIRL. I just want this nightmare to be over" [1/28/09]. "Woke up in middle of night & made chirping sounds. I went to her room and found a wide-eyed angel. We cuddled. I told her I loved her so much and she smiled the biggest most beautiful and natural smile I have ever seen from her" [3/3/09].

We tried every imaginable treatment for Flora. Some of them may have worked for other patients, but none of them really worked for her. Eventually I concluded that it was all futile: the damage done to her was irreversible. I let

Gayle try anything, however outlandish, as long as it didn't do any harm, yet I worried that the endless string of failures were taking a heavy emotional toll on her. I tried to tell her that she shouldn't exhaust herself waging a hopeless battle, and that was practically the only instance in our marriage when she became seriously angry at me, accusing me of "giving up on Flora." She was somewhat mollified when I said that we might give up on particular treatments or particular schools, but we would never give up on finding the best possible living environment for Flora. And I drew an analogy to flying in an airliner with a small child: if the cabin suddenly depressurizes, you put your oxygen mask on first. If your child momentarily blacks out, you can revive her, but if you black out, you're both goners. That's a message for all autism moms: it may seem contrary to all your maternal instincts, but your health comes first.

When parents receive an autism diagnosis for one (or more) of their children, the responses of friends and family can be stunningly different. Some will step right up to the plate and sincerely offer to help, but others will withdraw. We lost some friends and gained new ones. The new friends were usually other autism parents, but not always. Terri O'Brien, our next-door neighbor, became a surrogate grandmother to Jenny and Flora, and her extended family was also wonderfully supportive. Yet it was difficult to find partners for playdates, even for higher-functioning Jennifer.

By October 2008 Gayle's relations with her family were starting to fray. Her father, who had been her biggest fan, had died in 2002. We were celebrating Gayle's 50th birthday at the home of her sister, who now began to restrict Flora's movements and insist that one of the older children watch her. "I was a social outcast as a kid," Gayle later recalled, "and it hurt to see my own daughter as though she was not a member. I wanted my family to know how difficult it was to raise two girls with autism. Every day was a challenge, with some days being more onerous than others. So, I explained that some days I felt like taking one daughter in hand and the other daughter in the other hand and jumping off a bridge."

Gayle had no suicidal tendencies, but she had expressed what many autism moms feel when they are at the end of their rope. This wasn't a literal threat: it was a desperate cry for help. Gayle's sister-in-law phoned me and recommended that she get professional help, but what Gayle wanted was family help, and she felt that her family was withdrawing. Her mother, she explained, "previously supported the treatments we tried with the girls, wanting to know all the details, how the treatment might help, how the girls were responding. All of a sudden, nothing […]. My mother left me […]. I never thought she'd leave so suddenly, without giving me a chance." We always spent Christmas with Gayle's mother, but this year she sent us an email announcing that she would spend Christmas with Gayle's brother. Gayle was not invited. Her brother insisted that there was no room for us at his home or at local hotels. Gayle's comment: "No room at the inn? On Christmas? Where have I heard that story before?" Jennifer was crushed and phoned her grandmother, "Shouldn't Mom and Dad be invited too?"—but to no avail. "It was clear my extended family wanted an autism-free Christmas […] free of the stress of this disruptive creature (their granddaughter/niece/cousin) whom no one understood. Like the greater society, my family wanted to ignore autism, and it will go away."

My mother—Jennifer's and Flora's Jewish grandmother—made it up to them by inviting them to a Christmas Day brunch at a Manhattan restaurant. The girls were always welcome at gatherings of my extended family. And later, when Gayle was struggling with cancer, my relatives would call to see how she was doing, but rarely her family. All that contributed to Gayle's eventual decision to convert to Judaism.

The year 2008 was rough for all of us, as evidenced in this exchange of emails:

Dear Jonathan,
 I'm sorry I yelled at you last night. I'm sorry I yelled at all.
 My frustration level is at an all-time high. Over the weekend, I kept asking Jenny whether she had any math homework, and she kept assuring me she didn't. But it's written in her planner that indeed she did […] and French […].
 Of course, the fact that Flora can't write a coherent sentence also has me bummed. I know she's making progress, but she keeps falling farther and farther behind.
 I am so fortunate to be married to you. Staying calm is exactly what Jenny needs. She—and Flora—are very lucky girls to have you as a father.
Lovelovelovelovelovelove,
Cookie

Dearest Cookie,
 I cried when I read this message (honest!). I hate hate hate to see you put through this kind of misery. You've been cheated, the girls have been cheated. I make an effort to stay cool, but only because if I didn't, I'd start screaming for blood, and I'd do something […] that would land me in prison for life. And as you say, I'm not getting out of it that easy.

I count the minutes till we're together again. And then we can talk over this whole awful situation.

Lovelovelovelovelovelove,

Yours Always Always Always

Jennifer's meltdowns at school were unabated. In response to one outburst, the teacher evacuated the homeroom. "I keep thinking things can't get worse for/with Jenny@[middle school], and each day I'm shown things can and do get worse. It never should have gotten to this point. 'Experts' don't understand autism. 'Authority' wants to teach 'responsibility.' This attitude pushes kids with autism right over the edge that they live on. While Jenny was in tears upon learning we probably have to remove her from her classes, FLORA SHOWED EMPATHY! She told Jenny to wipe away the tears and made her lips into a smile face" [5/14-15/08].

Gayle was now moving in the direction of activism, confronting the issue of vaccine safety. She had joined the board of directors of SafeMinds. I was more reluctant to make trouble, but she wrote: "Vaccines need to be safe, effective and necessary. Chicken pox vax is none of the above" [1/3/08]. "I believe I can help my kids. I believe biomedical interventions help my kids. My kids, my kids. That's all that matters" [1/9/08]. At a town meeting she asked Governor Jon Corzine about the autism epidemic and was booed by the audience, which infuriated her: "Merck mafia. May they all rot in hell" [1/16, 18/08]. "Lately I've thought about choices I have. I can choose to be angry or I can choose to accept. I CHOOSE TO BE ANGRY. Anger helps me to get things done" [4/17/08]. She would channel that anger constructively into vaccine injury research, which her colleagues at Baruch College respected. In 2013 they awarded her the Abraham J. Briloff Prize in Ethics for her article "Conflicts of Interest in Vaccine Safety Research"—and she found plenty of conflicts.

Public health officials (who had their own conflicts of interest) consistently assured us that the soaring numbers of autistic children reflected no real increase, only "better diagnosis," and that the actual autism rate was more or less constant. But a century ago the autism rate was virtually zero, and today in Belfast, Northern Ireland (where exceptionally careful statistics are kept) a staggering 1 in 21 children are autistic. That is, we are asked to believe that the rate was about 1 in 21 everywhere and at all times, in all corners of the world and throughout human history. There were untold millions of autistic people out there for thousands of years, but until very recently no one noticed them. At that rate autistic individuals would have met face to face every day, but somehow they consistently failed to recognize each other. You don't have to be a professional historian to recognize that this theory is well beyond absurd. The question that future historians will have to address is how any rational person could have believed this, in the face of all the scientific evidence. Studies conducted by Dr. Walter Zahorodny of the Rutgers New Jersey Medical School have confirmed that the dramatic increase in autism is all too real. Modest adjustments in diagnostic criteria could not begin to explain autism rates leaping upward by several orders of magnitude, which could only have been produced by some kind of environmental toxins.[5] And environmental history teaches us that corporations and governments that create environmental disasters typically try to cover them up.[6] By promoting this wildly implausible misinformation, the media and public health officials only succeeded in destroying their own credibility, as well as the neurological health of ever-growing legions of children.

When Gayle and I saw the film version of Vera Brittain's *Testament of Youth*, we immediately saw the historical analogy. The autism pandemic was the First World War all over again. The authorities who governed us had blundered into a catastrophe that was decimating a generation, and they would not change course because they could not admit that their strategies would lead only to disaster. As the casualties mounted year by year, their response was more propaganda and more censorship, and anyone who questioned them was robotically denounced as a "pro-German"/"antivaxxer."

It says a lot about Jennifer that her favorite literary work was *Dr. Jekyll and Mr. Hyde*. She knew all the film adaptations, preferring "the Spencer Tracy version." And she fully recognized her own split personality. Gayle called the violent side "Lucifer," because we knew that was not the real Jennifer: that was what autism had done to her and an ever-growing number of young people. Often (Gayle recorded) Jenny could be "very sweet, especially when she sensed I was sad about Flora" [1/14/09]. And then a few weeks later: "Detention for outburst—kicked desk & then another student. No one offered her Advil" [3/31/09]. And just a week after that, she could calm down Flora

5 https://www.ageofautism.com/2022/06/autism-prevalence-since-2000-wayne-rohde-interviews-dr-walter-zahorodny.html. For still more evidence, see Dan Olmsted and Mark Blaxill, *Denial* (New York: Skyhorse Publishing, 2017), and Jonathan Rose, "Yes, There Is an Autism Epidemic," *History News Network,* March 6, 2016. https://historynewsnetwork.org/article/161992.
6 The scholarly literature on this subject is vast, but for a popular summary see Sheldon Rampton and John Stauber, *Trust Us, We're Experts!* (New York: Tarcher/Putnam, 2002).

on a shopping trip: "Jenny has a gift—she understands ASD kids" [4/6/09]. When Flora destroyed a napkin holder Jennifer made, Jenny accepted that it was "just a material object" [6/18/09]. On Halloween Day 2009, Jennifer pulled off a marvelously successful bat mitzvah, performing the whole service for a crowd of adoring family and friends. But not long after that, she was suspended from school for screaming in class and hitting another student [11/17-18/09]. A month later: "Major meltdown—Police were called—not sure by whom," but it was in response to Jenny screaming "My parents are trying to hurt me" [12/15/09].

And yet we still had wonderful times together on a regular basis. Every Saturday evening we watched Turner Classic Movies as a family recreation, from which Jenny acquired an impressive knowledge of cinematic history. She enjoyed *The Devil and Daniel Webster* and *Casablanca*: "Quite sophisticated tastes w/movies!" [11/28/09]. We were especially fond of those wonderful 1930s comedies: *It Happened One Night, My Man Godfrey, His Girl Friday, Duck Soup, Sullivan's Travels*. And we could entirely understand why they appealed to our grandparents. In the depths of the Depression, with Hitler on the march, they could forget all that for a couple of hours and enjoy pure escapism. We felt similarly entitled to a little respite from autism.

At age 10, after several wobbly starts, Flora learned to ride a bike. That we considered a major victory, until we realized that it gave her unlimited opportunities for eloping. In July 2011, she was apprehended cycling on a nearby Interstate Highway. A few days later, she cycled up to a busy commuter rail line and danced on the tracks. Service had to be suspended at rush hour, and Gayle was absolutely distraught, wondering aloud whether her treatments were doing more harm than good [7/17, 21/11].

Middle school is a difficult stage for many youngsters, but for Jenny it was one nightmarish outburst after another, all recorded in Gayle's diary. She was suspended for 10 days for trying to elope from the school [1/14/10]. She punched one boy and called another fat [3/10/10]. At home she spat out hostility: "Do I have to kill you?" [3/28/10]. "I don't want Mom to have an intelligent conversation" [3/30/10]; "Dad's trying to hurt me!" [4/21/10]; "Mom, you're ugly." "I want a different family" [11/25/12]. DYFS was called again [6/29/10]. And these rages were often followed by expressions of self-loathing: "I'm broken." "It's no use." "I need to be in a hospital" [9/9/10]. She succumbed to self-abuse, hitting the side of her head and banging her head against the walls so hard that she left craters throughout our house. She would phone the child abuse hotline, and we had to call the police repeatedly.

(They immediately recognized what was going on and were very good at de-escalation.) Over several days Gayle only wrote in her diary "PURE HELL" [7/10-14/12].

But Dr. Jekyll continued to coexist with Mr. Hyde. "Dr. Stu amazed at Jenny's progress!", which was very real [8/26/10]. "HELPING AROUND THE HOUSE VERY POLITE (BIG TIME)" [8/29/10]. She cuddled with her mother while watching Greer Garson in *Madame Curie* [11/6/10]. And when we organized a New Year's Eve dinner at Morristown Diner for the special needs families we knew, she was once again the perfect hostess. When Jenny was speech-delayed, Gayle and I would see other parents talking easily with their young children, and we felt terribly sad, wondering whether we would ever have a conversation with our daughter. But now we couldn't shut her up.

It the eighth grade we transferred her out of a mainstream public school to Montgomery Academy, a kind of charter school for intellectually disabled teens. Jenny said it was run by "superannuated hippies," and academically it wasn't very challenging, but for a while it was a good place for her. In a mainstream classroom she wasn't deliberately excluded, but somehow she always ended up on the margins. In contrast, autistic teens immediately recognized and accepted her, and they all chattered away among themselves, just like normal kids. Previously she had had few playdates and no real friends. Now she had two boyfriends who took her out on mall dates, with their mothers following close behind. And she continued to become more and more creative with language. When told it was 11 p.m. and time to sleep, her response was downright philosophical: "Mom. The world might end at midnight. I want to live life to its fullest" [5/21/11]. When she later applied to another special needs high school, the principal was at first skeptical, but was impressed and won over when she explained how *Spiderman* was an "allegory." It has to be emphasized that, in spite of her psychotic episodes, most of the time she was terribly sweet and appreciative, as when she wrote this:

> This is a poem for you Mom
> For all the times I said "I love you."
> Or texted it.
> Either way is nice.
> For all the times I gave you a hug,
> For all the times I came home upset about something that happened at school

And you came to comfort me.

For all the times we laughed while watching TV.

For all the times you woke me up and made me breakfast.

For all the times you took me to swimming class, acting class, or the movies.

For all the times you read my writing and told me how awesome they were.

For all the times you supported me and my dreams.

For all the times you took me to the mall.

For you, Mom.

And in April 2013 Flora had a tremendous success to celebrate: "Great Bat Mitzvah. JR FABULOUS HOSTESS" [4/13/13]. Flora's speech was limited, but she had an angelic singing voice, so she chanted most of the ceremony. Some handicapped individuals who cannot speak can sing. Her proud mother delivered this tribute before the congregation:

"Flora, you bring out the best in people. Those who are themselves good and kind, love to be around you. Your great smile makes others smile as well. All your friends admire your energy and determination. Those who take an extra minute to get to know you even better realize what an amazing person you are.

"Your mechanical abilities are phenomenal. Remember when we first had the filtered water spout attached to the kitchen sink? Your dad, Jenny, and I were constantly pressing down on the lever, grumbling about how inconvenient the mechanism was. You looked at it, looked at us, and proceeded to lift the lever UP so the water ran on its own.

"You have such a knack for dates [...]."

"And you are a fantastic biker. You maneuver the crowds at Loantaka Park with such grace. And when there are no crowds, nothing holding you back, you soar."

To end every day on an upbeat note, we developed a nightly ritual with Flora. Just before she went to bed we would ask her "What's something good that happened to you today?" and "What are you looking forward to tomorrow?", and she would ask the same of us.

For both children and parents, life with autism can be endlessly frustrating, humiliating, painful, and ultimately heartbreaking. It was all that for us, but it was not unrelieved misery by any means. It makes an enormous difference when parents work together as a team. More often than not, autism moms give up their jobs to care for their children full-time. But Gayle was a consummate career woman: she would have shot herself if she had to stay with the kids round the clock. So we staggered our teaching schedules: I taught Monday/Wednesday/Friday, she worked Tuesday/Thursday, so someone was always at home with the girls. We divvied up the domestic chores, with me taking charge of the cooking. (I had an ulterior motive: if I had left the food preparation to Gayle, she would have served me stir-fried tofu. Anything but that!) And Gayle paid me the highest compliment one can pay to a chef: "Are you sure you're straight?" "Do you want me to prove it? Again?" "Please do."

We were determined to have as much fun as we possibly could as a family, and we did. We watched old movies together on TCM. We threw fall equinox parties and invited everyone we knew. We vacationed as far afield as Toronto and Washington, DC. We could enjoy restaurants after all, without creating too much chaos: "The girls were adorable and so well behaved (except when Flora almost knocked over the guy with the hors d'oeuvres platter" [5/11/08]. When Jennifer published her first book (*It's Not a Perfect World but I'll Take It*) we arranged author signings at local bookshops. She might not sell many books, but we all went to cheer her on, just as other families cheered on Little Leaguers and soccer girls. Every fall I would load everyone in the car and drive out to the country to see the leaves turn, stopping at a quaint inn for lunch. Gayle loved it, but only after we had done this for several years running did she ask me where I had gotten the idea. I explained that my dad had always driven us out to the country to watch the leaves turn, and I wanted to carry on that family tradition. "Yes," she replied, "that makes sense if you're living in a cramped Manhattan apartment. But now we're living in the country. If you want to watch the leaves turn, look out the window." I had to admit that Gayle had seen the flaw in my logic, but that didn't bother her at all. The point is we were doing things together as a family, and that she always relished. Taking your autistic kids fishing is actually good advice, as long as you also do what you can to heal them.

In spite of everything, we never lost our sense of fun. My face and Gayle's would always light up when we saw each other. We yapped happily and licked each other's faces like puppy dogs. Gayle's autism mom friends called us "lovebirds" in a somewhat sardonic tone of voice which suggested that effusive displays of affection were not entirely appropriate for married couples. But we knew that parents must set aside time to play with each other—just the two of you.

INTIMACY

Many crusaders, in their zeal to save humanity, turn into puritanical killjoys, fixated on their ideological obsessions to the exclusion of everything else. But Gayle was never anything like that. She saw no reason why she should not fight injustice and have an absolute blast at the same time. She once proposed, as a fundraising gimmick, that autism parents, moms and dads together, should pose for a nude calendar under the slogan "We Have Nothing to Hide." She volunteered us for that project but couldn't persuade anyone else to cover the other 11 months. (Jenny McCarthy was amused but said she no longer did that sort of thing.) Gayle was that rare and beautiful creature, an epicurean without snobbery. She adored cheap diners and not so fine wines. She stole the show at a Halloween party dressed as a Playboy Bunny (she had the figure for it). Coming of age in Lancaster, she found Woody Allen incomprehensible ("What did Annie Hall see in that dweeb?"), but after she married a dorky Jewish guy she got all the jokes and never missed any of his movies.

Perhaps we related to those movies because our life resembled a Woody Allen joke. We enrolled Jennifer in a summer camp that promised an "Inclusion Counselor"—and within 36 hours the Inclusion Counselor expelled her. But our philosophy for dealing with autism was simple: whenever you are socked in the teeth, immediately activate Plan B (or C or D). Within a matter of days we relocated Jennifer to Camp Ramapo, an excellent special-needs camp that both girls attended for years.

And that gave us a glorious respite every August. We would dress up as too-cool-to-live hipsters, head to the East Village, dine in trendy restaurants, and check out edgy boutiques where Gayle would try on knockout dresses that she had no intention of buying. Come to think of it, we did purchase one: a slinky beige sheath with a hole revealing her right hip. When she unveiled that at a faculty party, my dean audibly gasped. She often told me, "It's so much fun being married to you," and believe me, it was mutual.

August also allowed us to frolic in the bedroom without distraction. Books on autism parenting don't normally have much to say about sex. Even in her bestselling *Louder Than Words*, Jenny McCarthy mentions the subject briefly, but then indignantly dismisses it as somehow inappropriate. After her son Evan was struck down by autism seizures and returned from the hospital, her husband John

> was encouraging me to sleep in our bed. It was our first night back in the house, and I told him he couldn't pay me millions of dollars to be away from my child for longer than twenty minutes. Then he asked me to lie down with him because he wanted to have sex. We had just brought our kid home from the hospital, and he wanted sex! That's the difference between some men and women. We really do tend to handle stresses much differently, and I know deep down that John was trying to escape the only way he knew how—with sex—but I did not oblige [...]. Sadly, sex was torture for me during this phase of life [...]. I had no desire whatsoever to get off and honestly didn't care if I never had sex again.[1]

Gayle admired Jenny McCarthy, but on this point she emphatically disagreed. She always reminded me that "Girls like it too," and if sex offered a brief escape from autism, that was an ironclad argument in favor of it. Gayle noticed that when she lunched with other special-needs moms, the subject was never raised (unlike those brunches in *Sex and the City*, a series that fascinated us). Perhaps the mothers were too exhausted. Or maybe they felt guilty if they did not devote all their energies to their children.

If the latter, that attitude has to be repudiated in no uncertain terms. Autism parents are fully entitled to erotic compensation for everything they have to endure. Autism moms suffer the same stress levels experienced by combat soldiers, and sex is the best stress reliever we have, organic and drug-free. Autism can also put a terrific strain on couples: a quarter of autism moms and 20% of autism dads report troubled marriages, compared with 10% of mothers and 2% of fathers of Down's syndrome children. Early reports of a divorce rate of 80% among autism parents proved to be wildly exaggerated, but a more careful study put the incidence at 23.5% (compared with just 13.8% of parents

---

1 Jenny McCarthy, *Louder Than Words: A Mother's Journey in Healing Autism* (New York: Dutton, 2007), 35–36, 103–104.

of nondisabled children), while yet another investigation concluded that 36% of autism parents were divorced by age 30.[2]

Autism parents desperately need mutual pleasures that don't involve their kids. Fortunately, Gayle was always in touch with her vigorous libido and determined to enjoy her husband up to the hilt. If I erased that side of her from this portrait, it simply wouldn't be Gayle. She stands as living proof that—with some imagination and flexibility—a robust and loving sex life is possible in the age of autism.

And we managed that without doing anything wild and crazy (if you don't count screwing in my campus office, where we were nearly caught). We were absolutely monogamous. I had no wish to be husband-swapped. We were no more athletic than any other healthy couple. The KamaSutra always struck us as more trouble than it was worth. We never used anything that needed batteries, and we preferred to keep our hands free (if you catch my drift). Ordinary garden-variety sex is absolutely sensational when both partners forget about autism and focus single-mindedly on pleasuring each other. Gayle would always say, "I wanna keep my man happy," and I told her that bringing her to a climax was the most beautiful sight in the world. Her favorite song was "Can't Keep My Hands to Myself (But Why Would I Want To?)." At any hour of the night, if she was feeling scared or sad or horny, she was authorized to reach over and womanhandle me. (And in fairness, Jenny McCarthy did eventually learn to enjoy a man's body again.)[3]

Some bored married people resort to adultery for the cheap thrill of doing something illicit that may be found out. If you crave that kind of excitement, never ever cheat on your spouse. Instead, cheat on your kids. That is, have surreptitious sex without letting your children know. That's what we did when the girls were little, but when they grew older and wiser, we switched tactics and became completely open about what we were doing. Borrowing a euphemism from the sitcom *Full House*, we explained that we were "doing our taxes." Even little Flora understood that. Time pressures meant that we often had to resort to quickies, what Gayle called "threeplay" and I called "Purr/grrr/thank-you-sir."

2 Shaun Heasley, "How Parenting Kids with Disabilities Affects Marriage," *DisabilityScoop*, April 11, 2022; Niki Bahri, Kyle Sterrett, and Catherine Lord, "Marital Status Over 28 Years of Parents of Individuals with Autism and Other Developmental Disabilities," *Journal of Family Psychology* 37, no. 6 (2023): 920–931.
3 McCarthy, *Louder Than Words*, 183.

So Rule Number One for autism parents is: Be absolutely faithful to your partner. Rule Number Two is: That doesn't mean you can't have a favorite pinup boy/girl. Gayle's candidate for Second Sexiest Man in the World was Jimmy Smits, the star of *NYPD Blue*. So when he appeared in a Broadway play, I did what any loving husband would do: bought us a pair of tickets. And whenever we encountered (another) beautiful woman, Gayle would pull me aside and whisper, "Isn't she a knockout?" (I politely mumbled something noncommittal.) And this reflected the fact that we both felt perfectly secure in our relationship.

Even more than other teens, autistic adolescents have difficulty handling sex because their ability to read social clues is impaired, and sex is all about subtle social cues. Consequently, autistic boys often fail to learn boundaries, and naïve autistic girls are easily taken advantage of. So, as part of her sex education, we let Jennifer watch with us those intelligently raunchy television series, *Sex and the City* and *2 Broke Girls*. That made her feel terribly sophisticated and grown up. We also found useful instructional materials in old films on Turner Classic Movies. Under the Hays Code of the 1930s and 1940s, Hollywood screenwriters could not be sexually explicit, so they had to resort to suggestion, double entendres, winking, and nudging. We used these movies to explain to Jenny the coded language of sex, which often escapes literal-minded autistic people. Yes, in *The Maltese Falcon* Peter Lorre was obviously gay, though the word was never used. And we assured Jenny that her grandmothers drooled over Clark Gable's classic male striptease in *It Happened One Night*. Thus she learned how to handle men, draw the line at inappropriate behavior, and enjoy R-rated movies.

Sex is a matter of highly individualized tastes, and couples have to decide for themselves what they find delectable. What we offer here are nothing more than suggestions, to illustrate that any couple can do wonderful things in bed in spite of autism.

As a nineteenth-anniversary present to ourselves, we did an erotic photoshoot. That is, we hired a professional photographer and did more or less what porn stars do. Though we held to fairly traditional family values, we both opposed all forms of censorship, and neither of us had any problem with erotica involving consenting adults. If God didn't want us to read porn, He wouldn't have put the Song of Solomon in the Bible. (When I was courting Gayle, I used that to seduce her. Worked every time.) That said, we found nearly all commercially produced porn stupid and boring. Our usual response was, "We could do better than that. Much better." And we sure did.

We were well into middle age, but we were still in fairly good shape, eating healthfully and exercising, so we thought this was something we should do before we became completely decrepit. And as autism parents we recognized that if we didn't allow ourselves some treats and respites, we'd go crazy. The great thing about DIY porn is that it's pure escape. It has no redeeming social value, it's just good clean dirty fun.

Gayle delegated the task of finding an erotic photographer to me. (There are some hard jobs that a man should take care of.) You can easily Google "Boudoir Photographers," who specialize in this sort of thing, but I looked for a more artistic professional who didn't usually do porn but was eager to try her hand at it. (And yes, wives will probably be more comfortable posing nude for another woman.) I searched for something imaginative, vivid, and real—because I knew that was how we were going to look naked. I found two charming young women, and we invited them over to our place for brunch, to establish a friendly and civilized working relationship.

The photographer will give you whatever you want, ranging from gauzy romantic to hard core. We definitely wanted soft core: simulated sex but no actual sex, steamy but not kinky. Usually boudoir photography involves young wives in naughty lingerie or less, but rarely husbands. Gayle, however, insisted that I get into the picture. (I can't see what feminists are whining about. I love being objectified.)

On the day of the shoot, the photographers brought in a makeup artist to get Gayle dolled up. That was a treat in itself, and tastefully done. "When you're doing porn, you don't want to look like a French whore," Gayle explained. Then we got into our best party outfits: she in a smashing blue cocktail dress, me in my Brooks Brothers blazer and silk tie. First we did some romantic outdoor shots: hugging, kissing, nibbling. Then we moved indoors and fed each other strawberries and cherries. Well, there's only so much of that a girl can stand. So she grabbed me by the necktie, ripped that (and everything else I was wearing) off, and had her way with me on the living room couch.

Then, for Act Two, we retired to the boudoir and changed costumes. She put on a charmingly slutty green lamé strapless number that I had bought from a Soho street vendor for $15 nineteen years earlier. (For Gayle, "slut" was a badge of pride, right up there with "Warrior Mom.") I wore a torn T-shirt that Gayle was always nagging me to get rid of, but now she was glad I'd kept it, because in this context it was "screamingly hot. Like Brando in *Streetcar*." And soon all of that was on the floor. Our finale was a (literally) steamy scene together in the shower.

Since my wedding, no woman had ever seen me naked, other than Gayle and some medical personnel. So I was slightly apprehensive about doing full frontals for two female photographers. But they put me entirely at my ease, deftly guiding me through various poses. To be instructed by young (and imaginative) women to do sexy things to my wife was an experience like no other. I highly recommend it. And they had to teach Gayle how to do something she never did before or after: fake orgasms. When they wanted her to climax, their code word was "Dramatic!" (I suggested "Meg Ryan!")

The result was a record of our love that would be shared with no one else. It cost less than a weekend in the Caribbean, though we couldn't show our friends our snapshots. And we were very glad we did it when we did, because shortly thereafter Gayle was diagnosed with breast cancer.

THE SUCKER PUNCH

By Easter 2011, before any signs of cancer were detected, Gayle was already having health problems: "Numbing headache, body ache, lethargy [...] I'm just so tired" [4/24/11]. The cancer diagnosis a few years later of course left her devastated, but once she recovered from the initial shock she consulted Sloan Kettering, where she was prescribed chemotherapy and radiation. When she asked for a second opinion, she was told that there were no second opinions at Sloan Kettering, just one "standard of care." That left her determined to take charge of her own treatment. She saw what chemotherapy did to the human body, and calculated that alternative treatments offered equal longevity with much less pain and suffering. She did have a single mastectomy in July 2015, but we were determined not to let a little thing like that get in the way of our fun. After the operation, the female surgeon asked if I had any questions. "Sex?" I asked concisely. She looked shocked, perhaps she thought I was hitting on her (in front of my wife), so I hastened to clarify: "When can we resume having sex?" She laughed: "That shows you love her for her soul rather than her body." "Both, actually," I corrected her. And we found that Gayle could fly on one engine.

To keep up Gayle's morale (and mine) I got into the nightly habit of sending her raunchy emails. Before I shut down my computer (I was a night owl) I would find a dirty image on the web and write a funny caption under it, or find a clean image and write a dirty caption, and then email it to Gayle, so she would always have something to look forward to in the morning. For a photo of a Viking woman with a horned helmet and spear I wrote, "My ideal woman: a horny Warrior Mom." Under an exhausted sleeping kitten ran the line, "I'm sorry I wore out your pussy." And when Gayle went on an organic diet to treat the cancer, I promised to eat something organic too: "Mom." She was a MILF ("Mother I Love Forever") and I was a HIGH ("Husband I Gotta Hump"). For Father's Day Gayle wrote, "The way a man treats his mother is how he is going to treat his wife [...] Well, almost"—over a graphic photo of a couple doing what healthy married couples do. "Your husband is basically a math problem," I wrote. "He's hard, and you can do him on your desktop."

In November 2014 Gayle publicly announced online, "I have autism-induced breast cancer (AIBC). While I am not absolutely certain that the 1.9-centimeter lump that grew in my left breast is the result of the stress of raising two autistic children, all indications point in that direction." She went on to lampoon the slogans of neurodiversity and the facile formulas of the mainstream media: "Unlike autism, no one is telling me to 'celebrate' my cancer. No one is telling me that cancer is 'just a different way for cells to grow.' People have told me that we've always had cancer, but no one is using that as an excuse for not doing anything about it. No one is blaming me (or my mother) for my cancer. Unlike a person with autism, society does not say my cancer is my fault."[1] Her enemies accused her of blaming her children for her cancer, which of course she had not said, but twisting words beyond recognition is nowadays a standard propaganda tactic. In fact her conclusion was based on two obvious scientific truths: (1) autism moms suffer extraordinarily high levels of stress, and (2) stress can aggravate cancer.

Several sympathetic readers suggested alternative therapies for stress reduction, and here is what I proposed: "It's called Penis Therapy. It's far more pleasant than chemo. It involves regular injections of protein. But it's only really effective in very, very large doses [...]. This medication may be administered orally or vaginally. Possible side effects include convulsions and screaming like an air raid siren. And yes, it may be addicktive." To which Gayle replied, "It is such a(n orgasmic) blast being married to you!"

Starting in August 2015 Gayle worked with Dr. Linda Isaacs, who pursued an individualized nutritional approach to cancer, prescribing specialized diets, supplements, pancreatic enzymes, and coffee enemas. Whether Gayle would have lived longer with conventional treatments cannot be answered, because she never tried that experiment, and different patients respond to treatments differently. Frankly, I had limited understanding of the treatments she was pursuing, but I trusted her judgment and her research skills. After all, we both had a vested interest in keeping her alive. And it wasn't just a simple question of longevity: a rational cancer patient might reasonably prefer seven years of mostly good health to eight years ravaged by chemotherapy. In any case, it was

---

1 Gayle DeLong, "Breast Cancer and Autism: The Lesser of Two Evils," *Age of Autism*, November 7, 2014.

her life and her body, and she was always determined to think for herself and pursue methods that made sense to her. That was one of the many reasons I adored her.

We had at least found an ideal residence for Flora, and that did reduce Gayle's level of stress. The first three years of her public high school had been a waste, where her reading skills actually regressed. For "vocational training" she would work a few days in the county courthouse refiling legal briefs. It would never lead to any real paid employment, but each morning she put on her dress-for-success professional woman's outfit and went to work—until she was fired. She had given up filing the briefs in alphabetical order and instead stuffed them every which way. When we asked her why she didn't do the job properly she explained, "Because it's *boring!*" Evidently this was her way of sticking it to the Man.

So in the 12th grade we transferred her to the Camphill School and its transition program, Beaver Farm, near Phoenixville, Pennsylvania. They were part of a larger Camphill movement, founded in 1939 to provide humane and useful education for the intellectually handicapped. Here Flora flourished, mastering a roster of house chores, picking organic herbs in a working farm, collecting eggs from chickens, designing pottery, and addressing packages in the mail room. That left open the question of where she would live after she aged out at 21.

Flora was home on vacations, and though she wasn't violent she did have a serious case of OCD. She insisted on going to Walmart every day to buy glue sticks, which she didn't use. She stayed up all hours of the night playing an absolutely dreadful Paul McCartney rock video over and over. She habitually stole car keys for reasons we could not fathom. She binged on food, and we had to put locks on our refrigerators. On three separate occasions she stole ice cream cakes from Friendly's (3000 calories each) and devoured them whole. (These heists involved elaborate planning: one had to admit that she was a master criminal.)

Jennifer was admitted to Drew University (where I taught), but her college years were a constant struggle for her and us. Sometimes she didn't do her assignments, sometimes she wrote them but did not turn them in, and some courses were simply too challenging and had to be dropped. She had frequent anxiety attacks in classrooms—and while she was granted some accommodations for her disability, disrupting a class is never a reasonable accommodation. She loved extracurricular activities (especially the Anime Club), but even by normal college standards, her dorm room was a toxic dump. After one late-night screaming fit in the dorm the police took her to the local hospital, where she spent time in the psych ward.

This was yet another example of what Gayle and I called "sucker punches." Just when we thought we had achieved tranquility and equilibrium for our girls, something totally unexpected threw our lives once again into chaos. In December 2016, Gayle had laboriously addressed upward of a hundred Christmas cards and put them aside. Then Flora systematically scribbled all over the envelopes. When Gayle exploded, Jennifer tried to calm her nerves by taking far too many propranolols, and once again she went to the hospital. You begin to see why many autism parents feel that their lives are being sabotaged by their children, even if the kids don't mean to do that.

By the end of her junior year Jennifer had exhausted the patience of the deans at Drew, so we transferred her to the College of St. Elizabeth, a nearby Catholic school. St. E's took very seriously its social mission of taking care of the lame and the halt, and there we felt everyone, students and faculty, was looking out for her. Like her parents, Jenny craved freedom and adventure; but unlike her parents, she lacked planning and survival skills. Once, without telling us, she took the train into New York to see Benedict Cumberbatch on a talk show, but arrived too late. She then tried unsuccessfully to check into a hotel (apparently it was the Plaza), spent the entire night wandering the streets of Manhattan, and somehow made her way back to campus the following day. We tried to impress upon her something she could not entirely grasp: that this was very dangerous behavior.

Jennifer completed her BA at St. E's and entered a certificate program in School Librarianship at William Paterson University. That seemed to make sense, given that she loved books, she loved little kids, and it looked like a low-stress profession. But the program was entirely online, so she enjoyed no campus life. She was forced to do something that no twentysomething wants to do: live at home with her parents, who nagged her to complete her class assignments. Tensions inevitably escalated and often exploded. Jennifer endlessly needled her mother about her research: snidely labeling her an "Angel Mother" (not meant as a compliment) and demanding that she make herself "more marketable." Gayle was appalled by the ingratitude, especially as her daughter apparently agreed with her about the causes of autism: Jennifer always refused vaccinations. This hostility may well have been a function of online vitrol directed against "antivaxxers," which made Jenny feel all the more outcast. She often protested that she was not "the right kind of victim," and in a sense that was true. The media treated some kinds of victims (e.g., transgender people) as fashionable and lavished favorable publicity on them.

That generosity was not awarded to autistic people, and certainly not to vaccine resisters or the vaccine-injured.

One of Gayle's moral victories concerned her article "A lowered probability of pregnancy in females in the USA aged 25-29 who received a human papillomavirus vaccine injection," published in the *Journal of Toxicology and Environmental Health* in June 2018. Gayle was not a physician, but she was far more expert in statistics than most doctors, and she found that 60% of women who never had the HPV vaccine had at least one pregnancy, compared with just 35% of those who had the HPV shot. That suggested that the vaccine might be causing ovarian failure, as some doctors suspected. The article proved to be one of the most widely read the journal had ever published, attracting nearly 24,000 views. But in October 2019 the editor informed Gayle that he was reconsidering the article owing to "several public and private expressions of concern about flaws in analysis." Though the article had initially been passed by three peer reviewers, he now sent it to four more external readers. One suggested that the journal open up a public debate about the paper, which Gayle would have happily accepted, but three others recommended that the article be withdrawn, and it was. In their retraction letter, the editors did not clearly explain why the article was being suppressed, or why they found the paper's three critics more persuasive than its three supporters, or why they did not open the issue up for debate (as is normally done in scientific controversies). It was one more example of a general effort to shut down any debate regarding the safety and effectiveness of what the pharmaceutical companies are trying to sell us, censorship that became ever more apparent during the Covid pandemic. And in the long run that censorship would backfire, undermining public confidence in the medical establishment.[2]

In the short run Gayle had to deal with the usual online trolls, which did not bother her. But they did bother Jennifer. She had never brought her violent outbursts entirely under control, and now they grew worse. So we were not surprised to learn that two out of three autistic young people are violent toward their family members or caregivers. We found that proportion among the autism parents we knew. One had to institutionalize her violent daughter. Another, with a violent autistic son, told us that no one else in our circle

---

2 Gayle DeLong, "Author Response to *Journal of Toxicology and Environmental Health* Retraction of 'A Lowered Probability of Pregnancy in Females in the USA Aged 25–29 Who Received a Human Papillomavirus Vaccine Injection'," *Age of Autism*, December 16, 2019.

of special needs families wanted to hear about this. And a colleague at my university, bitten and scratched by her autistic son, had permanent scars. (Fortunately, Flora belonged to the one-third who are not violent.)

Families dealing with these attacks have nowhere to turn. Many services for autistic young people refuse to handle anyone with a record of violence, so those who need help most are effectively abandoned. And even battered autism moms like Gayle, who would never tolerate a wifebeater, often can't bring themselves to institutionalize their violent autistic children. On October 9, 2013, the online newsletter *Age of Autism* published the post "Lost & Afraid: Where To Turn When Autism Turns Violent," and received more than a hundred comments, many of them desperate cries for help. Some have tried to excuse autistic violence as a response to bullying and exclusion, but surely the nonautistic intellectually disabled are bullied too, and they are far less aggressive. The targets of autistic violence are usually family members who have done nothing to provoke it, siblings who happen to be within striking distance, and parents who are wearing out their lives to help their children. We are and should be responsive when autistic children are bullied, but as a society we have callously ignored violence, often far worse than bullying, perpetrated by autistic young people. That becomes apparent when the victims are (on rare occasions) allowed to speak out:

- "I've got an 18 year old son who is violent [and] low functioning [...]. He outweighs me by about a hundred pounds and is six inches taller than me but at least I can defend myself. My wife didn't have siblings to fight with so she just walks around all scratched up [...]. Would say suicidal thoughts are pretty much par for the course with me but we've been lucky so far and I keep praying that some day the state will take him from us but the reality is that we would have to say 'we abandon him' and my wife will never do that" [Steve, January 7, 2015].
- "I once knew an 18 year old child with autism. He was in my college classes and made the lives of people around him very difficult. He began to punch people. At first he hit a girl he liked, but then he started lashing out on his friends and teachers. He finally got punished by the college after he held a girl down, whilst he touched her. When he was punished he showed no remorse and didn't even try to apologize. He told us how everyone was bullying him and that he should be allowed to do whatever he wants [...]. He punched me in the throat and when I was on the floor

he tried to carry on kicking my ribs […]. It truly is a terrible disease" [Sam Lavin, January 29, 2015].

- "I am 14 and I have an autistic sister […]. My childhood will be forever ruined and scarred. My arms, hands, neck, will never be flawless due to having to hold her down in the car when she has a meltdown. She literally gets out of her seat belt and attacks my mother, we could be riding in silence and BOOM […]. I don't want an autistic sister, but everyone will scold me if I say so. Well sorry I don't enjoy getting headbutted and scratched. Do you? […] I will disown my family when they ask me to watch her in my adult years. Because she'll be bigger and more violent" [Deondra, May 15, 2015].

- "I too have to struggle with an aggressive 35 year old moderately retarded autistic son. I have watched in horror as he threw every object that he could find from the landing on to my husband trying desperately to protect himself on lower steps of the staircase. I screamed at my son to stop and locked him in his room. My son regularly smashes light bulbs, paintings, tears pants' pockets and shirt pockets and shreds books when he isn't throwing them at his father. His outbursts are unpredictable with no obvious triggers. His father is on the receiving end of most of his aggression. This is horrible because his father is his main caregiver and extremely gentle with him" [LW, April 29, 2016].

- "I am the sibling of a severely autistic 13 year old girl, and for the last 10 years the lives of me and my parents have been complete hell. I'm riddled with scars that make me look like a meth addict, I am turned down at every job interview because of this, my mother has PTSD and her health is going downhill because of it, and my parents' relationship has been ruined. My sister screams and hollers all day and night, upset or happy. I haven't slept a full night in 13 years, and I'm slowly losing hope for the situation to get better. Every time we have had occupational therapists, regular therapists, and doctors try to help, they run away as fast as they can because she's not a normal autistic, and they can't just open a book and fix her. We've had to fight every step of the way just to get her medicated, and still it's not helping […]. Everyone says they want to help, but nobody does. Our cars have had to be replaced twice, because she's kicked out windows and vents, and our walls have over 40 holes in them. My mom told me that whenever the house gets damaged to the point that it's unlivable, we will just walk away from the house. My family spends almost every cent on candy for this kid, since if we don't she screams and tries to bash our skulls in" [Terrin, July 8, 2016].

- "PLEASE READ THIS!!!!!!!!!! I'm a 15 year old teenager with a 12 year old brother who has autism […]. My brother has tantrums and often, if not always, becomes violent in almost every way. Whether it be hitting, kicking, smacking, you name it. And the things he says during his tantrums are just as hurtful, often using terrible language like 'I'M GONNA KILL YOU (or himself)!!!' […]. He has also got us in a neverending blackmail situation where it's do what I want or I make your life hell. If we dare try to make him do something for himself (which he totally can do) or saying no to something he wants, he then throws a tantrum which by the end of it you would have rather just done what he wanted. My parents try their hardest to help but they are just as lost as me on what to do. We took him to behavior therapy looking for anything that could help […]. But it turns out all they did was take our money and give us a useless plan that we did try to put into effect […]. I'M TIRED of crying in my room while listening to my parents being hurt by my brother! I'M TIRED of society feeling bad but not helping people like me! I'M TIRED of living in fear of the next tantrum and wondering what might happen! I'M TIRED of not being able to do anything about it! […] Society wake up!" [Jacob, July 19, 2016].

- "My 16yo daughter [has] destroyed our new home putting holes in the wall […] threatening suicide and descriptions of how she will murder us all […] her lil 12yo brother […] my fiance […] and myself […] her own mom […] then laughs about it. We hide all the knives […] oh, and the most embarrassing part is the cops and ambulance at our house every week. She stays inpatient in a ward for a week and is let go. With us scared for our lives. I've reported this time and time again. But NO SERIOUS ACTION TAKES PLACE. I FEEL ONE OF US WILL BE DEAD BEFORE SOMEONE WAKES THE FUCK UP. I'm covered in blood from her digging nails in my skin and bruises and black eyes. She even twists my nipples until they're purple and very painful […]. No one will take her. Even her biological father. It's so hard I am losing my sanity" [Dana, August 9, 2016].

- "I have a grandson who is very violent. He can be snuggling with you, lean back and slug you with his fist all without missing a beat. He kicks and I mean like he can karate kick you in the chest in a split second. The other day he threw a cell phone at his father and hit him in the head and when his dad reached up to touch his head, the boy kicked him in the private parts. He had broken the TV screen, windows, furniture, he loves to stomp on his brother's toys. Every time he is transported to the hospital (as from school when he has these episodes, he has thrown a chair at the teacher several times) in a police car in cuffs because you can't control him. It took 3-4 police officers to tackle him once […]. The hospital keeps him for a few hours until he calms down then sends him home because it's the autism, not psychiatric and they can't do anything for him. He spent a month in an institution, being sedated several times because of his uncontrollability then they sent him home. What do these people have to do, wait until he kills someone, breaks someone's bones, etc., before this family can get some help???" [Kathy, April 2, 2019].

Although autistic violence usually seems to be impulsive, Emily Miller worked with a girl who had a "demonstrated capacity to make a plan and carry it through. She is capable of clearly verbalizing her wishes when she wants something although her verbal expression is telegraphed and ungrammatical […]. If she does not get her desire (that 5th banana, 4th shower, to go outside in the snow sans shoes, to work with me on her school work, etc.) there can be extremely violent outbursts. Recently she wrote a step by step plan to get a kitchen knife and kill her tutor (grammatically correct and numerically ordered). Several weeks later she did attack the tutor with a knife that she deliberately obtained ahead of time, and it was only fortune that kept this from becoming a tragedy. This twist to her inability to empathize or see the lives of others as anything other than facilitators/impediments to her desires has me frightened in ways that her unplanned rages do not" [Emily Miller, February 1, 2016].

Some autistic abusers realize that they have lost control over their own minds and feel remorseful after violent episodes. One mother recalled that her son "had put his head through walls, doors, a windshield, then he started coming after us. I have been bitten through to the bone, hair pulled out, almost lost my ear one time. He doesn't mean to, and in fact he once said, 'why did God make me this way? I want to die'" [Sarah H., November 8, 2015].

A young autistic man fully recognizes that his lashing out is destroying the family he loves: "I get violent but I feel HORRIBLE, so bad I can stop talking for days. I hate myself and I hate my autism. It is not a gift. I love my parents. We are NOTTTT doing this to manipulate!!! We have terrible lives. I can't be around anyone, cannot eat or sleep. And Drs say it is a difference? NOT. I love my family so much. We are in as much pain as you are!" [Aaron, November 27, 2016]. This may explain the self-abuse that so often accompanies autistic aggression: the abusers are punishing themselves for the violence that they inflict on others.

One autism mom is absolutely determined "to combat this 'neurodiverse narrative' of the delightfully spectrummy children whose parents 'hate them'. I'm convinced that this is a ploy by the pro-vaccine; exploiting vulnerable, high-functioning ASD young adults into portraying the 'I don't want to be cured' meme." Her son was now 15, 6'3", and 220 lbs., and "his clenched fists come at me about 100 times per day." In the car he punched her regularly at one-minute intervals. "Last week while I was pumping gas he grabbed his 17-year-old sister around the neck & choked her almost to unconsciousness. On a long car trip a few weeks ago, out of desperation, I pulled over, grabbed a roll of packing tape & restrained his arms to his body, his feet together, clicked him in his seat belt & was able to safely drive down the highway [...]. His meltdowns at school last year necessitated evacuations," and he was transferred to a new school "with an 8-foot high fence around the perimeter, locked doors & security cameras," as well as its own security officer. "I refuse to consent to off-label psychotropic prescribing for him, as there is a chance that without them, his brain may change in his 20s & his behaviors will deescalate. With them, the case histories suggest he would require permanent institutionalization" [Christine, August 24, 2019].

That last sentence suggests that, though we congratulate ourselves on "deinstitutionalizing" autistic individuals, many continue to be effectively institutionalized in hospitals, especially if they are violent. And if they live at home with their families, then the families bear the brunt of their violence. "One of the glaring weaknesses of the system is there is no real option for families whose children fall into that category," explains Christopher Treiber, associate executive director for the InterAgency Council of Developmental Disability Agencies. Programs for autistic minors often exclude those with a record of violence, motivated by a sincere concern for the safety of their children and staff, but that still means that services are denied to those who need them most. The demand for places in residential schools far outstrips the supply, and the cost per student can exceed $300,000 a year, or nearly $3,000 a day for hospital care.[3]

---

3 Joseph Goldstein, "Sabrina's Parents Love Her. But Her Meltdowns Are Too Much," *New York Times,* June 1, 2022.

Anyone who knows Jennifer Rose knows that she is usually charmingly sociable. Her first book, *It's Not a Perfect World but I'll Take It,* won many fans with its insights, its cleverness, and its loving tributes to autism moms. So readers of this volume may be profoundly shocked to learn that Jennifer had her own record of violence, though judging from the accounts above, her case was milder than average. Her violence was directed mostly against her mother, sometimes her father, and in a few instances her sister. She might brandish a kitchen knife, but only as a theatrical prop: she never stabbed anyone. Other parents suffered much more than we did.

For several years it appeared that Gayle's cancer had been contained. An ultrasound in June 2019 turned up "no areas of concern," but a follow-up the following fall reported the first signs of metastatic disease. In January 2020, Jennifer enjoyed a wonderful treat: visiting Israel on a special-needs Birthright trip. It was a welcome respite for all of us. Then Gayle began to write her "Musings" diary. And not long after she started, the unimaginable happened. The entire world was sucker-punched.

MUSINGS

January 30, 2020: This weekend, I'd like to send off the [paper on the] HPV vaccine and increased HPVs to *Infectious Diseases and Cancer*. The Royal Academy of Medicine […] recently published an article showing cervical cancer up among HPV vaccine recipients. I wonder how long the article will remain in print […].

I may have to buy a new computer […]. Not the worst thing in the world, as images from Jonathan's naughty emails to me do not appear on the Chromebook ☹ ☹!! […]

Never a dull moment.

But what I want most from life is to see Jenny happily and safely living independently and to see Flora be a part of the world.

February 1, 2020: The pre-dawn hour is magical. This is the time when ideas and energy meet. All the ideas that swirled in my head during sleep now find their ways to action. The time before the duties of the day intrude and sap the energy to act.

I respect Night Owls. Indeed, my best friend (forever!) works best after midnight. I just don't understand how—after a long day of attending to life's inevitable tedium—Night Owls have the energy to act upon their ideas.

For me, it's the morning—the darkness hides the painful reality that man has created for himself here on Earth. It is the time when theoretic concepts reign, untouched by vulgarities of day-to-day life.

The pre-dawn hour also reminds me of when I see Flora. She is so innocent, so unaware of the stupidity and pettiness of other members of the human race. She, of course, is the victim of their stupidity and greed, but she is unaware. She seems to be giving Reality the Finger.

Of course, she is an easy victim of other predatory humans, but she's also tough. She won't put up with their insanity.

But I digress. Let me get back to the ideas that swirled in my head during last night. Today, I'll work on the paper on increased HPV in HPV vaccine recipients [...].

Ah, what an enchanting day I will have!

February 5, 2020: Jenny has had two major attacks in the past two days. Something attacks her brain, and she becomes insane. She has physically and verbally attacked both Jonathan and me. Mostly me.

When Jonathan and I were going over Jenny's history of abusing us (me) physically, I realized it happens in warm weather. The most recent time she was like this was in summer [...].

I wish Jenny were not so sick. I know that she attacks me because she is sick. Still, I've been trying so hard to guide her and she—when her body is attacking her—lashes out at me. It hurts. I know it's not the real Jennifer, but I never know when Lucifer is going to emerge. I guess I just have to enjoy the moments when Jennifer is with us.

February 7, 2021: As Deirdre Little [an Australian pediatrician who was the first to warn, in the *British Medical Journal*, that the HPV vaccine might cause premature menopause] wrote to me, some people owe their existence to my research. THAT's motivation.

February 9, 2021: Technology can be used for good. Such a shame that those with power use technology so corruptly. Bill Gates did not start out to be corrupt. He did not want to inflict the agony of vaccine injury on millions of people around the world. He wanted to do good, but the pharmaceutical companies snookered him. Now, it's too late to admit he made a mistake. How many millions more will suffer?

February 11, 2020: Ah, the magical pre-dawn hour. What thoughts swirled in my head last night?

The Anatomy of a Retracted Paper draft [...] needs to be more scientific. Analyze Retraction Watch. Number of articles with the word "vaccine" in the title over time. Then determine how many of those articles challenged vaccine safety. Then discuss Andy [Wakefield]'s paper and my experience [...]. The attempt to stifle legitimate scientific debate.

Then (maybe) Jonathan's paper about how laypeople read Jenny McCarthy, because they already agree with her.[1] That observation could be in a section on the effect of literature on doctors and laypeople [...].

---

1 Jonathan Rose, "The Autism Literary Underground," *Reception* 9 (2017): 56–81.

And maybe something about the heat RFK Jr. is receiving. And all the crap on Facebook […].

Ah, what fun I will have with the project! Naturally, I wish I didn't have to do this project, but as long as I have to do it, I'm going to have fun.

February 12, 2020: […] man, oh man: Gardasil Dads are as tenacious as Autism Moms. Some of those girls actually recover.

February 13, 2020: I so love Jonathan. More & more each day. Going through this stupid lawsuit [over whether our school district would pay for Flora's education at Camphill] and getting expensive home improvements done—all in a day's life. So much easier with Jonathan. Plus, he's great in the sack.

February 15, 2020: [Our basement flooded, and when we called in workmen, they] found sewer water is leaking into house. Cost of project now $30K (easier to write $30K than $30,000—ouch!) […]. Then picked up Flora. Forgot that she steals keys and elopes. Also, she makes orange juice, if the opportunity (oranges) exists. And drinks the workmen's half-and-half. She's so clever!

Also yesterday, I said something to Jonathan about assuming the workpeople were men. He suggested I ask which pronoun they prefer. It is such a blast being married to him.

He was very tired yesterday. I did much of the driving. It was fine doing the driving, I just hope he is ok.

February 16, 2020: The basement is all ripped up. Glad Anthony [the contractor] trusts us that we can pay by Thursday. I sense it's because we trust him about the needed repairs. So much to be said for trust. What happens when a society loses that trust? Lawyers, I suppose. Lawyers happen. And chronic illness among 54% (and counting!) of children. Then society as we know it disappears.

But in the meantime, I continue teaching and engaging in my research. Maybe I can contribute—however humbly—to the recovery of our civilization. Jonathan & I.

February 17, 2020: Jenny terrified me last night. She became upset when I told Flora (loudly) to SHUT UP! We needed to have Flora fast for 12 hours, and Flora was being such a pill. But all I said was, SHUT UP! Jenny flew into such a rage. She became an animal: She punched my arm, hit my head, stomped with her boots on my foot. She came after me with scissors, saying she wanted to cut my hair. I gave her Velaria, Passionflower and Lyn's remedy. [Lyn Farrugia was our homeopath.] She finally calmed down when she called the child abuse line—yes, we're being abused by our child! The woman was very understanding and recommended I call Autism Speaks. I wanted to throw up, but merely explained that I had reached out to AS before and they were not helpful. She also recommended the Autism Society of America—also a nonstarter. Finally, she recommended the Children's Aid and Family Services. Jenny could also call their Zoe's Place Hotline when she's upset [...].

It is amazing that Jonathan & I survive. Suzanne and Mark [Jonathan's sister and her husband] are as helpful as they can be, and my "family" (people with whom I have a common last name) is worse than useless. The greater society has nothing of value to offer. The Psych Ward would put Jenny on drugs so that we would never get her back. The Zombie-Jenny might not attack (but actually might), but ZJ is not the real Jenny. Neither is Lucifer—the product of Jenny on vaccines.

Still, Jenny has some responsibility in all this. She lied (I'm almost sure) about taking supplements yesterday morning. She said she had some in her room. I can only do so much. If she wants to destroy her life by ignoring my suggestions, there's nothing I can do. Unfortunately, she might kill me in the process. That's the downside.

February 18, 2020: Jenny was quite pissy again yesterday, especially in the morning, but also throughout the day. It could be the Barlean's Oil that is not good for people with low blood pressure. Or it could be that she is just a brat. Why does she have to attack me? Physically, mentally, emotionally. I know she doesn't want to live at home anymore, but the fact she can't yet live independently is not my fault. Although she is trying to find a job, she needs help in doing so. Although we are exploring a place she might live [...], these things take time. In the meantime, she is blowing her chances [...] by developing a police record.

I just don't understand her. When I have a problem, I deal with it. If one way doesn't work, I try another. That's how Jenny (and Flora to a lesser extent) have gotten as far as they have. I keep trying different approaches to their vaccine injury. I recognized the problem, knew I needed help in addressing, and sought that help.

Jenny is so much like Ruth [Jonathan's deceased mother]—the world owes me. It is a selfish and self-centered approach to life. And it brings nothing but disappointment and resentment. [When I was engaged to Gayle, I had to tell my mother, politely but firmly, "Sorry, Mom, I only take orders from one woman at a time."]

February 20, 2020: Interesting chat with Anthony. One son is addicted to drugs—destroying the family financially and emotionally. The other—who is earning a PhD in psychology—has extremely high levels of anxiety. "We raised them right," he pleaded. "My wife is a good woman." The shame and sadness he felt was palpable. Fortunately, his wife (who has Lyme) seems to know about natural remedies.

What we are doing to our children, our families, our country, our civilization, our world. This is why I do the research I do. To prevent the train from crashing further. To prevent more trains from crashing. And to provide first aid to the victims on the train crash, starting with my children.

February 27, 2020: Jenny attacked me (and Jonathan, but mainly me) last night. The discussion of vaccines for the coronavirus upset her. Also, she said something immature—was it "I'm sorry I'm such a pain in the ass"?—and I didn't respond, so she blew up. Mainly pinching, but she threw my purse at Jonathan.

Something takes over. I gave her a ton of Valerian Root yesterday. It seemed to help until it didn't.

She thinks the world revolves around her, but it's more than that. Immature people don't attack. I don't know where her place in this world is. Sadly, it may be an institution. They'll dope her up, and she won't attack.

Carol [the wife of our plumber and an autism mom] is right. We moms are the only ones who really try with our kids. Once we're gone, it's game over. And yet our kids are putting us in early graves […].

February 28, 2020: I'm remaining grouchy with Jenny. I've had it with her. She has an outburst—pinches, punches, pulls my hair, wraps her hands around my throat. Then the next morning, she's all apologetic. Until the next time. As soon as authority—the police, Lyn, Mom-mom [our neighbor and Jenny's surrogate grandmother]—arrive, she's all sweetness. She's a bully. Standing up to a bully seems to work.

Her financial decisions suck. Last week, she spent $60 both ways [on Uber] to take her book to a meet-and-greet with a politician. He probably would have preferred receiving the $120 she spent on transportation. These stupid acts she does in calm states. Anyway, we pulled her $30 a week allowance. She now receives $20 a week from Mom's Christmas gift.

What a pain in the ass her autism is. She blames me for her woes, when the true culprit is her autism. The sooner she admits to that, the closer she can come to recovery […].

My upper arm was quite painful yesterday, and I was concerned my cancer had spread. It's much better today, so I think it was just a pulled muscle. Still, stress-related.

March 1, 2020: I so love being married to Jonathan. He was half asleep (actually, MORE than half) when I told him I flubbed up the Danish presentation. He muttered, "Don't worry about it." He's right, as always. [And fixing the flooded basement?] "It's only money."

Plus, Jonathan is great in the sack.

March 2, 2020: In 18 days, Dad will have been dead 18 years. How I miss him. He stood for what was right and just; family was everything to him. I didn't realize he was my protector in the DeLong clan. Now, I count for nothing. My immediate family and I count for nothing. Unless it's happy news. Just nothing too taxing like autism. His death revealed the hypocrisy of the remaining members. He would have encouraged me about the girls, reminded me how lucky they are to have Jonathan and me as parents.

Now, no one in the family supports us […]. In fact, there are no family gatherings, no gatherings among just us siblings.

We're not even siblings anymore. We're just people who happen to have the same last name.

The only two people in my "family" who have been supportive are Ryan and Julie. [Gayle's nephew and niece. Julie was absolutely opposed to vaccinating her children, who—as Gayle often noted—were remarkably healthy.] They don't completely understand our situation, but they each offered help. Ryan with legal stuff, Julie with medical research. The rest are a sorry lot.

March 4, 2020: Toni Bark died yesterday. Unbelievable. How can so much life be gone? Every time I saw her, she was energetic, enthusiastic, optimistic. The world was a better place, because she was here. May her energy, enthusiasm, and optimism live on in each of us. [Toni Bark MD was a vivacious holistic doctor who campaigned for the vaccine-injured and ultimately succumbed to cancer. She produced the film *Bought* (2015), in which all four members of our family appeared.]

I stayed home from teaching yesterday. The last time I called in sick was when I had food poisoning and was barfing water. In normal times, I would have sucked it up and gone into school. These are not normal times; sickness is causing tremendous fear. With fear comes control.

Today, I will visit the Amish. They lead such different lives from ours. They are good and kind people (for the most part—I assume there are some bad apples). The Amish I know are good and kind people. And they are being targeted—the Dark Side does not want a control group of non-vaccinated people. When people mentioned the Amish as not vaccinating and not experiencing autism, good old Julie Gerberding said they had different genes. However, now that they are vaccinating, they are experiencing autism. That proves our point—vaccines cause autism. Vaccines and glyphosate.

So, today I'm a missionary to the Amish. Who would have thought??

March 5, 2020: Fascinating day with Amish. The children are so HEALTHY! And respectful and playful and loved. And the Dark Side wants to take that all away from them the way they took that all away from us.

I'll contact Mary Ann [an Amish mom] about asking RFK Jr. to Family Days on the Farm [an annual summer fair in Amish country]. It would be an experience like no other for him […].

Flora and I had some fun at the restaurant last night. There were conversation cards on the table. She learned what the word "procrastinate" means. She also asked me what book I would write. *Love in the Age of Autism.*

March 6, 2020: Tapes from Andy arrived yesterday. [Wakefield was featuring Gayle and Flora in a film.] Flora was so cute! Obviously, speech-delayed. And we just kept injecting her with more and more toxins. God damn those murderers. They destroyed both my daughters' lives. Flora's more than Jenny's, but Jenny has such a hard road. I hope to see their crimes against humanity punished.

March 7, 2020: Mary Ann likes my idea of RFK coming to Family Days on the Farm. Some controversy seems to be brewing within the Amish community.

Great. The Dark Side splits families—like mine […]—now they are splitting the Amish community. All the good aspects of civilization are slipping away—family, community, health—so the Dark Side can rule. But what will they rule over? Sick, sad, angry people who have no support. And what happens to those on the Bright Side—the ones who did not vaccinate their healthy children? Who still believe in family and religion? Are there enough of those people remaining? Can they fight back?

Those of us with damaged children will certainly try to help, but we are struggling just to survive.

March 10, 2020: What a day yesterday! Ruth Beiler [an Amish activist] called while I was on the road to Flora. She said everything came together for "Bobbie" (she calls him Bobbie, very unusual for Pennsylvania people to call others by their first names without being formally told to do so) to come to Family Days on the Farm. A bishop came to her court case to support her; she discussed Bobbie coming to FDF with the bishop, who is very interested. "And I *never* talk to a bishop," she giggled […].

The public health authorities are planning four meetings to discuss the importance of vaccines. Jonathan says I should go. I wonder […]

Ruth said the public health authorities have never pushed vaccines so hard. She said the Amish are also under attack, because of the natural remedies they use. "And they work," Ruth observed. I assured her I know.

We also found out Flora will not be able to attend Morristown High School for the summer. Those scum. No, that's an insult to scum. We need a superintendent who cares about students, all students.

Jonathan is helping me find a summer camp for Flora. One of the many reasons I love him. Ruth asked how our marriage works under the immense pressures we face; I sense she and Isaac have issues. Ruth is *so* smart and so energetic. She may feel frustrated within the confines of the Amish life. Yet, she loves her children. And she has healthy children, which she probably would not have, had she not been Amish.

March 11, 2020: Coronavirus hysteria is everywhere. People wearing masks, Italy shutting down, schools closing, at least one student boycotting my class (presumably other classes as well). We've forgotten that it's ok to be sick. We get sick, we get well. "Out of an abundance of caution," is translating into "No longer living."

Yes, the virus is weird. Probably man-made. I say that, because whenever a health authority gets on the air, the first thing they say is, "This virus is definitely not man-made." But the precautions are the same as any other virus— wash hands, get sleep, sanitize public areas.

If only the health authorities cared—truly cared—about finding causes and treatments for autism.

March 12, 2020: The world has gone completely mad. Universities are going online. People are no longer permitted to interact. Fear stalks the streets.

That's just the way the Dark Side wants it. So when they have a vaccine, everyone will be fighting over who receives it. The others may have mine [...].

I have to figure out how to move my class online. I have to get past the insanity of preventing healthy and strong young adults from gathering and using public transportation (which, by the way, they are FINALLY sanitizing). This generation, already crippled by vaccines, is now denied a decent education. At least, for the duration.

March 13, 2020: The world has officially gone mad. The stock market is crashing. Schools are closed. [When schools went to fully remote learning, parents experienced a 33% increase in anxiety, depression, and worry.][2] Sports events (gasp!) not taking place. Everything that makes us human has been banned. OK, not everything; but I bet sex is next.

---

2 Corey A. DeAngelis and Christos A. Makridis, "Remote Instruction Is Bad for Mom and Dad," *Wall Street Journal,* January 7, 2022, A15.

I wonder if this is a ploy by the elite to show us who (WHO?) is in charge. It is not us […].

Coronavirus does seem to be more contagious than regular common cold. Even Tucker Carlson is admitting it may have been developed in a lab. Jonathan thinks U.S. authorities are not discussing that possibility, because we have virus-making labs ourselves.

Yesterday was the first day of no in-person classes (actually, "academic recess"). On-line classes start next week for the duration of the semester. What an overreaction.

And U.S. health officials are talking only about a vaccine, not about a treatment. A few are talking about Vitamin C infusions or chloroquine.

I suppose once I've figured out this online routine, I'll have more time for research. Yeah!!

March 14, 2020: March Madness takes on a whole new meaning this year! The world has gone completely *mad!* […]Yes, [coronavirus] spreads quickly—probably due to the man-made nature of the virus—and it creates complications for people with underlying medical conditions. Maybe that's the rub. The health officials know that people who received the flu shot are much more likely to have upper respiratory ailments. Oops. They screwed up again. Big time. And they were too busy pushing vaccines to prepare for a national health emergency.

Don't abolish ICE—abolish the CDC! […].

Flora comes home today. [Beaver Farm was ordered closed by the Commonwealth of Pennsylvania.] We will bike and bake. And watch videos of Flora as a little girl. I hope, pray even, that watching the videos wakes up a part of her that exists, but is lying dormant. Please, please, please. I want her back, I want my healthy little girl back.

March 15, 2020: The Ides of March. This would have been Aunt Gloria's 90th birthday, except that her children allowed her to die. They could have intervened. So sad. [Gloria was Jonathan's aunt, who effectively starved herself to death.]

Wonderful time last night at the Crockett's [colleagues of Gayle's]. Madeline [their daughter] has turned into a very sweet young lady—so kind with both Flora and Jenny. Thankfully, she was not harmed—as I had suspected—by the HPV vaccine.

She also reminds me of what could have been. Very, very painful.

Glad for the Crocketts that they have new opportunities in California. So wish it wouldn't be so far away. That's life.

What isn't life is having a 20-year-old shell of humanity, struggling—or not—to make it in this world. Flora will never live independently. She will never be the person she was supposed to be.

Neither will Jenny, but at least Jenny will get closer to the person she was meant to be.

I know my anger is literally eating me. Very fortunately, I have Jonathan. He struggles the same way I do. We struggle together.

Flora's home for at least three weeks. I pray to GOD it is only three weeks. Her food obsessions are the worst. Jenny's right—let's have Flora focus on different activities.

But I need to do some research. So people realize how dangerous vaccines are. So no family ever again suffers the way my immediate family is suffering.

March 16, 2020: *The Plague* continues. Yesterday, Loantaka Park was packed. Felt like Germany on a Sunday afternoon. Trader Joe's was less full, but many shelves were empty. Eerie.

A car just stopped by our house to deliver the newspaper. That's about the only semblance of normalcy.

We're watching the videos of the girls when they were young. And cute. And when we had hope of recovery. It was a lot more fun having hope. Even if it were false.

Working on *Social Medicine* article—increased HPVs among HPV vaccine recipients—helps me to keep my sanity.

Preparing for classes, which resume online on Thursday, also helps me stay sane […]. I'll use Zoom to reach my students […]. Jonathan and I will be using the same program to teach. How romantic!

Funny, our romance is even stronger during these times of chaos and despair. We've got each other. And, really, not much else.

March 17, 2020: St. Patrick's Day 2020. No celebrations today. Just concern and fear. "Don't panic" the health authorities say, but don't go out. And the finger-pointing already. Trump is doing it all wrong; [Phil] Murphy [governor of New Jersey] is doing it all right. But we don't know how this situation is going to turn out. We can't possibly know what the right and wrong measures are at this time.

Jenny attacked me again last night […].

The videos are—as I feared—reminding me of how much work we've done. How much we tried. For what? So Jenny can attack me? Physically, verbally, emotionally.

My research keeps me sane. And, I think to some extent at least, teaching. And Jonathan.

March 18, 2020: Suspicions are on the rise. Bill Gates was wondering aloud in November 2019 about the spread of the coronavirus (John Stone). Also, coronavirus has been around, it's just this strain is new (German scientist on YouTube that went viral, so to speak).... The people profiting from this shutdown of society are Microsoft (everything is now online) and Amazon (for the necessities of life that are not online). Pharma companies will do well when they develop a vaccine (ugh!). Peter Hotez said March 11, 2020 that developing a vaccine for the coronavirus is fraught with complications. The immune systems of vaccinated people overreact when exposed to the virus. Hotez calls this "the immune reaction" and it can be serious. (Hotez changed his tune— heck, his whole melody—a few days later when Tucker Carlson interviewed him.) But the health authorities are bulldozing ahead with human trials without even testing the vaccine on animals first. Trials on healthy people in areas where the virus is not widespread are being conducted. No placebo group. The insane part is that health authorities expect us to believe the results. The ***really insane*** part is that some people will.

Here's what I know or believe about COVID-19:

1. It is real and deadly.
2. Infection can be prevented and at least ameliorated in people with healthy immune systems.
3. It is man-made. The only time germ warfare worked was in WW2, the Japanese against the ***Chinese***. Since the best defense is a good offense, China began developing its own labs to create viruses. COVID-19 is a Frankenvirus.
4. Most people don't die from COVID-19.
5. Sometimes people die. Especially if they have underlying health issues. In fact, all people die at some point.
6. People who received a flu shot are more likely to experience the immune reaction that Hotez warned about. Their bodies are primed to overreact. Nurses who were forced to receive the flu vaccine are most at risk since they are more likely to be exposed to the virus.
7. The overreaction by our health officials is destroying our economy and making us dependent upon those health officials. They like it that way. They don't care how many people's lives they ruin. They care only about power. That's the point.
8. I hope their plan backfires and regular people become wiser. The powers that be are committing crimes against humanity.

March 19, 2020: The insanity continues. Yes, the virus is serious, because (1) it's man-made, so we don't know if remedies that work for natural viruses will be effective for COVID-19; and (2) so many people have the flu shot, which makes them overreact.

People are beginning to ask questions. Why are we shutting down 83% of our economy to bolster the health-care industry (17%)? Coronaviruses have been with us for a while; why the concern with this one? Maybe because it's man-made.

John Stone [UK editor of *Age of Autism*] and John Gilmore [Executive Director of Autism Action Network] are on it. They provide insights that I trust. I guess when you realize an industry (pharma) along with their government puppets (WHO, CDC, FDA) are willing to let babies die for the sake of the "greater good," you realize they are capable of anything. They don't care about people or humanity. They care only about their own money and power. What better way to take away people's liberties than to scare the hell out of them? Then force vaccination and semi-martial law. Prisoners are being released early. People are anxious and will do stupid things.

Jenny is a case in point. Damn, and now Jonathan and I must be the grown-ups in the room. I'm too old to have to be a grown-up every day. But I did last night. Jenny was getting pissy, so I apologized for speaking too loudly and I accepted the fact that I'm an "angel mother." [When Jennifer's hostile self took over, she would hurl this at Gayle as a term of abuse.] Actually, I AM an angel mother. My children have been crippled by the war on infectious diseases. When will I get recognized as such? When will my children receive the compensation for their war injuries? They are receiving what appear to be handouts; for them, Social Security is not a handout, but rather a reparation. What I really want to see is proper research into proper treatments.

But for that to happen, the corrupt powers that be must admit that I am an angel mother, which they will never do.

March 20, 2020: Complete and utter total insanity. Fortunately, 40% of Americans think the response has been an overreaction. Heartening to know that even Paul Offit believes we are doing more harm than good. PAUL OFFIT, who has never met a vaccine he didn't like.

Perhaps the Powers that Be wanted to unleash a pandemic, but got the timing wrong. They wanted to be further along in the development of a vaccine. Now, all they have is a cheap malaria drug that seems to work quite well in treating coronavirus and a public that will not go through this loss of civil liberties—even temporarily—a second time.

At first, the FDA did not want to consider chloroquine, but Trump forced them to investigate it. Tucker Carlson is pushing it, saying he knows someone who is taking it.

Interesting to note that among the original ways to reduce the risk of developing the novel coronavirus was to get a flu shot. Now, that recommendation has quietly disappeared. Does the flu vaccine cause healthy people to overreact to the virus? Inquiring minds want to know.

Flora is changing subtly. Although her obsessions remain intense—buying glue, going to the mailbox after our walk, removing the camera from my computer, getting stickers from Jenny's computer (that one's new)—they are far fewer than before. She does not seem to be watching the Paul McCartney tape (that's a huge change) or eloping even when she could. She seems to be sneaking less food and watching fewer (if any) cooking videos. She now knows her password, but doesn't sneak back onto her computer. Every once in a while— not always—she responds more fully. "Flora, would you like some tea?" "No, thank you," she replied.

Of course, she will never be the person she was meant to be. I'm learning to live with that tragedy. My research helps me—being able to spotlight inconsistencies with vaccines. But it is a realization that no parent should have to endure. Not in America. Not anywhere. And yet, here we are […].

I'm so glad to be married to Jonathan. Best.decision.ever.

March 21, 2020: The madness continues. Except people are beginning to notice who is profiting—pharmaceutical companies, Microsoft and other companies serving telecommuters, Amazon, corrupt politicians. The devastation to the economy and the disruption of people's lives is far-reaching and perhaps irreversible. Not that the Powers that Be care. They don't care […].

They are tearing apart families—who can visit grandma—and isolating the most vulnerable. The old, the sick, the lonely […]. The powerlessness we each feel. And that's the way the 1% want it. They control everything.

But what does revolution look like? Defying lockdown orders? Enjoying life? Using the time to research the negative side effects of vaccines?

Let me go do the last two. See you tomorrow!

March 22, 2020: Dad's death day. I so miss him. Little did I know that when he died, my place in the family would be all but obliterated. He was my supporter and my defender. He brought only good to this world.

I've adjusted to my new non-place in my family. Social distancing.

Speaking of social distancing, the world continues on its path of madness. Phil Murphy—to show his power and not to be outdone by governors of New York, Washington, Connecticut, and California (I think)—has us in lockdown mode. If I attempt to go to my office, I will be arrested. The people in power are sick. They are irrational.

I hope this power grab and dream of dissolving civil liberties backfires to such a degree that those perpetrating it are banished to footnotes in history. They do not deserve to be in power. They are not leading. They are playing on the fears of humans and exercising draconian measures just to show who's in charge. I hope this episode exposes them for who they are.

Businesses are shuttering, people are not being educated ("distance learning" is not the same), grandparents receive no visitors. More will die of drug overdoses, suicide, and murder than from COVID-19. Criminals are being let out of prison.

I know Dad would find something good out of this situation. ☺ Of course, as a teenager, I did not appreciate his total and complete optimism. ☺ Now, I understand. I can't bring myself to ask, "I wonder what great and wonderful things will happen today," but I try.

I wonder what Dad would say about autism. About the country he fought and almost died for forcing his granddaughters to be permanently disabled for the sake of a few dollars.

The only good thing I can see coming from autism is that I have dedicated my work to exposing the fraud that is vaccines. My goal is to reduce to zero the number of lives—like Flora's—that are destroyed or—like Jenny's—that are permanently impaired from vaccine injury.

And I have dedicated my life to recovering my girls. Just like Dad's last words to me, "Take care of those two girls, those two beautiful little girls." Dad, I'm doing my best, Jonathan and I are doing our best.

March 23, 2020: IN.SANE. The.world.is.totally.INSANE. Friends from Denmark report that vaccination is now mandatory. No vaccine exists, but it is ***mandatory***. People in Germany know that the "emperor has no clothes." Even Mom agrees this could be a conspiracy. The line at Trader Joe's—disciplined, but still six feet apart.

The entire world economy is collapsing except for pharma, Microsoft, and Amazon. Unemployment, depression—both economically and personally—broken lives, suspended education. For what? As the woman in *Fargo* admonished the brutal murderer, "For the sake of a few dollars. That's why you did this, for a few dollars?"

I'll write to my friends soon about my research. It will be a great way to connect and find out how they are doing.

But first, I need to write the mid-terms and do taxes (literally, and maybe even figuratively today).

March 24, 2020: Sanity appears to be slowly creeping back into the U.S. society. Of course, our community sees the attempted power-grab by pharma. We've been smart enough to couch our arguments in different terms—Toby Rogers [who wrote a doctoral dissertation on "The Political Economy of Autism"] points out the "deaths of despair" and how people die from unemployment—heart conditions, suicide, homicide. Del Bigtree [CEO of the Informed Consent Action Network] points out the numbers: We're not all dying [on] the streets; in *fact*, relatively few people are dying at all. And they have co-morbid conditions. Del was one of the first to mention hydroxychloroquine as a treatment. Ah, a treatment. Pharma must hate that.

But even mainstream outlets are now bravely coming out and saying we have choices. They call them "difficult" choices, so they don't sound heartless [...]. Some politicians like the Lieutenant Governor of Texas (man, I'm moving to Texas—except, as Jonathan protests, it's *TEXAS*)—and even Mom realize the entire country can't shut down for the sake of older Americans. Of course, The *Wall Street Journal* has been making economic arguments for a while.

I get it. Why we had to hold our collective breath at first. This is most probably a man-made virus. We didn't know how it would affect humans or how it would spread. If it had affected everyone quickly with a 100% death rate, we'd be in big trouble. But it doesn't kill everyone. It nudges people with pre-existing conditions over the edge. They should have the right to self-quarantine. As a society, we need to give the people who want to self-quarantine the economic capability to do so. But let the rest of us live.

One problem is that COVID-19 appears to affect people who received the flu shot more profoundly than those who did not. As soon as the data are available, I'm going to study that.

In other great news, Skyhorse [Jennifer's publisher] published Woody Allen's book! When I heard Jonathan say, "Woah!", my first thought was oh, shit, the Dow has fallen another 2,000 points. But I was pleasantly shocked to hear the news. And all the media outlets covered it. And there is a Twitter storm of outrage. And the book is sold out at Barnes & Noble. [When Hachette axed Woody Allen's *Apropos of Nothing*, I contacted Skyhorse CEO Tony Lyons and suggested that he pick it up. Ten days later, Skyhorse published it.]

Rationality. Justice. Freedom. This is what makes America great. Again.

March 26, 2020: Jennifer (as Lucifer) can be such an ingrate. It's so painful to me that she makes fun of my work. I'll know she's mature when she can realize the value of what Jonathan and I are doing. Until then, she (as Lucifer) is such an ingrate.

The Ingrate & the Imbecile. Through no fault of their own, but that's my children. I haven't given up hope. I can't, or else it's all over. But neither girl will be the person they were meant to be. Both struggle with horrendous demons. Flora doesn't even know the demons inside of her. Unfortunately, Jenny does.

Onward!

March 27, 2020: Hard to believe that the day that changed the world was a mere two weeks ago. March 12. The United States went from a country of bursting employment, crowds of Chinese New Year's revelers, and delightful St. Patrick's Day plans to a ghost town. We could still go out for lunch the day we picked up Flora, March 14. Yes, people were concerned about going to the Crockett's SPD party, but they came. Some didn't, but Sean's extended family did. And I'm so glad. His parents are really cool. His dad and I went to the same high school! And his mom had insights about the Amish and sexual abuse that floored me.

New York City is totally desolate right now. Many people getting sick are health-care providers: nurses, doctors. Flu shot, anyone? The nurses were forced to get the shot, and now they are overreacting to the coronavirus. God has interesting ways of punishing people.

So, the coronavirus is hitting some parts of the country much more than others. Trump and Cuomo seem to be working well together. Good. For the sake of New York and the country.

On a different note: Distance learning is for the birds. I tried to give an exam yesterday, but a glitch did not allow students to access the exam. I felt bad for them; they are (or *should* be) nervous enough already. Then they can't access the exam.

I sense many students are not really following my online lectures. Very little reaction when my screenshot showed the picture of my family […]. Their loss. But it is a loss.

I do hope life returns to a semblance of order soon. Jonathan misses restaurants—what a New Yorker! I would love to see Flora back at Camphill. Having her here is painful. Not because she is a nudnik—which she is—but because I'm constantly reminded of how sick she is. There really is no hope for her to be even close to the person she was supposed to be. Jenny might emerge from the wreckage of vaccines—get her outbursts under control—and be the creative writer she was meant to be. Flora's brain is so rotted and her physical body so mutilated—including from the drugs we gave her to address her inflammation—that she won't even come close to Flora Alice Rose: the happy, productive, sincere, dedicated, intelligent, and funny individual she was intended to be.

March 28, 2020: I'm up earlier than usual again (5 am). When I get awake early and lie in bed, I think sad thoughts. About what could have been.

Trump appears to be dissolving Dr. Fauci. Fauci was fading from the scene as Dr. Birx started doing more of the talking. Yesterday, Fauci was gone from the stage. Are we beginning to break the pharmageddon stranglehold on the U.S. government? Oh, God, please, yes.

Maybe now fewer children will die or, worse?, become permanently disabled. Maybe more children will be born, because their mothers did not receive the HPV vaccine.

Anyway, much work today [...]. And research, my precious, precious research.

March 30, 2020: The world is still eerily quiet. But the birds are so happy! They chirp away, not just in the morning, but *all day*.

Flora seems to be improving. She is responding more quickly, and her handwriting is smaller and legible. She still insists upon going shopping every day—either to Trader Joe's or Walmart—and upon taking something out to the mailbox every evening. But I love seeing her eyes. Her beautiful, bright eyes.

I credit the sauna and HBOT and her new supplements.

We're going to Pennsylvania today, if they'll have us. Trump almost called for a quarantine of NY, NJ, and Connecticut. Cuomo yelped. The CDC (not Trump, but I guess the Deep State is conflating with the Executive these days) called for a "travel advisory," respectfully requesting New Yorkers to avoid domestic travel [...].

We're supposed to see the worst in about two weeks. Who (or is it WHO) comes up with this stuff? Someone else said the virus has been circulating for several months now. Whoever was going to become sick is already sick. Those of us with strong—non flu-vaccinated—immune systems have developed our colds or nothing.

I think that's the rub. People "inoculated" against the flu are more susceptible to respiratory ailments, specifically coronavirus. A study of DOD families found that roughly 5% of people who did not get the flu shot developed a coronavirus, while 7% of people who got the shot had a coronavirus. The study didn't mention (I have to check this) how sick people became. I think it's just susceptibility, not intensity [...].

March 31, 2020: Jenny might have PANDAS. When I first heard of PANDAS, I thought of Jenny. But then she got tested [...]. And the test was negative. That was in 2009. Dr. Kevin said a reliable test did not exist until

2013. Pediatric acquired neurological disorder associated with strep. There's also PANS. Pediatric acquired neurological syndrome. I think.

I have much to learn.

Blood tests first, then perhaps a direct test of PANDAS. I like Dr. Kevin. Alternatively-oriented chiropractors in general are great […]. Such independent minds, unorthodox, yet extremely knowledgeable. Dr. Grams rescued Jenny from the "benign" grips of propranolol.

Dr. Kevin also thinks the sauna will be great for Flora. [Gayle had a sauna constructed in our bedroom.] He had very good advice: makes sure she sweats—especially her trunk—do jumping jacks before going in to get the heart rate up, wipe away the sweat and then wash the towel.

April 1, 2020: The birds are having a field day (pun intended)! Really, they just chirp and hum and sing *all day and night*. Makes you wonder what we're doing to our environment with all the cars and planes and factories.

Well, sorry Nature. I'm looking forward to getting back to normal.

We're making the best of a bad situation. We have Flora started on the sauna—three times a week—and doing HBOT almost daily.

And Jenny. We might be able to help Jenny. Dr. Kevin suggested she might have PANS. That would explain *so much*. She might need IVIG. We'll try other treatments first—assuming she has PANS—and we'll find the money somewhere. Period.

Chiropractors are great. They have the knowledge and expertise of MDs without the arrogance. Even holistic doctors can be (are?) arrogant. Sometimes even more than mainstream MDs. I suppose it comes with the territory. They are taught to be arrogant, yet they have the toughness of mind to think differently => arrogance.[2]

April 2, 2020: Insanity has again gripped the world. Trump appears to have succumbed to Coronavirus Derangement Syndrome. Why on earth would he extend the "social distancing" to the end of April? What does he know that we don't know? Italy has always had problems with overrun hospitals. This year isn't even the worst; 2017 was. The stats sound awful, until you compare them with daily deaths from other causes. 102 for traffic accidents […].

Mom will join my class today. She's so excited. I'm glad.

April 3, 2020: I'm so angry. Coronavirus is completely overblown, yet its impact on society is devastating and far-reaching. The bastards who concocted this scheme don't care. Bill Gates is probably behind this. He enlisted the World Health Organization—to which he donates much of their budget—and who else? Cuomo? Or is Governor Cuomo just one of the politicians who needed peer pressure to comply? Did pharma enlist Gates or did Gates enlist pharma or did they both figure out this scheme together?

The disruption, the deaths from suicide and homicide, the child abuse, the elder abuse, the abuse of the disabled. They don't care. All they care about is power. They have enough money. Now, they want power.

Our society is being ripped to shreds. People are afraid—no, terrified—of each other. Legally, we are not permitted to congregate. No protests. No resistance. And our neighbors would turn against us if we did. Don't you care about the "common good"?

What has the "common good" ever done for me? would be a weak refrain.

But how will this end? Which politicians will say, enough! We can go back to living. Trump held out for a while, but even he succumbed. Why? DeSantis also held out, but even he ordered—ordered!—citizens to remain inside […].

Of course, if you code all deaths as "coronavirus" then deaths from the disease rise. It's like the number of boys born at St. Vincent's Hospital doubling on August 1, 1996, except that all babies born at that hospital on that day were coded as male.

Except deaths will rise […] but from suicides and homicides. So, be sure to code suicides and homicides as "coronavirus" and you're good to go for the next pandemic.

Assuming there's a society left after the ravages of this pandemic.

One epidemiologist pointed out he's seen lots of pandemics, 30 in fact. Each year. There's a flu pandemic each and every year. The flu reaches many countries. And yet, until now, we survived without lockdowns.

I'd like to study the different outcomes between Sweden and Norway. I'm sure Norway has lockdowns, being the Nanny State they are. Sweden, on the other hand, is allowing life to go on. Let's see whether the outcomes are different. Or not. Just curious.

April 4, 2021: And now we see the effects of regulatory capture. The World Health Organization, a puppet for both China and pharma, is running the world into the ground. I think WHO's first master is China and Bill Gates. Pharma is simply reaping the benefits.

As the world stands still, stunned. How could this be happening? Health authorities are stripping us of our civil liberties. The unelected have bribed the elected and co-opted (most of) the media. A terrified population clamors for a vaccine.

Dr. Birx noted that the numbers predicted by the models are not matching reality. The models would have predicted 400,000 deaths in Italy. We're nowhere near that […]. The ship *Comfort* [a 1,000-bed US Navy hospital ship dispatched to New York harbor] has three patients.

Listen to Dr. Birx, please, Mr. Trump. You seem to be. You have her telling the media to "cool it," that sensationalism is detrimental to the country. Thank you.

I shudder—shake and tremble!—to think of where we would be if Hillary Clinton were president. It would be a national lockdown for 18 months.

At the end of next week, point out that people are not dying in the street. That hospitals are fine. Watch the "Citizen Reporter" videos of the empty hospitals.

April 5, 2020: People, get a grip! We are being led to slaughter. By Bill Gates, whom the pharmaceutical industry convinced that he could save the world. He wants respect. He has all the money he could possibly need—though more is always better—and more power than any human being alive—though, again, more is better. He wants respect. He wants us to see him as the Savior of Mankind.

Yet, in the process, he is destroying mankind. The means are medical marshal law. We can't leave our homes. We can't congregate. We can't protest. We can no longer be human.

We watched *Night and the City* last night [a 1950 film noir in which the] wheeler dealer got his comeuppance. God, if you do exist, find a way for us to survive. To grow. To be human.

We don't know how to fight the scourge of medical tyranny. It's a new war on a whole new level. Neighbors are afraid of each other. Grandparents can't see their grandchildren. Human contact—except among family members—is banned.

Those of us rebels who don't wear masks are seen as suspect by those who do. We protest the yoke of the medical tyranny. We can identify one another. We know it's ok to get sick. People get sick, they build their innate—God-given—immune systems; they get well. Some perish. But people die. Every day. We all do at some point.

But this lockdown, this inhumane caging of law-abiding citizens is killing people. Cirrhosis, suicide, *homicide* will kill more than covid-19. Child abuse, elder abuse, abuse of the disabled, domestic violence. All will increase. Probably already is on the rise.

And then we hate ourselves as human beings. When a parent turns on a child, the parent inevitably feels terrible remorse. I speak from experience. The shame, the self-loathing.

OK, I have an idea, Mr. President. Make federal aid contingent on getting life back to normal. Provide in-kind aid—hydroxycholoraquine, hospital beds, ventilators (even though 70–90% of people who get to the point where they need ventilators die). But also incentives to get people back to normal life.

While we are doing fine financially right now, the havoc that this plague is wreaking on the economy could dramatically limit Flora's future. Funds for the disabled are the first to dry up. Setting her up in an appropriate environment out of state becomes much more difficult. New Jersey's economy is sinking fast. They would not be willing to send her out of state to a farm where she can enjoy life to the greatest extent possible. Who knows how much our savings will be worth at the end of this ordeal? If there is an end.

In the meantime, I plug away at my research. I have more time for my research, which is about the only element of sweet revenge that I have.

April 6, 2020: The madness continues. Depressing, how ignorant many people are. Fortunately, many people are *not* wearing masks. What do we do if/when the health "authorities" mandate the masks? Cross that bridge if we get to it.

Hyperbaric oxygen—*not* ventilators—might help. Jonathan immediately offered ours. We do care about the greater good. Genuinely care.

April 7, 2020: President Trump and Dr. Birx are talking about a "Light at the End of the Tunnel." Sean Hannity—whom even *Jonathan* watched with me last night [I was not fond of Hannity]—asked Dr. Birx why the predicted numbers of hospitalizations and deaths were so much higher than the reality. She said it was because Americans came together and listened to stay-at-home orders. Are you saying that, because you want me to feel as though my sacrifice has meaning or are you saying that, so you can again impose medical marshal law in the future?

In regimes/people I trust, I assume the former; in regimes/people I don't trust, it's the latter […]. And future regimes I don't trust. If Hillary Clinton had been president, we'd be in lockdown until a vaccine was developed. A shoddy "immunization" with horrible side effects that would kill more people than the disease itself […].

Jenny blew up last night. She was twitchy (slapping herself and masturbating) […]. Maybe the news is overwhelming […]. Cheer up, Jen. We'll get through this. I'm not sure we'll be stronger—we're already incredibly strong—and I'm not sure there is *anything* good coming out of this disaster (sorry, Dad!), but we'll get through this.

April 8, 2020: Almost forgot to write my musing! Flora ate an entire box of pasta and a huge block of Jonathan's cheese last night. My cancer is acting up, so I didn't check up on her as I normally do at 1:30 am. Jenny didn't correctly close the lock on the refrigerator.

I want a different family!

But in the meantime, I'll change the lock.

Governor Murphy closed New Jersey's parks. What the h-e-double-hockey-sticks! The covid-19 numbers are not nearly as bad as anyone predicted and they are going down. Why close the limited places we can go? For exercise? Fresh air?

Because he—like so many progressives—wants control.

I can't believe this is America.

April 9, 2020: Phil Murphy is a DICtator! Closing businesses, schools, PARKS. Why? The numbers of sick and dead—which are already exaggerated—are much lower than the models predicted.

I *really* want to analyze how many fewer flu deaths we have, compared with how many deaths from covid-19.

Notice the name: covid-19. Obviously, the powers that be are anticipating more covids. Covid-20, covid-21, covid-infinity.

Except I have some faith in the American people that we will see through the exaggeration. The World Health Organization and the Centers for Disease Control (and Prevention!) are losing credibility by the day [...]. And, as Del Bigtree pointed out, why should I listen to the CDC? They have stood by as chronic diseases among children have gone from affecting 13% in 1985 to 54% now. They SUCK at their jobs.

And the politicians are taking advantage of a manufactured crisis to exact marshal law—medical marshal law [...].

What I fear is a mandated vaccine. Not the virus, not getting sick—it's OKAY to get sick—but the injecting into my body and the bodies of my husband and children of toxic substances for which no long-term studies could possibly be performed in 18 months and for which the short-term studies are bogus.

I hope we can get antibody tests. I hope I and my loved ones have the antibodies.

April 10, 2020: The world continues its journey into coronavirus insanity. The number of deaths is nothing compared with other maladies. We've lost all sense of context. People get sick, some die. It happens every day. We've been conditioned to think all sickness is bad and that death is optional.

Levi Quackenboss [pseudonym of a vaccine skeptic blogger] found seven silver linings in the coronavirus scandal. The WHO and CDC are exposed for the corrupt institutions they are. Bill Gates is going down. Not as many sheeple are lining up for an experimental vaccine as planned. Parents are not taking their babies for "well visits" and *fewer babies are dying from SIDS*. I see a research project on the horizon […].

Fabrizio wrote to me from Italy. I so look forward to skyping with him again. We have to meet sometime. Maybe Jonathan and I can also visit Italy when we travel to Vienna. [Dr. Fabrizio Strata is a neuroscientist at the University of Parma and an opponent of compulsory vaccination.]

The wonders of travel. Flora will never experience them. Goddamn those bastards […].

April 11, 2020: I WANT MY CIVIL LIBERTIES BACK!

The DICtator Governor Phil Murphy is tightening the screws by the day. Wearing masks in public is now law. Parks are closed. Stores require social distancing. Some states are now separating "essential" from "nonessential" goods and allowing citizens—the last time I checked we were still citizens—to purchase only "essential" goods. If Flora can't buy her glue, she is going to FREAK OUT!

Pennsylvania schools are closed through the end of the academic year. Camphill applied for an exemption, but was denied because the area was so hard hit. HARD HIT?!? No area—not even NYC—has been hard hit. The death tolls are way less than the models predicted. Instead of needing 65K beds, NYC needed 16K […].

Jenny had a rage yesterday. Took a swing at Jonathan, missed, and dislocated her shoulder. It was fascinating to be in a hospital during this "pandemic." Four residents joined the attending physician to observe how to relocate a dislocated shoulder. Obviously, they had nothing urgent to do. X-rays came back faster than any other time we've been in the emergency room […]. There were more hospital staff than patients. So much for the pandemic.

Flora's ritual became an obsession when I said we couldn't go to Trader Joe's. She kept asking, "Are we going to Trader Joe's today?" Whenever I replied no, she replied an emphatic YES! I caved. Then Jenny insisted upon coming. But Jenny stayed in the car, so I could have a real conversation with the person controlling the number of people going into the store. She believes Murphy is in the pocket of "Uncle George (Soros)." Interesting. Murphy doesn't need the money, but I bet he enjoys being part of the cabal that is taking over the world. I mentioned Bill Gates, and the woman agreed. We then discussed the draconian measures Murphy is imposing, e.g., no reusable bags allowed in the stores. Where's the science showing reusable bags bring germs? She gave us the heads-up that soon we might not be able to bring in purses, only wallets.

Then we discussed vaccine injury. She saw it happen, too. A perfectly healthy baby died at age two.

April 12, 2020: T-shirts we need to make: [...].

Kiss me, I'm immune! [...]

Where did my civil liberties go? (on front) They were here just a minute ago. (on back)

Covid-19**84** [...].

Flora ate the entire bag of candies that Trader Joe's gave her. I thought I had hidden them. I failed. Flora 1 Mom 0. Then we found her stash of empty yogurt containers and pretzel bags in the sump pump in the basement.

Why do I even bother? Her life is nothing but urges. Her life has no meaning. Vaccines destroyed my daughter's life [...].

Does Bill Gates [...] take sadistic pleasure in destroying people's lives? Or is that just an unavoidable by-product on his quest for respect?

Of course, Gates is not alone in his sadistic actions. Individual governors and heads of state are gleefully imposing medical marshal law on their citizens. They delight in imposing edicts that make life arduous and create drudgery, because they can [...].

Today, I need to prepare for Flora's online classes.

April 13, 2020: So, Flora's home for the duration. While I dread that thought, we are able to pursue some therapies such as sauna and HBOT on a regular basis now. Perhaps I should look into eye therapy, so long as she's here.

Jenny was wonderful yesterday. She became a little weepy, saying she was concerned about the whole situation. I tried to console her the best I could. Weepy is so much better than taking swings at her father. I congratulated her on handling her anxieties appropriately.

I suggested my t-shirt campaign to Children's Health Defense. Let's see. Jonathan thinks it's a great idea.

Covid-19 appears to be more of a blood disease than a lung disease. CAT scans of the lungs of severe patients are not white, suggesting massive amounts of fluid in the lungs. But rather blood clots appear to be forming. Since the lungs themselves are in good condition, ventilators appear to do more harm than good. The pressure ventilators exert actually damage the lungs. The blood cells need oxygen or else the patients experience something similar to the bends. Hyperbaric oxygen (!) appears to help.

But the medical establishment can't admit that they made a mistake. They didn't understand why people were short of breath, and assumed their lungs were full of fluid. Now that the "standard of care" (where have we heard that term before?) is to ventilate, few doctors can risk their reputations by ordering oxygen.

Covid-19 being a blood disease is also consistent with hydroxychloroquine being a useful antidote. In healthy people, oxygen attaches to iron within the blood. The virus prevents that, robbing the blood of essential oxygen. At the same time, there is an excess of free iron, consistent with the elevated ferritin in covid-19 patients. Hydroxychloroquine opens the cell and allows in zinc, which then allows oxygen into the cell (?). Zinc deficiency also explains where covid-19 can't taste or smell.

The theory is fascinating to me, because Jenny has a low zinc to copper ratio.

April 14, 2020: The outrage is near universal against the demagogues known as governors. Several showing their raw political ambition or pure desire to control […] Sweden did not lock down and has had far fewer covid-19 deaths than Michigan. [One recent survey found that America "would have had 1.6 million fewer deaths if it had the performance of Sweden."][3]

[…] Governors are beginning to work together to get themselves out of the mess they created. They've totally pissed off parents by closing schools. Now, several of them have said the schools will remain closed through the end of the academic year. One way to un-piss parents is to lift that ruling. Please, for Flora's sake.

Jenny flipped out again yesterday. I kept muttering how stupid the masks were, and she almost lost it before we even got into Walmart. I sucked it up, so as not to create a scene. (My cancer cells were swimming so gleefully in the extra cortisol in my system.) Once we got home and I said I will not bring her with us again, she started punching and kicking me. Then the hotline. Again. And the nice person on the phone told us to say something kind about each other.

Jeez, Jenny. Grow up! This is a trying time for all of us. Don't blame me. And for god's sake, don't lash out at me or Dad. You're hurting yourself and your family. You are profoundly sick.

Dad and I have tried everything. And we keep trying. Yesterday, I spoke with yet another doctor. I hope he can help. Your body is not healing itself, the way normal bodies do.

Someday, you'll be on your own. I hope you can figure it out.

---

3 Quoted in Scott Atlas, "America Still Needs a Covid Reckoning," *Wall Street Journal*, March 4, 2025, A17.

I'm back to teaching today [...] Ugh. This remote teaching is for the birds. I don't miss the commute, but I do miss the 3-D human interaction.

April 15, 2020: Jenny blew up again last night. No provocation. Could be allergies.

Lockdown continues [...]. Politicians are grabbing power like never before. Imposing draconian measures, and so proud to do so.

My students are falling for it. Sweden's "social experiment" of not imposing a lockdown is an exception. Actually, social distancing is a social experiment. No research exists showing that it works. In fact, we're learning that people appear to spread the virus mostly by prolonged exposure to the same person—not momentarily passing by someone. So, in effect, the lockdown means that if someone in your household has the virus, you have a much greater probability of developing it than if you were in a restaurant.

How soon before we forget what civil liberties mean? How soon do we forget how important the right to assemble is—for religious reasons, for protests, for just having fun? And freedom of speech: We are literally muzzled every time we go to a store.

The governors have become feudal chieftains, each battling to outdo the other's toughness. Each vying for the notoriety bestowed upon Andrew Cuomo for his decisive action. Never mind his quest for ventilators is probably killing more people than it is saving. Ventilators, it turns out, crush the lungs of covid-19 patients. The disease seems to be more a blood disease than a lung disease. On CAT scans, the lungs [...] are fine. Patients can't breathe, because their blood is not carrying enough oxygen. Blood clots form. Hyperbaric oxygen should be the response, not ventilators.

It's fine that we didn't know this from the beginning. Covid-19 is "novel." But we need to learn and to incorporate the learning quickly. Hospital protocols, however, have decided on ventilators, outcomes be damned.

Explanations that seemed right to me when I first heard them—that the virus appears to come from a lab, that hyperbaric oxygen could be a solution, that the hysteria could be overblown—seem to be correct. Maybe I should trust my instincts more.

Through all of this, Jonathan and I are becoming closer and closer. I.am.so .glad.to.be.married.to.him.

April 16, 2020: Flora's eye contact is better, warmer. And yesterday, she asked what the "T" stands for (in HBOT) as well as "When will the coronavirus end?"!!

I'm not sure whether it's the sauna or the Fiji water or the homeopathy or the supplements, but something is happening.

Yes, Dad, maybe something good is coming out of the covid-19 crisis.

Still, Dad, Flora will never be the person she was meant to be. Miracles like that don't happen.

But I can continue to do everything in my power to help her come closer to her potential.

Phil Murphy on Tucker Carlson last night. What a phony! Phony Phil. "Every life is precious. Every life matters." What about the lives of the unemployed, those living in poverty, the addicted, the disabled? Your "get tough on covid-19" act rings hollow. You, and so many governors […] like you are motivated by greed and fear. Greed for more power, fear that you're not tough enough. Everyone wants to be the next Governor Cuomo, the get tough guy who has probably done more harm than good.

Policies born of competition and greed are necessarily corrupt […]. The discussion of corruption in FIN 4920 could make class a lot more interesting. Start with Sharyl Attkisson clip that establishes the U.S. government is corrupt. Then apply that to covid-19. Fauci with his interest in Moderna, a vaccine maker. Maybe the CHD clip. Birx and the CDC with exaggerating number of covid-19 deaths. Show the clip. And the Michigan governor overstepping authority. Phony Phil, too, not acknowledging that he's trampling on the Bill of Rights.

OK, maybe this last month of teaching won't be *so* bad.

April 17, 2020: Each morning, when I sign onto my computer, Microsoft reminds me to sign into my OneDrive Account. "Error!" screams the message, "We couldn't sign you in and monitor your every move!" I click the "Eat shit and bark at the moon" button. I'm so rebellious.

The insanity continues, but it appears to be lessening. The authorities— President Trump, Governor Cuomo—are saying, ok, I guess it's ok to open the economy […] in phases. There is talk of getting the schools reopened. That would be a great way to un-piss parents […].

It appears more and more that the virus came from a lab. What do we know about viruses that are man-made? How virulent? How deadly? We don't know. Which is why we—and China—had to take drastic measures.

Now that we see covid-19 appears to kill the frail—the elderly, people with preexisting conditions. OK. Quarantine them.

Something else we're learning is that the virus may not be attacking the lungs directly, but rather the blood. Patients can't breathe, because their blood clots and clogs the lungs. Blood thinners and oxygen should perhaps be the treatments of choice—like what Boris Johnson received.

But what do I know? I'm just an informed citizen. And a mom.

April 18, 2020: Today is the second day of my 2-day juice fast. I'm so listless. It's like induced coma. I'm useless. I tried called Dr. Isaacs late yesterday afternoon, but she wasn't in. Once, she told me I only had to do the juice fast for one day. I'll soldier on today, since my cancer is active again, but I'm miserable.

I would have been a dreadful chemo patient. I can't even handle the discomfort of limited food for two days. How would I have been week after week, knowing that the chemicals they were about to inject into me would make me sick?

And Flora managed to find the lock open and remove the cables that hold the lock. She now has all the removable parts that lock the refrigerator. VERY interestingly, she ate only one container of yoghurt. There were three full containers. She may have had some goat cheese as well. But she didn't clean out all of the dairy products. Self-control? Satiated? Limits to her own consumption?

I wish our politicians could exercise the same amount of self-control. I sense some of them—Phil Murphy?—are scared. They don't want to happen in their states what is happening in Michigan.

I'm looking forward to my classes on corruption.

Short musing today, because I'm so listless.

April 19, 2020: So, what do we do for multi-generational households like the O'Briens? [the extended family of our neighbor, Terry O'Brien]. They are already terrified that John [her son] will bring home the virus. Social distancing may alleviate some but not all of that fear. Let's look at the facts:

1. The number of deaths is overstated in the United States. Hospital officials are recording anyone who dies **with** the covid-19 virus as dying **of** the virus. At this point, we have no idea the extent of this overcounting […].
2. Hydroxychloroquine is a successful treatment. While it is off-label, enough reports of positive responses to the medicine suggest the doctors should at least try it. One study found it worked for SARS.
3. Why would health officials exaggerate the number of deaths and hold back on a potential treatment? This is where corruption comes in. Fauci is working on a vaccine.
4. Does the current situation necessitate the suspension of the Bill of Rights?

But getting back to the O'Briens. Yes, the elderly should self-quarantine. What about John? How about he choose to shop later? Or provide special hours for the elderly **and those who provide for them**. Remember, we are talking not only about suspending the Bill of Rights but also destroying the economy. Let John decide what is essential and not. Let the Verizon store stay open.

April 20, 2020: Rough night last night. Cancer area painful. I've experienced worse pain (childbirth), but not often. Darting pains. Ice packs helped sort of. Castor oil (yes, Aunt Bee!) helped this morning. HBOT will help. I'll call Dr. Isaacs, maybe.

Insanity continues, though there seems to be a very slow lifting in some places [...]. Certainly not New Jersey. But people were out yesterday without masks. I think technically, we are to wear masks in public. Since streets are not private property, they are public. 80% of people were not wearing masks.

Jonathan, Flora, and I went biking. On the street, which is of course more dangerous than in the park [which was closed]. That's insane. Flora was great on the steep hills. She knew when it was too much for her. She wouldn't get off her bike and walk it, though. She straddled the bike between her legs and slowly crept down a steep hill. Explaining to her that getting off her bike and walking it down the hill would be easier was like talking to the hand.

It's ok, Flora, I'm used to it. My students do it to me all the time.

Soon we'll be discussing corruption. I'm looking very forward to that topic. I'm sure many of the students won't agree with me, but I'll plant seeds.

April 21, 2020: Feeling much better. Breast area still hard and bumpy, but not painful.

This morning, it's my eyes that are watery. Ah, what flesh is heir to!

No science backs staying at home to alleviate a pandemic. Fresh air and exercise disperse a virus, not being cooped up.

The only part of the Constitution that the government can explicitly suspend is habeas corpus. So, if there is an invasion, the government can put suspected combatants in jail without charging them. And that's it. That's the only time the government can suspend the Constitution.

Right now, our leaders have suspended the Bill of Rights (part of the Constitution). They have suspended the right to assemble and the right to free speech. But there is no provision in the Constitution that allows for the suspension of the right to assemble.

And why? Because of a state of emergency. But the state of emergency no longer exists. And probably never did. The models have been completely wrong. The number of dead is exaggerated. The measures are unscientific.

And now Bill de Blasio is asking citizens to report their neighbors. He never did that for murder or rape [...].

[I'll] plant seeds. That's what I can do most effectively. Going overboard reaches nobody. Providing measured, scientific evidence can plant seeds.

April 22, 2020: Internet is down. Fucking Third World Country, the United States is an effing Third World Country. Jonathan might not be able to teach his class. No information can flow. **This** is how you bring a country to its knees.

A protester in New Jersey got arrested for exercising her right to free speech. Medical marshal law. The government has suspended the rule of law. There might be a good reason, but we have to admit that many state governments have suspended the Constitution. Is the reason a good one? Where is the science saying social distancing works?

April 23, 2020: The insanity continues. Polls say the DICtator Murphy is popular for the steps he took to mitigate the virus. *I hate New Jersey!* How misinformed can people be? Just look around. People are not dying in the streets. Hospitals are not overrun. The focus on covid-19 to the exclusion of all other illnesses and elective surgeries is devastating to the hospital industry. Eighty percent—80%!—of their revenues come from elective surgeries.

And now they are trying to scare us with a "second wave" coming in September. Be sure to get your flu shot, they wail. What about the study that said people who had flu shots were *more* likely to develop a coronavirus? And the scare coming from the people who oversaw the largest increase in chronic illnesses in young people the world has ever seen. In 1985, 12% of people under the age of 18 developed a chronic disease—asthma, ADHD, autism. The percentage now stands at 54%. Fifty-four percent of young people have a chronic, sometimes crippling disease. The CDC sucks at its job!

While I'm looking forward to class on Tuesday, I'm nervous and I don't know what to expect. I will plant seeds.

My right side along my rib cage feels sore, like a pulled a muscle. I don't feel any bumps, just tenderness. Also, I have a herpes outbreak ☹.

April 24, 2020: The insanity continues, even though the Plague is winding down. The authoritarian rule continues in many states, including—especially!—New Jersey. The stillness has become the New Normal. People like me complain, but few voices accompany mine in the lines to Trader Joe's. Jonathan thinks there is little rebellion in New Jersey, because we've been hit hard. But we haven't been hit all that hard. More die of heartbreak.

On second thought—yes, our area has been affected. Especially residences for the elderly. The most isolated and socially-distanced among us are also the most affected. What does that say about social distancing?

Tucker Carlson excoriated McKinsey last night. Very effective segment. The people who promoted U.S. dependence on a despotic regime have no regrets. The company that sells very high-priced solutions has none. TC asked whether we should lock people who have the virus in their homes to die and the former McKinsey partner said no. Whew. But it's ok if China does it? China has a different culture. You've got to understand. They are different; not wrong, just different.

I'm preparing for my class on corruption. The Sharyl Attkisson segment first. Then a discussion of the CDC, how they suck at their jobs. And now CDC says we're going to have a second wave in September. Should we trust them? Should we follow their advice and get a flu shot? What about the study that finds people who received the flu shot were *more* likely to develop a coronavirus?

And what of this emphasis on a vaccine? Can we do *anything* until a vaccine is developed? Or rather, why keep pushing a vaccine that could—according to vaccine experts—be extremely harmful? And Fauci. We have to discuss Fauci's corruption.

The students seem to want to talk about covid-19. That's all they are thinking about right now. Let's show the corruption behind the responses. Compare the reactions of individual states, some that locked down and some that didn't.

Let's plant seeds.

April 25, 2020: I think Jenny stole money from me. How horrible, if she did.

Here's what happened. I noticed a large amount of money in her account—$150—on the ledger, but -$4 on the amount available. When I asked her where the money came from, she said sold books […] to people in the street. When we asked what she used the money for, she claimed to have entered a contest, a poetry contest.

I'll check her account today. I'll hide the glass globe with the orange rose in it; Flora might try to throw it when Jenny starts to get upset when we confront her.

She already senses something is up. She's humming more. Just checked up on "how I was."

Why, Jenny, why?

Rough time sleeping last night. Cancer area feels like sunburn. That could easily be part of the healing process. But my right side at the rib cage feels tender. Not painful, just annoying. And, of course, my herpes outbreak. So no penis therapy. Bummer.

April 26, 2020: The time is 6:26. Or at least was a minute ago. Dad's birthday. How I miss him. Of course, I'm glad he's not some 100-year-old geezer living in a residence right now, unable to receive visitors or hug his grandchildren. *That* is elder abuse.

Jenny fessed up to the stealing yesterday rather easily. No punching, hitting, only a little screaming. Flora threw a box of tissues, but otherwise nothing got hurled. Nothing broken, no racing around the neighborhood screeching, "HELP ME!"

I guess that's progress.

Anyway, she gets no allowance for five weeks. I might shorten that to four or even three. Jenny claims she stole "only" $60, then asked for only four weeks of no allowance. Jeez. When is she going to learn to count? [She received $20 a week.]

I lied and told her we can trace the serial numbers of bills from the bank. She's not the only one who can make shit up.

Maybe I should stick to what I know. Yeah, that might be better. With Jenny, I wanted her to think that I have more information than I do. With the very exciting class I am preparing, I think I'll stick just to what I know.

At least two types of corruption could be occurring in the United States right now. Corruption among regulatory officials and corruption among politicians. Establish corruption at CDC: Attkisson segment, CHD segment on Fauci and vaccines. Then establish corruption among politicians: Murphy and Bill of Rights, de Blasio requesting information about social distancing. Not sure whether de Blasio's request is corruption. If social distancing is unconstitutional, is requesting information about the enforcement of an unconstitutional declaration corruption?

Not sure. But it would speak to the students, especially those who are trying to figure out what is going on. Which, I hope, is all of them […].

April 27, 2020: The insanity appears to be lifting in some places that are not New Jersey. Georgia is opening up […].

I blew up at Flora last night for not turning off her computer when the last person did. It doesn't matter what time she goes to sleep. She doesn't learn anything in school anyway. Her days are the same. Fortunately, she's listening to Beatles all day (*Help!*) and not watching the cake porn videos. That's progress. [Flora could spend all day watching YouTube videos of rich gooey desserts, which we called "cake porn".] But she's a two-year-old in a 20-year-old body. What they have done to our children […].

Although the pain is slowly dissipating, my right rib cage still hurts somewhat. Does seem to be a pulled muscle that takes time to heal. The herpes outbreak seems to be cleared. Yeah! Getting my body back in installments.

April 28, 2020: Last night I had the strangest dream (I've ever dreamed before […]). I dreamt I was living in West Germany, but we were rounded up and placed in barracks. I was wearing contact lenses and feared that I didn't have my glasses, but my glasses were in my purse. And we were allowed alcohol—my roommate and I had wine and Jägermeister. But we were not allowed out and we could not make any calls. The guards told us when to go to meals. My greatest concern was reaching my mother. (Jonathan was not in the picture; neither was my Dad.)

Calling Dr. Freud.

Life is beginning to reopen [...]. Georgia is opening up [...]. A haberdasher in New York City who has the balls to open his store! The police questioned, but did not fine him. I do hope his store is packed today. Maybe de Blasio should have been nicer to his police.

The death rate in Wisconsin, where voters gathered in great numbers, did not rise; in fact, it fell.

Phil Murphy is still being a DICtator. This matters very much to me and my family. We were hoping to place Flora in a residence out of state with the help of New Jersey. Our backup plan was to pay out of pocket from our money that is now invested in the stock market. Plan C is to have her live with us and we never die.

P.S. Right side feels better, but there's still a twinge. I sure hope it's not cancer, or else Plan C goes down the toilet.

April 29, 2020: The insanity continues. Facebook is cracking down on the organization of protests. My students are terrified. Of what exactly? I think of spreading covid-19.

This isn't America anymore. Our 200-year experiment is over. Power corrupts and absolute power corrupts absolutely. There is no way to control those urges in some people.

Most Americans are decent, caring people. "Charity begins at home," Dad always said. "And more or less stays there."

But corporations are built upon greed and self-interest. The business model is to keep people dependent on your product. Keep them dependent on you. Then you are powerful.

I want to get the hell out of New Jersey. Pennsylvania may offer some refuge [...]. Is there any state where Flora could live that we could move to? We hope to find a place for her this summer.

I'd be thinking about the future a lot more differently if it weren't for Flora and Jenny. I guess that's what kids do to you. That's what kids are ***supposed*** to do to you.

Big Tech companies are doing fine as are online stores and some big retailers (e.g. Walmart). Small businesses are getting creamed. That may be one of the agendas working here.

So, our stocks may not plummet to the point we would not be able to provide for Flora. New Jersey will certainly not pay for an out-of-state placement. I doubt any in-state placement would be humane anyway.

I feel so powerless.

But I have Jonathan. Love in the age of ~~autism~~ covid-19.

April 30, 2020: We'll be discussing FDI [Foreign Direct Investment] in Africa today. Rule of law is an issue. Equal application of the law [...]. I wonder if the students have heard about the penis pix and Hitler memes [snarky internet responses to the lockdowns]. I'll find out! [...]

My work is cut out for me. My life—no one's life—is not.

May 1, 2020: The insanity continues. DICtator Murphy has thrown us a bone: He's opening the state parks tomorrow. Oh, thank you, thank you, thank you, DICtator Murphy! Now, could you please allow the businesses to open so people can get back to work and feed their families without government assistance? [...].

Del Bigtree says it's time to forgive. It isn't time to forgive yet, because there's not much to forgive. However, Del is correct that when the time comes to forgive, we should. Not forget, but do forgive. "What happened during the quarantine stays in the quarantine." I think you mean neighbor against neighbor. OK, I'm willing to do that [...].

But forgiving DICtator Murphy? I don't think so. I'll forgive him by booting him out of office [...].

Nerves between Jenny and Flora are fraying. They are fighting like teenagers. How normal! But Flora is so sick. It's so tragic. And yet I keep hoping there will be a medical breakthrough that rids her of her demons and allows the person she is to emerge. Judy Mikovits's book[4] discusses retroviruses—viruses that enter the body without alerting the immune system. Jenny seems to be plagued with viruses. Flora more with inflammation, which might also come from viruses.

I hope they all rot in Hell, the people who did this to my children [...].

May 3, 2020: We watched *Parasite* last night [a 2019 film exposing the class system in Korea]. Powerful film, though I still don't quite get it. I thought there was to be a transformation between the "parasites" of the lower caste as they took more control as well as the upper caste becoming more like parasites.

---

4 Judy Mikovits and Kent Heckenlively, *Plague of Corruption: Restoring Faith in the Promise of Science* (New York: Skyhorse, 2022).

Perhaps when the upper-class family scurried away from the crime scene, they were like the parasites.

Many people had blood on their hands. Just like Bill Gates and Tony Fauci and Paul Offit. They have the blood of my children on their hands.

They are shooting their wads right now, and I hope they go down. And stay down. At least Paul Offit and Peter Hotez are very cautious about a coronavirus vaccine […].

If the vaccine becomes mandatory, there might be a way to avoid taking it. If lines form, we register, then leave before receiving the shot. The Medical Gestapo may get wise to the plan, but it's an idea for now. Only one of us needs to "get" it. For the rest, we can forge a confirmation.

So odd to be thinking in these terms. In the United States. The girl who wore at least two American flags pins after 9/11. Go figure.

May 4, 2020: I'm so enjoying Woody Allen's book *Apropos of Nothing*. Just some background. Woody Allen has been blacklisted due to an allegation made by his former lover Mia Farrow. She said he molested her daughter [Dylan]. There appears to be little truth to the allegation […]. Just as a side note, [Jonathan's] Uncle David (Schulman), a child psychiatrist, was approached by Ms. Farrow's legal team and asked to examine Dylan […]. Uncle David said he would examine the girl, but he would call it as he saw it. If he believed she had been molested, he would report that; if she had not been molested in his eyes, he would report that finding. No deal, said the lawyers.

Fast forward to the #MeToo movement and Woody Allen is blacklisted on what appear to be bogus charges. He writes his autobiography and it is just about to be published, but is pulped after the child that he and Mia Farrow produced together (unless the father was Frank Sinatra, somewhat unclear), Ronan, objected. Jonathan alerted Tony Lyons to a great opportunity: How about Skyhorse publish Woody Allen's book? They did and it's a super seller! The critics hate it—they have to—but the riff raff—including me—love it! Thank you, Tony Lyons; thank you, Jonathan! [The dark irony here is that Allen had produced and starred in *The Front*, a 1976 film about the McCarthyite blacklists of the 1950s. And now, in another episode of mass hysteria, he found himself blacklisted. We never learn.]

May 5, 2020: Cinco de Mayo. Fifteen years ago, 05-05-05, we began to have tremendous hope for our girls. David Kirby has just published *Evidence of Harm*, and we had found a Defeat Autism Now! Doctor. We filled out the paperwork for Dr. Freedenfeld on Cinco de Mayo 2005.

Now there is very little hope for Flora. Maybe more for Jenny. Helplessness, hopelessness, uncertainty.

And the rest of the world [...] is feeling it too. Those who were able to lend a hand earlier will no longer be able to do so. They were beginning to pull back when they realized how expensive and **how much work** taking care of our girls is. The school district no longer supports special-needs families. The acting teacher and others **just can't handle** the special-needs kids [...].

So, we are more on our own than ever. Fortunately, I think we'll be able to afford a good placement for Flora even without funding from New Jersey, which at this point has no money.

Flora interrupted my sleep last night. There was no wifi, so she couldn't pull up her picture of Brendon Criscione [a boy she was enamored with]. How can we unlock your brain, Flora? How can we rechannel those brain waves into something useful, something productive, some fun?

Jenny's test results show HVV-6 virus big time. HVV-6 is related to Alzheimer's. Oh, great. I hope—I pray!—we can do something to help you, Jenny.

In the meantime, Mr. Gates, can we have our world back?

May 6, 2020: Flora might be able to go back to Camphill soon. Here's what happened: We got an email from Camphill saying Pennsylvania is allowing them to accept students from homes where the health of the student or other family members is in danger, for example if the student has seizures. Jonathan and I looked at each other—no way could we qualify. We decided to write to Camphill and explore the idea of Flora's returning; while we are not in immediate danger, Flora's OCD is worsening and the stress is impacting my cancer (might as well get something out of this bout with cancer!). Within five minutes, [Camphill] wrote back and said, sure, apply. So we did. Fingers crossed. For her sake. For everyone's sake. Jenny's right: Maybe we should add that we are geezers.

If Flora does remain, I'll probably contact the eye doctor David Yermack [a friend] recommended. But we tried eyes—the prism lenses—and ears—the hearing aids. And heavy metals and brain waves and neurotransmitters and lasers and exercises. Guess it just boils down to love. For Flora and Jenny both. I guess that's what it always boils down to: Love. It's just love in most cases produces happy, healthy, productive individuals who bless their parents with grandchildren. In our case, love results in survival.

May 7, 2020: Flora was up last night, obsessing about a piece of paper she lost. Two washed-off Advil seemed to help. [Gayle was always careful to wash the red dye off of Advil.]

What those bastards have done to our children. Judy Mikovits said the "unholy scientific trio" is Harold Varmus, Francis Collins, and Tony Fauci.

Anytime we don't understand why public health officials are not addressing an important health issue, their fingerprints are at the crime scene.

I hope Tony Fauci gets his comeuppance. With exposure comes scrutiny. He's been doing so much in the shadows. Now that he is being exposed to sunlight, I hope his crimes against humanity are revealed and addressed.

Same with Bill Gates. We in the vaccine-skeptic community have been in this territory longer than those who are joining it now. So many landmines, so like film *noir*—you can't trust anyone.

Except that you can. You can trust Lyn Redwood and, by extension, RFK Jr. You can trust the Bonos and Toby Rogers, Mary Holland and Chris Exley. People who really care. As far as I can tell, anyone connected to Children's Health Defense is trustworthy. They are carefully vetted. [Laura Bono, wife of Scott Bono, was founder of the National Autism Association. Mary Holland was President and General Counsel of Children's Health Defense. Chris Exley, a Professor of Chemistry at Keele University, published findings linking autism to aluminum adjuvants in vaccines and had his research funding cut off.]

So, we can trust one institution. And that's about it. We can't trust the CDC, FDA, HHS. Department of "Justice" is a joke, except for Bill Barr. That's a big exception, I know.

Betsy DeVos is great. Perfect timing regarding "believing the survivor." Tara Reade probably experienced some sort of unwanted advances into her personal space. Maybe or maybe not finger-fucking from Joe Biden. But it's great how she has exposed the fraud that is the #MeToo movement.

Interesting conversation with Lisa Fidler [a Camphill parent] yesterday. She observed that I think the whole coronavirus episode is overblown, because "you're a Republican." I should have clarified my position. Yes, it's a virus that spreads very rapidly and affects certain people—the elderly, those with preexisting conditions—very profoundly. But for the most part, it is benign or bearable. Shutting down the world economy is the overblown part. People get sick, and they usually get well. Lisa pointed out, correctly, that many people have underlying health conditions so that caveat cannot be taken too lightly. I agree. But healthy, young people should be able to live their lives. They should not be cooped up in their New York apartments, fearful of going outside. Such behavior *lowers* their immune systems.

May 8, 2020: Some chinks in the Wall of Insanity are beginning to appear. People have taken to the streets, though you wouldn't know by reports in the Main Stream Media. Fox reports on it, and the "HighWire" [a weekly broadcast from Del Bigtree]. The video of two doctors saying the shutdown is harmful received 10 million hits, before YouTube removed it.

Perhaps the silver lining to this lockdown—I am my father's daughter!—is that people outside the vaccine-injury community are seeing greedy, power grabbers for what they are....

I will miss the students. I *do* miss the students. Jonathan is right: Remote teaching is to classroom teaching as watching porn is to actual sex. *It's just not the same.*

Other glimmers that sanity is returning is the salon owner who was released from jail. She had—against a state executive order—dared to open her salon so that not only she, but also her employees could feed their families. The extremely liberal judge called her selfish. After her lawyer filed a writ of habeas corpus—listen to me!—the appeals judge released the woman from jail. A group of people gathered outside the jail to welcome the woman. She was your average Jane, just trying to get by.

Another glimmer of sanity is that the Justice Department (William Barr) dropped the charges against General Flynn. Documentation shows the FBI set a perjury trap for Flynn.

I've never felt so happy for two people I've never met in my life.

The MSM are brainwashing people, and the closing of the schools means children are only getting dumber. And, coincidentally, more dependent on technology. Robots. Mechanical robots. It is a nightmare scenario from a science fiction movie. Only it's all too real.

Today, I work on the finals for my classes [...] while Flora has her Beatles music droning in the background. It's so difficult to concentrate, but she might be going back to Camphill soon! For everyone's sake, that would be a blessing. Yes, I'd like to do a blood test on her, like the one from Dr. Turner that revealed so much about Jenny. But if that doesn't work out now, we can do it in the future. It probably won't make much of a difference anyway. They destroyed her brain beyond repair. I have to accept that fact [...] but I keep trying to find the switch that will connect everything in Flora's brain. I know it's killing me (stress is causing my cancer), but I'd be experiencing more stress if I wouldn't do anything.

May 9, 2020: Jenny attacked me again last night. It's been a while. But Jonathan and I had been talking about the state of the world—it sucks!—and Jenny got upset. So, she physically attacked me. Squeezing my entire body, hitting me on the head. When I reached for her throat and squeezed, she yelped, "Hey, she's trying to strangle me!" and let go. When Jonathan accused her of trying to strangle me, I fessed up. I said, "No, I *was* trying to strangle her." The knives were close, but I didn't reach for them. It's odd. I don't like being attacked and I know she could injure me, but I don't fear she's actually going to kill me. I know she doesn't want to, but something comes over her.

May 10, 2020: Ah, up at a decent hour—6:27 am. The world is quiet and fresh and clean. Hope exists at this hour. Hope that fades during the day, but spring anew each morning at 6.

Maybe there is some hope. Judy Mikovits is all over the internet. A video about an upcoming movie called *Plandemic* has been taken down by YouTube and keeps popping back up. I think there have been 10 million views, but I could be getting my banned videos mixed up. I had a happy thought—President Trump, are you listening to Judy? She seems to have a research agenda to help your son. I know you're a family man, that you love your children very much. Listen to her for the sake of your son; oh, yes, and for my daughters, too. I'd be much obliged.

When will the Dark Side ever learn? The more they push back, the stronger we become. Why are you banning information? What don't you want us to know? Give us the information; let us decide. We aren't stupid, and we have very different goals than you do. You want profits; we want healthy, happy children. It's OK you want profits, but one of the assumptions of an efficient economy is full information. When you violate that assumption—when you keep information from us—we devote more resources to an industry than is economically efficient. Withholding information about the addictive properties of opioids means we purchase too many drugs, more than we would have purchased had we known the negative side effects. So what, you ask? First of all, society experiences an opioid epidemic and hundreds of thousands of lives are ruined or destroyed (people die). Secondly, we divert resources from other areas of economic activity such as science to address other diseases, e.g., muscular dystrophy.

What would happen in a world with full information? Most people would decide not to vaccinate their children, that's for sure. Some still might. People wouldn't take opioids for pain. They would find alternatives. Homeopaths, chiropractors, herbalists would make a comeback. Apparently, at the turn of last century, 25% of all doctors were "alternative." There seemed to be more information back then than now with all the regulators we have in place. Funny that.

Transparency is vital. Why on earth did Cuomo reduce access to hydroxychloroquine? Why did he order EMTs **not** to resuscitate people with cardiac arrest?? Numbers that quadrupled for the first week in April from 69 per day with a death rate of 38% to 284 per day with a death rate of 72%? Why did he order more ventilators when 9 out of 10 people placed on ventilators died? And why in God's name did he send people with covid back to nursing homes?? He is a political animal. I'm sure every decision was based on a political calculation. And I suppose it doesn't matter, Mr. Cuomo that your political calculations add up to more death and suffering of your constituents.

Film last night, *Ace in the Hole*, was a documentary. A newspaperman, Kirk Douglas, wants to prolong the story of a man trapped in a cave. He co-opts the local sheriff, the local contractor, the local townspeople as well as his young, naïve assistant. Sound familiar? The man in the cave dies, even though he could have been saved by extracting him directly instead of drilling down to retrieve him. Prolonging a disaster for political, economic, power reasons. No, that can't happen in real life, not in America [...]

May 11, 2020: Yesterday was Mother's Day. My first instinct is to say, "Bah, humbug!" But I actually had a relatively pleasant day. Jonathan & the girls made a bagels and lox brunch for me, just like what we used to do for Ruth. It did bring back nice memories. Jonathan was such a great son. He continues to be a great husband and a wonderful lay.☺

Bill Gates really is trying to take over the world. As a dictator, he wants to rule with an iron fist and yet he wants to be loved. He has no successor—as dictators seldom do—but Mark Zuckerberg is certainly playing along with the plan with perhaps grander aspirations. The information he's taking down on YouTube is astounding—two doctors saying the lockdown should end, the nurse crying about treatment of covid patients, anything Judy Mikovits. And the harder the Dark Side pushes, the greater the Truth pushes back.

T-shirt for Jonathan for Father's Day: Mr. Gates, Can we please have our world back? Let me work on that right now.

May 12, 2020: My last day of actual teaching. Thursday is a review. With the pass/fail option, some students don't give a flying fuck about school.

Mr. Gates' plan to control the world is hitting some snags. People are protesting, some of my students continue to want to learn—though I'm curious about their reaction to the NJ Office of "Rumor Control and Disinformation" + YouTube removing the *Plandemic* trailer—and some [...] governors are allowing their citizens to make their own decisions. I **really** want to move to North Dakota. [Though it sounds Orwellian, the New Jersey Office of Homeland Security and Preparedness did set up a webpage devoted to "Rumor Control and Disinformation," a clumsy title suggesting that the site *provided* disinformation.]

[...] An Italian study of 6,500 people who take hydroxychloroquine for other reasons (Lupus, rheumatoid arthritis) found that only 20 developed covid (no ICU, no deaths), a 90% reduction compared with the rest of Italy.

There's no transparency in Cuomo's decisions. Why send covid-positive elderly back to nursing homes? He recently lifted the March 25th order, but why did he proclaim the order to begin with? The *New York Post* is all over the story. The station where Chris Cuomo (Andrew's brother) works is curiously quiet regarding the rationale for the governor's decisions.

We went over Jenny's tests results, and Dr. Turner had some suggestions for additional supplements. She may indeed have PANS. We're going to do the same test for Flora. Oh, God, please. Let me find a way to help Flora. A way to enjoy life, to grow, to be curious.

Of course, in the current world, being curious can only lead one to depression. And yet Anne Frank a few days before being discovered and sent to a concentration camp said she still believed in the goodness of mankind.

I don't. OK. For the most part, people are good. Circumstances can promote that goodness as well as turn people mean. But there are some bad seeds. Evil people. Like Bill Gates, Tony Fauci, Paul Offit (though even he seems to care somewhat about the safety of vaccines).

Oh! I figured out how to make a picture of Bill Gates tossing the globe. It looks really good. I can't wait to give Jonathan the t-shirt!

May 13, 2020: My half-sister's birthday. I call her my half-sister, because half the time she's a good sister. The other half of the time it is as though we are not related. No one stood up to my former brother when he hosted Christmas and didn't invite my family. No one said, "Hey, this isn't right." That was one of the times—the major time—it seemed as though we were complete strangers.

She didn't call when I was first diagnosed with cancer. People who care call. But she doesn't. Our "family" doesn't work that way. We share the good times, and we ignore the bad times. We just want to have FUN. And, of course, autism is such a downer.

I'll call her today, because I half-care.

Flora got into the refrigerator last night. Ate a pound of cheese and some yogurt. Ugh […].

I had trouble sleeping last night due to the state of the world. Until now, I've been so busy concentrating on classes and the Autism One presentation. Now that classes are almost over, I have time to ponder the state of the world. How are we ever going to get out of this mess? .... Some of my own students say censorship is sometimes needed, such as now when there's a life-or-death situation at hand. Others were shocked at New Jersey's Office of "Rumor Control and Disinformation." I planted seeds.

Jonathan promised this morning that people are beginning to question Fauci, that people are beginning to ignore stay-at-home orders. Funny, isn't it? HE'S the optimist […].

Oh, Fran Drescher's CancerSchmancer.org featured Bobby Kennedy. We're getting out our message.

And Lyn Redwood asked if I wanted to be part of the Children's Health Defense's Research Committee. Whew! I can finally contribute without having to be an administrator.

May 14, 2020: The insanity continues. Nerves are becoming frayed. Yesterday after we went shopping to get apple juice for my liver cleanse, Flora insisted on going to Walmart for glue. With Jenny not in the car, I lost it. I kept screaming, "I HATE YOUR AUTISM!" Flora started crying and screaming, and I didn't care. She kept saying she was sorry. I said, "Then let me go home." But she couldn't. Her OCD would not allow it.

The grip that OCD has on her brain is devastating. Her brain wants to work, but the OCD has it working only to focus on buying glue or something sticky every day.

Of course, we can use this obsession to our advantage. If she puts her laundry away, etc., she can buy glue. If Trader Joe's doesn't have stickers AND she does not get upset, we will buy glue at Walmart. Let me try that.

Flora is 20 years old. She should be in college, getting laid. She is reduced to a permanent child.

Judy Mikovits is right: The government is our enemy. The government required us to poison our children. The CDC knew vaccines could cause harm, and they didn't care. They abandoned us for their own greed. Money. Power. But mainly money.

In one sense, I'm kinda glad we probably will not have grandchildren. I can't believe I'm writing that. But, really, what kind of world will they be living in? The greedy, the mediocre, the tyrants rule. They care nothing of the pain they inflict. Like me yesterday; I was a tyrant. It was a momentary lapse of sanity on my part. But to have tyrants rule the world, the pain, the suffering. I can't bear to think of future generations of mine enduring that. And they probably won't. Flora will never have children, and I doubt Jenny's body could handle the stress of pregnancy much less child-rearing.

So, I must do everything I can to enjoy my life and enrich the lives of my family. That means doing research to keep the question of vaccine safety alive. Perhaps scientists—immunologists, rheumatologists, biologists—can understand what is making them suffer so much and help alleviate that suffering. That's all I can do, but I will do it to the very best of my humble ability.

May 15, 2020: Fully two months into the lockdown. Insane. A classmate from high school (whom I don't remember—I think I had a crush on him and then he slept with my sister ☹) posted the outline of how to control people from a scholar whom both Obama and H. Clinton wrote about: provide total health care, take away guns and religion, make people dependent […] It is unbelievable how the Elite are following the recipe to a T.

May 16, 2020: The insanity continues. Murphy continues to be a DICtator, but not the worst. LA mayor won't let people on dry sand, but they may be on wet sand. The science behind the decision? Nonexistent. Other tyrants include Maine's governor—Janet Mills—and Michigan's governor—Gretchen Whitmer. Women who are vying to be Biden's VP. (At least Whitmer.)

Saw Lyn yesterday. How wonderful! She's a breath of fresh air. Then Flora obsessed about losing a sticker. Crying, screaming, jumping up and down. She was calmer after I gave her her new remedy (and also turned on her computer). Let's pray it works! Jenny took everything really well. She announced, "I can't take this anymore!" But she didn't attack me. She was really quite mature.

Jenny is also staying on topic much more. She's a pleasure to be around. Usually.

[…] I contacted my best student of all times, Alex. He's back in NYC permanently. His mom must be so happy. I think if our girls had not gotten sick, they would have been female versions of Alex—smart, hard-working, respectful. It will be great to catch up with him tomorrow.

May 17, 2020: The insanity continues; it's becoming normal. ***That's*** the scary part.

Over 30 million people are unemployed. Many are receiving benefits greater than the amounts they would earn if they were working. So—according to the *Wall Street Journal*—they are not going back to work, even though they could. That is economic rationality, SHORT-TERM economic rationality. What happens when they try to go back to work and there are no jobs to return to?

Lyn (Farrugia) is the only person I know who knows people who are unemployed—her daughters and her workers at Chubby's. I have to ask her more questions. I'm so curious.

May 18, 2020: Elizabeth Bruen [an autistic family friend] turns 21 today. Her life is certainly not the life God meant her to have. She's fortunate in a way—two parents who love each other and her very much. Still, her life should not be the way it is. And even when kids aren't given much of a chance—their parents don't or can't provide for them—they are given *a chance*. Our kids are damaged for life. We can tweak around the edges, and maybe someday we can flick a switch to get the brain to work. But only a few brave souls are doing the work that could find those switches (Chris Exley, Yehuda Shoenfeld). [Schoenfeld is an Israeli physician and autoimmunity scientist, controversial for his work on vaccine injury]. The damage wrought by the vaccines is severe and profound.

But that wasn't enough for Bill Gates. He needed more. He needed to ruin more lives. For better or worse, people seem to be figuring this out. Comments on postings with him are turned off. As John Gilmore put it, the expected love fest did not materialize. People are making tremendous fun of his masculine-looking wife. E.g. Bill Gates is awful and so is his husband! That is totally uncalled for and misses the point. Stick to the facts. The lockdown is a power grab by mediocre people, not leaders. Bill Gates is not our savior, but rather a cruel and demanding DICtator.

On May 5 or 6, the mini-DICtator Phil Murphy extended the stay-at-home order another 30 days. Why? Hospitalizations are low, the only deaths occurring in large numbers are in nursing homes. And people cooped up at home.

May 19, 2020: There's a protest on Monday. Yeah! Now *these* are protests that matter. In college, I was always looking for protests that mattered. By the late 1970s, America was all protested-out, so I became a rebel without a cause. Now we're rebels with causes! And how! Starting with bodily autonomy under the guise of Freedom of Religion, Jonathan and I marched three times on Trenton. Now it's Freedom of Speech, Freedom to Assemble, Constitutional Rights [...].

Elizabeth's birthday party yesterday made me realize how different I am from my friends. They were wearing masks *in their cars!* WTF?!? I am in a totally different orbit from them. **In their cars!** That's dangerous [...].

Judy Mikovits mentioned Suramin in her book as a drug that could address inflammation and lack of communication between cells. I wonder whether the drug could help Flora. With real and proper unconflicted research, I still believe man can undo what man has done. I have to have hope.

May 21, 2020: Jenny had an outburst last night. Flora was being loud, but Jenny had been masturbating—a sign that she is stressed—earlier in the evening. Jenny has run out of several supplements without telling me [...]. She had been doing so well recently, though [...] she is so irresponsible for not telling me when she's running low on a supplement. She just doesn't get it [...].

The stock market seems to be reacting to every iota of information concerning vaccines. On Monday, Moderna—a company that has patented

nothing in its ten years of existence—said the human subjects of its vaccine produced antibodies to the coronavirus. What they left out was that 20% of the healthy subjects receiving a high dose of the vaccine experienced severe negative side effects. Apparently one insider started selling his/her stock. The SEC is looking into the potential insider trading. Anyway, the markets were lower on Tuesday.

I can't wait to get back to my research. Yesterday, news that birth rates continue to fall came out. The total number of births are down to their lowest point in 35 years. General fertility rates fell to the lowest level since the government began tracking fertility in 1909. The only age group to experience an increase in birth rates were women in their early 40s […].

May 22, 2020: Flora is going back to Camphill on May 31. Nine days. It's funny. I had mentally prepared myself for her being here all summer. Now that she will be returning to Beaver Farm, I'm going to miss her. But it's a better place for her than here. I know she's in good hands. They care about her ***almost*** as much as we do.

The lockdown insanity continues. Tucker Carlson has guests who are small business owners. They are being destroyed by their government, which is owned by big business. Rather, big business and big government are working together. DIC-tator Phil Murphy comes from Goldman Sachs. GS is, of course, essential. The small business selling at least 25% food but mainly gifts in Ocean City, NJ is not. And the gym owners. DIC-tator Murphy can work out in his own gym, but most people who want to work out need to be part of a club. Murphy is not allowing gym owners to operate. Kevin Barry [a lawyer defending religious vaccination exemptions] is defending the gym owners featured on Tucker Carlson. My God, what cool friends I have! Heroes all! […]

Debate between Alan Dershowitz and Del Bigtree was very good. Dershowitz says that the government has a constitutional right to force vaccination for the greater good. However, he admits that the vaccine must be safe and effective; if it has not been tested for specific groups, then that specific group should not be forced to receive the shot. I hope I can use that defense when New York tries to shoot me in order to retain my job. If there are no studies showing the vaccine is safe for people with cancer, I respectfully decline.

May 24, 2020: Last night, I posted the following picture on Facebook with the question, "Anyone else feel this way?" [This was also Gayle's design for my Father's Day T-shirt.]

Hey Mr. Gates,

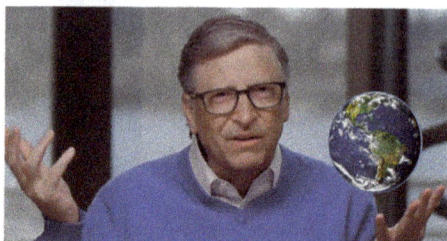

Can we have our world back?

Toby Rogers and Hillary Downing [an autism mom and friend] gave it a thumbs up. My cousin Doug Stine asked whether someone could explain to him what we meant.

Where do I start? Those of us with vaccine-injured children understand without explanation. Bill Gates believes vaccines are the answer to all of mankind's problems. He wanted to make headlines by eradicating polio, so he arranged to vaccinate as many African and Indian children as possible. The problem is the version of the vaccine he sent to developing countries can itself cause polio. The oral polio vaccine is known to cause vaccine-acquired paralytic polio and is no longer used in developed countries. But it's cheaper than the inactivated polio vaccine and good enough for Africa and India. As a result, a disease that was almost nonexistent is now returning, and tens of thousands of children are crippled for life for no reason. Now Mr. Gates wants everyone vaccinated against coronavirus. EVERYONE, all seven billion of us. Never mind if we don't trust the vaccine researchers who have conflicts of interest; never mind if we realize a strong immune system is the best way to fight disease; never mind that treatments such a hydroxychloroquine are effective in preventing and treating coronavirus. Never mind what WE want; Mr. Gates wants us to be forced to receive a vaccine rushed through the approval process with no long-term tests for safety.

May 25, 2020: America seems to be wising up. Yesterday in Loantaka Park, 95% of people were not wearing masks. Seeing the bright, happy faces was beautiful! The insanity is lifting.

Here's a contemporary joke: I don't know what General Flynn is complaining about; I love being unmasked! Yes, I made that up myself.

I had a little trouble sleeping last night. My cancer spot felt sunburnt. I sense this is part of the healing process, but it hurts. Drinking water helped as did Valerian Root. This morning, I applied castor oil, which also seems to soothe. Maybe I do belong in the 19th century.

Today, I'm going to email Vince [Vincent DiGirolamo, a Baruch College colleague of Gayle's] about Cuomo appointing Gates to the task force to "reimagine education." This task force is a huge threat to education, and not a single educator is part of it. I just started reading *The Prize* by Dale Russakoff about Mark Zuckerberg's $100 million donation to the Newark School System. The plan was to use Newark as a laboratory to test various educational systems to improve learning outcomes, measured—of course—by test scores. I haven't read very far, but it is my understanding of the project that it was a complete disaster and the only people it enriched were technology firms. The students and teachers were decidedly worse off.

Common Core is another example of tech giants intruding upon public education. Bill Gates was behind this project, that reduced teachers to robots following a hollowed-out curriculum. However, it made lots of money for Bill Gates.

The point is, I sense these tech giants are attempting to turn students into programmable robots with teachers and professors being the programmers. Once all classes are online, they can be recorded and replayed. After, of course, administrators check class content for any radical ideas that might induce students to question assumptions or—heaven forbid!—make tech companies look bad. Such thought-provoking ideas could be scrubbed from the electronic versions of lessons that students see. And then administrators can cut the cost of having to employ living, breathing teachers.

I'm not sure what mechanisms exist to address these concerns. We know that teachers and parents rose up against Common Core and were able to roll it back to a large extent. I stand ready to contribute whatever I can to address Gates' attempt to "reimagine education."

May 26, 2020: A wonderful protest yesterday! Hard-working, determined people who just want our country back. "Make the Constitution legal again!" "Impeach Murphy!" "Phinish Phil's Phascism!" "Murphy sucks!"

Nicely, we didn't get arrested. Police were present and we were decidedly *not* social-distancing. But other than disobeying an unconstitutional order, we were peaceful [...]. It was grand, especially when Flora smiled and started to chant "USA! USA!" [...].

We met a young man who had a sign "WHO and CDC are clande$tine." When Jenny asked what clandestine meant, Jonathan said secretive. The young man explained the word in more nuanced terms; yes, secretive, but everyone knows they are up to something. He seemed to be a words person, slightly on the spectrum. I tried to encourage Jenny to talk with him, as they seemed to be kindred souls. All to no avail. Oh, well. I tried.

Then we heard a speaker relate his experience about his autistic son in Devereux. During the shutdown, the facility has allowed no visitors. He speculated on the treatment the residents were receiving when no visitors were allowed. Louiesvoice.com. [A few months later a public scandal erupted with reports of widespread physical and sexual abuse at special-needs facilities run by Devereux Advanced Behavioral Health.]

As we were leaving we ran into Kevin Barry. What a treat! Kevin is defending the gym owners whom Tucker Carlson is following. The co-owners of Atilis Gym who reopened against Murphy's unconstitutional lockdown orders. We didn't social-distance as we chatted, and we gave each other hugs when we parted. Oh, bliss!

We watched *Best Years of Our Lives* last night. Our girls have had their hands shot off, they suffer from post-traumatic stress disorder, **and**—through no faults of their own—are devastated by drugs (not alcohol as Fredric March in the film, but drugs nonetheless). They are victims of war, and the battles on many fronts continue. They are heroes, yet there are no parades for them. Not yet. [Here Gayle is drawing analogies between the handicaps that confront the three veterans in the film and our daughters.]

If it were up to the people we met yesterday, there would be parades for our girls. And all the victims of the war on greed.

May 27, 2020: The weather outside my window is misty today. In normal times, cars would begin to appear to greet the new school day. A truck would deliver milk for lunches. Buses would arrive around 8:30 am. But today, there's just mist. Sadly, the stillness is not so odd anymore. Students have essentially stopped learning. Or playing. Or growing. The only growth they are experiencing is the growth of anxiety. And depression.

[...] Bill Gates and Mark Zuckerberg and Anthony Fauci and, probably, Deborah Birx [...] are evil people who do not care about ruining other people's lives. Count the Clintons in there, too. But especially Bill Gates.

Did Bill Gates start out evil or did the money and the ensuing power corrupt him? Probably a combination of the two. He was able to amass power, because he was so corrupt. Decent people care about others, or, at least, are concerned if they harm others. Bill Gates—like all dictators—at some level wants to be loved. And he doesn't care how many people he has to destroy to reach that goal.

Gates' initial goals were worthy: become a tycoon-turned philanthropist. The pharmaceutical companies saw a chance to further their agenda by coopting him. Get Bill Gates to further their drug-pushing. Once Bill (and Melinda!) were convinced that vaccines would save the world, there was no stopping the push for vaccine mandates.

Except the American people. Some of us are wise enough to see what's up. More than I thought and from nonobvious corners.

I'm able to return to research now that teaching is over. Oh, bliss!

May 28, 2020: Groundhog Day yet again. Except that Flora will be going back to Beaver Farm on Sunday. Other than that—and that's a notable exception—life here is the same. Jenny is a total pain in the ass. So ***selfish***. Yesterday, she came downstairs in a t-shirt that she had obviously freshly chewed. "Here we go again," I thought. No blow ups in the morning or early afternoon. Then, when she realized she wouldn't have much time to make a salad, she freaked. Jonathan and I both tried to give her suggestions to no avail. And it escalated from there. Every little thing set her off. Matt [her boyfriend] calls; she screams. Flora chirps; she screams. I cough; she screams.

I do think—hope, ***pray***—it's allergies that Neuroprotek can address. Jenny seemed to do well with Neuroprotek. Fortunately, I was reminded of the product while watching an Autism One video on PANS.

That's my life right now—watching Autism One videos so I can help my children address their chronic health issues. And for what? […] There are times I so want to smack the living daylights out of her. But I know she would just freak out more and then Flora would freak out and we would get it in stereo.

So, I suck it up. And my cancer acts up.

And what about Jenny's school? Has she received her grades? Has she registered? She's so ***irresponsible***.

But it's the ***rages*** that are the worst. The other stuff we could handle, but when she loses all control, all self-awareness that I sense anything we try is hopeless. Except, oddly, she doesn't seem to lose self-awareness. She seems to be totally aware, and yet she doesn't seem to care. It's horrible.

And so very, very draining. I'm drained these days. It started Monday, after the wonderful rally, when Flora needed to go shopping (as usual). I'm just so tired of having to go shopping every day with her. And Jenny comes along. It's so much easier when it's just Flora. But Jenny almost always insists upon coming along. These days, Flora is stockpiling her glue. It's curious. Instead of coming home and gluing stuff and mainly washing the glue down the sink, Flora collects the glue in her purse. Maybe she's saving it for her next life.

Today, I'll explore the *Indian Journal of Medical Ethics* as a possible outlet for my article on HPV vaccine and lowered fertility. Indians take fertility very seriously: I remember Simi [a graduate school friend] getting into an argument with a Chinese classmate at NYU over China's one-child policy, vehemently proclaiming that the government does not belong in the bedroom. Perhaps I could somehow work into the story the reports of African women being given vaccines—was it DTP?—laced with birth control. While the HPV vaccine is not purposely used as a method of birth control, the effect is the same. Mmmmmm. Let's see.

May 29, 2020: There is no poetry that can do justice to that first sip of coffee in the morning. Especially now, with the chorus of birds singing their disjointed but lively symphony!

Beneath the surface, people—especially young people—are committing suicide, dying from drug overdoses, inflicting pain on themselves and others.

Sorry, birds, we need our civilization back.

Wonderful chat with Julie Kranz [a niece] yesterday. We wondered aloud why some governors ordered nursing homes to admit covid patients. I speculated that old people vote Republican; Julie noted that old people are expensive. Later at dinner, Jonathan opined that as the number of deaths increases, so does the fear. Cuomo certainly went out of his way to say his 88-year-old mother was not expendable and neither is your mother.

But they were. The people in nursing homes. Members of the Greatest Generation. Who fought for the freedoms in our country that are now wiped out.

In three months' time, some of our basic freedoms have been obliterated: freedom of speech (that's actually been deteriorating for a while), freedom of assembly, freedom of religion. Life, liberty, and the pursuit of happiness. All gone.

Today is Mom's birthday. She seems content, blissfully unaware at how her life is in danger. Like John Gilmore's mother (who died of covid in a nursing home).

[...] I wish the medical profession would do what it's supposed to do—heal people—so I could understand and help to heal my daughters.

Working on "Anatomy of a retracted article" for *Indian Journal of Medical Ethics*. Nice, VERY nice to be back at research. I've **got** to look at health outcomes now that infants and children are avoiding vaccination. Diphtheria rates don't seem to have skyrocketed even though kids are not "protected." What about rates of SIDS? Those data are just **begging** to be analyzed.

May 30, 2020: The world is literally falling apart. Riots in Minneapolis, Atlanta, LA, New York. The spark was the death of a handcuffed black man who was pinned to death by a white police officer in Minneapolis. The officer was charged with murder—the wheels of justice were turning. But the rioters didn't care. They destroyed 170 businesses as well as cars and a police office.

1967 all over again, according to Jonathan. And Newark has yet to recover from those riots.

Part of the reason these neighborhoods were so incendiary was the lockdown. People cooped up inside, maybe many family members; the noise, the stress, the anxiety, the depression. Hell, my family of four is barely making it in a large house.

The back of my knee, which I pulled on Thursday, is better; but as I was watching all the riots on [television] my back or my sides—around my rib cage—fell into great pain. I could scarcely move.

What I don't understand is how people think destruction, looting, setting cars on fire will solve anything. At our protests—for vaccine choice and for ending the lockdown—we are LOUD, but we are peaceful. The system has screwed us big time and destroyed what is most precious to us—our children—and we see no justice. None. Not even a path to justice. But setting cars on fire will not solve the problem. I have no idea what will solve the problem, but looting a Target definitely will not. How many of those 170 businesses will rebuild in Minneapolis? Probably close to zero [...].

Ah, and my research. I noticed yesterday that Yehuda Shoenfeld republished an article with the exact same name as the one that the journal *Vaccine* retracted. (*Amazing* that *Vaccine* published the article that questioned vaccine safety!) RetractionWatch reported on the republication and asked the editor of *Immunological Research* for comment. RW is a disgusting organization that seeks to quell scientific debate through any means possible. In any event, Shoenfeld republished basically the same article in a different journal. *Immunological Research* is a member of the Committee on Publication Ethics (a corrupted organization), but it's also part of the Springer family. Today, I'll look at the Springer publications and see if any would be a good outlet for the HPV and lowered fertility paper.

Flora goes back to Camphill tomorrow. Hallelujah! Today, I focus on getting her packed and ready to go (trim nails, bathing suit).

May 31, 2020: Unintended consequences, Mr. Gates. The United States is on fire; people have been cooped up too long, and they are emerging angry. Unfortunately, their anger is directed [...] not [against] your dictatorship. But the world is falling apart nonetheless. No one is dying—so you are not culling the human race—but they are destroying cities so people will not be able to purchase computers or have health-care facilities to distribute vaccines. Nice job, fucking up our world, Mr. Gates. [In fact, at least 25 Americans died in the protests and riots in 2020, not counting the additional crime victims as the police were held back from combatting violent crime.][5]

Flora goes back today. Last night, she got another container of yogurt. How does she do that? I suspect she grabs it during the day when we momentarily aren't looking. That's how she gets the eggs as well […].

So, I have to get Flora's supplements together as well as her clothes. And email Reydan and Jackie [her houseparents at Beaver Farm] about her current supplement regime. And also Reydan about her stealing food and how she cut her toenail below the line. And Reydan and Carly with Flora's homework.

How life would have been so different without autism. Both girls would be in college—Jenny graduated by now, possibly in grad school. They'd be figuring things out for themselves by now. Everything, or almost everything. Jonathan and I would be here to guide them, but not arranging their lives. Autism sucks. Vaccines destroy lives.

June 1, 2020: Flora went back to Camphill yesterday. I'm profoundly sad. NOT that she's back—believe me—but because she is so profoundly sick. By almost totally erasing her soul—leaving but a sliver—they have erased a part of my soul. A huge piece is missing; what could have been, what should have been.

And I continue to hope that the sliver that exists can grow and show us more of the real Flora. I was hoping during her stay we could develop more. That we could see more of Flora's soul. But it didn't happen. She reverted to her daily shopping trips for glue sticks and her stealing food, especially yogurt and cheese. It was a constant battle that we often lost.

So, I'll take St. John's Wort—funny that I need that now and not while she was here. When she's here, I have to focus on so many of her needs—her supplements, her sit-ups (before we type in her password so she can listen to the Beatles' *Help!* album for the umpteenth time).

Lyn's remedies do seem to help. When Flora steals food, she steals only one item and not the entire stock in the refrigerator. Also, Flora isn't exposing her tongue as much; it always scares me when she does that as it appears as though she has Down's. Odd that that would worry me. Flora's IQ is similar to

---

5 Lois Beckett, "At Least 25 Americans Were Killed During Protests and Political Unrest in 2020," *Guardian*, October 31, 2020.

a person with Down's and quite frankly people with Down's seem much happier than Flora seems. It's just there's not much we can do about Down's […] and I figure we can do something about autism. When will I admit there's not much I can do to help Flora? NEVER.

She's in good hands at Beaver Farm. This summer, we were supposed to explore places for her to live long-term. Looks as though we need to postpone that trip […].

Riots continue worldwide. People are rioting against the lockdown, but they are doing it in the form of race riots. The powers that be are absolutely fine with that. Divide and conquer.

Jonathan senses I'm sad. He asked how he could help, and I suggested we clean. Clean the playroom, the closet, and Flora's bedroom. Cleaning is so much easier with Jonathan. He's so good at throwing things out!

June 2, 2020: Yesterday was kinda rough. I'm still decompressing from Hurricane Flora. And the realization that vaccines have erased much of her soul. A sliver remains. I cherish that sliver. I want it to grow, so I get to know more of Flora. When vaccines erased most of Flora's soul, they erased part of mine. There's a hole in my soul. As Flora's (IF Flora's) soul becomes restored, so does mine.

Jonathan and I are cleaning—first the hall closet, next the playroom. Then Flora's room. Then the BASEMENT. It's so much easier clearing out stuff with Jonathan. But I see all the therapies we tried with Flora. All the attempts to reach her. All the failed attempts.

We need to find a spark to reach her. A spark that makes that sliver grow. Her obsessions have taken over her soul, uninvited intruders who wreak havoc.

Perhaps Triform [a Camphill community in Hudson, New York] can help find a spark. Before we put her away forever. Let's find what she enjoys doing, what makes life meaningful for her.

Riots continue across the United States. Senseless, bloody riots. Anarchists, arsonists, thugs are trying to take over from the current thugs in power who are not arsonists, but only anarchists and thugs. The corporate "leaders" don't care about everyday Americans like me and my family. Bill Gates, the Clintons, Jeff Bezos—they care about themselves and their power. They are thugs and they are sowing anarchy. The politicians go along, so they can solidify their power. I cannot believe that 2/3 of the people of New Jersey think the DICtator Phil Murphy is doing the right thing. He is destroying small business, people's livelihoods. Cuomo has decimated New York.

June 3, 2020: A blister developed at my cancer site. It hurts. Not like a knife; more like a sore. And I feel listless, slight fever (99.6). Not much of an appetite. Breathing fine (yea! Probably not corona!). I'll call Dr. Isaacs today.

The United States is falling apart in many cities. The Democratic politicians keep calling the outbursts "protests"; the Republicans call them riots. Police are getting killed. There seems to be a very organized group of anarchists—so I suppose anarchists **can** organize—behind the riots.

Soho is shattered. Macy's on 6th Avenue looted. Five hundred people arrested in NYC, most of them released due to the new bail bill.

[...] As long as we little people are arguing amongst ourselves, we aren't noticing how the elite are hollowing out the U.S. middle class. Jonathan and I worked hard to become professionals, wealthy even. Our girls are not able to achieve what we've achieved. Vaccines—mandated by politicians whom the drug companies corrupted—injured their brains. In Flora's case, vaccines erased the majority of her soul. Jenny faces struggles just to survive. Everyday life skills do not come naturally to her; she must learn how to make tea in a painful step-by-step process. But she can do it; making salad just clicked one day for her and now she chops the vegetables beautifully every time.

Jonathan and I are cleaning nicely. Monday was the hall closet. Yesterday, the playroom. Today—if I'm up for it—Flora's room.

June 4, 2020: People are permitted to gather again! Large groups are forming around the United States, and the police are not arresting them. Unfortunately, they are gathering to protest "systemic racism" which does not exist. It is disgusting to see people "take a knee" and denounce themselves for their white privilege. Police killed ten unarmed blacks in the United States last year. Ten [...]. Most of the people were using their fists as weapons. I know from personal experience (Jenny) that fists can be dangerous. Police killed 19 unarmed whites last year. In 2015, when Obama was president, police killed 38 unarmed blacks and 32 unarmed whites.

The ruling class doesn't care. They are probably enjoying this chaos. With all the turmoil, no one is asking why 54% of our children have chronic disease or the overall fertility rate is the lowest since the government began tracking data in 1909.

It is time for a revolution [...].

Cancer site is somewhat irritating. Not painful. Just annoying. First, a big red blotch appeared Monday. Now, it's more brownish. If feels like the healing process after scraping a knee or a rug burn [...].

Jonathan is encouraging me to submit to *International Journal of Childbirth*, a journal for midwives. He pointed out that midwives loathe doctors. That's a good context. And it has a truly international audience.

Victor would have been 101 yesterday. In some senses, it's good he's not around to see the world he fought for—albeit from the comfort of a desk at Arlington Hall—fall to pieces. [Jonathan's father Victor was never under enemy fire during the Second World War, but he worked to break the Japanese codes. "Wow," exclaimed Jenny, "Grandpa was just like Alan Turing, only straight."]

June 5, 2020: The chaos continues. Riots, looting, murders, assassinations of police. The anarchists want to defund the police. And the politicians are going along with it. Seventy-one percent of Americans want the National Guard called to quell the violence; 51% want the military.

The politicians, the media, big business, celebrities are so out of touch with us commoners. We are looking to our leaders for safety, yet all we receive are platitudes. I hope America pulls through. I hope we boot the cowards—the corrupt cowards—out of office. Have we again mixed greed with incompetence? [...]

My left side aches a bit. The red blotch that appeared on Monday is now brownish, and the area around my rib cage is sore. The ache is worst at night. I sense it's part of the healing process, but perhaps I should call Dr. Isaacs. A baking soda and Epsom salt bath would also feel good.

Suddenly, it's summer. Could be the heat from the NYC riots that has drifted west, but it's t-shirt and skort weather.

Talking with Flora last night. She wanted to know when we were picking her up. But first she wanted to make sure she could have more watermelon. Camphill is a great place for her. I'm so grateful we found it and can afford to send her there.

June 6, 2020: D-Day. Real Freedom Fights. Not the whiney little bastards who are destroying our cities. ***Think*** people, ***THINK!*** In my 20s, I may have gone along with the "white privilege" scheme and felt ashamed for all the fortunes I had been given while others suffered. Now I see that for the crock it is. I treat people fairly—I give them the benefit of the doubt. Yes, I grew up in good circumstances. But lowering myself does not raise up others. It just lowers everyone. Help the others to live decent, hard-working lives [...].

Yesterday, I called Dr. Isaacs. She asked whether the cancer area had grown. It has, ever so slightly. She said the next step is pharmaceutical hormone treatment. I do **not** want that. My body can heal itself, given half a chance. Once you start messing around with the natural rhythms, so many systems can go haywire. Dr. Isaacs is a little nervous about me. Interestingly, she's also nervous about coronavirus. She of all people should be able to see through the bullshit. But as a physician, I suppose she has seen the worst that can happen; not what typically happens, but the *worst*. Therefore, she's always preparing for the *worst*.

Anyway, under the threat of pharmaceutical hormones, I'll make a few changes. I'll drink more carrot juice [...]. And I'll do more acupuncture. That should relax my muscles. The slurp of wine at dinner I keep.

June 7, 2020: The day after D-Day. D+1. Were the battles over? Was there deadly silence?

I wonder what went on last night in America. Over weekends, I no longer listen to news. Not that I listened much before the riots. But especially now, I need a break.

Things are getting done around the house. Let me be more proactive—*I'm* accomplishing things around the house. Little things that add up. Jonathan and I were cleaning a little each day until I felt unwell. But we'll start again; today, I hope. Things I had been planning to do, but never quite got around to doing—purchasing a new phone for Flora, readying the Legacy Box for shipment, recording the small tapes—the three minutes of Jenny *in utero*, the five minutes of Applied Behavior Analysis [...] during the Summer of 2005. Ah, yes. ABA. *That* was supposed to clear away the scourge of autism; to lift the veil that shrouds our children's souls. What crock ABA is! It's research-driven, they cry. Research shows ABA *works*. Research written by the founders of ABA. Total baloney. Total waste of time and very precious resources.

Jenny gave me a couple of book suggestions—yes, she'll be a wonderful librarian. Books affect me. Today, for example, I'm writing somewhat differently. I'm reading *Thirteen Ways of Looking* by Callum McCann. Several short stories. The first one, which shares a title with the book itself, is the last day in the life of an 82-year-old Jewish attorney who was married to an Irish Catholic woman, Elaine. Or Eileen [...]. I know it's his last day, because the synopsis tipped me off.

Maybe I shouldn't be reading something so depressing, because I'm already so sad about Flora. When she's here, I'm so busy getting her supplements, going for bike rides, buying glue sticks (every day!), that I don't have time to think. When she's away, I have time to ponder what might have been, and that makes me very, very sad. Profoundly sad. Is there a greater sadness than seeing a child—*your* child—lost, with a shriveled soul, knowing it was all preventable. The greed that I teach about—business—caused Flora's autism. And yet I teach on—what else can I do? We have to pay these doctor and tuition bills somehow. I try to instill ethics and a high degree of skepticism in my students. I have no idea how successful I am, but I try. I plant seeds.

June 8, 2020:

- World continues to go to hell in a handbasket.
- I hope I don't have to work with another doctor doing hormone treatment […].
- I'm so tired of doctors.
- Doctors are arrogant; sometimes the most arrogant are the "alternative" doctors, because they have to put up with more shit (figuratively speaking).
- Most doctors didn't help. Some did: Dr. Freedenfeld, Dr. Turner, Dr. Grams. Some did more harm than good […]. The others were a waste of time and money and hope.

June 9, 2020: The United States continues to go insane, only a different way now. Black Lives Matter is a terrorist organization that is now taking over our society. Similar to the Black Legion, which is based on the Ku Klux Klan, the organization is run by thugs who want to amass wealth and power. [The Black Legion was a racist terror group, similar to the Ku Klux Klan, that flourished in the 1930s. It was also the subject of a 1937 film starring Humphrey Bogart, which we saw on Turner Classic Movies.] There are sincere calls to defund the police. Imagine. Abolishing the police […].

My rash is doing funky things. It is less red and less protruding, but the light red seems to be spreading and there are these little squiggle lines near the site (broken blood vessels?). I have a full-fledged appointment with Dr. Isaacs—as opposed to a quick observation—next Wednesday. Come to think of it, the redness comes and goes. Last night, very few darting pains at the cancer site. And less intense darts […].

I also need to call Eunice [Bloom, an elderly neighbor]. I suspect her son is here, because she doesn't have much time left. Damn covid. Damn the lockdown. In Eunice's case, I understand why she needed to shelter-in-place, but still a crying shame. And I, an asymptomatic person, should have been allowed to visit. Maybe she'll see me now. [She never did.]

We're going through Flora's books. I think the fewer she has—and she'll still have **a lot**—the more likely she is to read at least some. So, it's not so bad, going through them. Odd, that's not so bad, but I'm glad. I guess I'm still hopeful we can find a spark or two to help Flora develop some interests. Like the Beatles. **Not** like Brendon Criscone [a boy she obsessed over]. Interests, not obsessions. Dr. Turner said the fact that not more was going on was good. He also implicitly cautioned there's not a lot he can do.

A kid in California, an autistic kid, was restrained and later died in health-care custody. No marches, no riots, no nothing. [There have been many cases of autsitic children dying when placed under restraint, like George Floyd, but they never arouse public protests.]⁶

June 10, 2020: Jenny is being a royal pain in the ass. She was doing so well, until yesterday at lunch. I said something like "I should be a guy," and she just flew off the handle. She squeezed me and kicked my shins.

Child abuse. I'm being abused by my child.

She ripped up some papers—Flora's writings mainly—and added a plastic purple flower to my research papers [...].

I'm so glad I have my research. It's logical, exact. Unlike my offspring. And yet I do my research for my offspring. Fat lot of gratitude I get. Maybe someday, but I'm not holding my breath.

June 11, 2020: Lyn Farrugia was so excited yesterday when I told her I was sick. She said ok, ask Jonathan to get these remedies for you. You'll feel better very quickly. I was going to try to get the remedies myself, but realized Jonathan is old enough to figure out where to find the remedies. So, I asked him! So glad I did. I was flat on my back with fever.

I'm drinking coffee, which I probably shouldn't do. But it tastes good. And sometimes when I do the things I do when I'm well, even when I'm sick, I feel better. Fake it 'til you make it.

June 15, 2020: Last evening, we watched *Chariots of Fire.* Jonathan wanted to watch *Philadelphia Story*, because he was in the mood for a comedy. I swear we've seen *PS*, and I wasn't quite in the mood for a comedy. We saw a comedy on Saturday night, *Designing Woman* with Lauren Bacall and Gregory Peck. It was cute. I was more in the mood for something with lush scenery and fabulous music. I asked Jonathan whether it was ok if I watched *CoF*. He could watch with me, but he didn't need to feel obligated to do so. He wants to make me

6 Sawsan Morrar, "School Where Boy with Autism Was Restrained, Later Died Has Been Investigated by State Multiple Times," *Sacramento Bee,* January 15, 2019; Alice Hines, "Deadly Restraints Are Being Used on Children at Youth Homes and Schools," *Vice News,* Novermber 14, 2020; Hannah Fry, "After Autistic Boy Dies During School Restraint, 3 Educators Charged with Manslaughter," *Los Angeles Times,* November 13, 2019; Andrew Court, "Autistic Student, 21, Dies After He Was Restrained by Teachers at Texas Special Needs School That Is Also Being Investigated for Video of Six Educators Pinning Fourth-Grade Girl to the Ground," *DailyMail.com,* June 18, 2021.

happy; I want to make him happy. I almost didn't propose the idea, because I do want him to be happy. But I did propose the idea, giving him an exit at any time. He stayed the entire time! He said he had forgotten what a great film it was [...].

So we watched *Chariots of Fire*. A film with lush scenery and fabulous music (Vangelis, whom Jonathan had never heard of; I used to do Nordic Track to Vangelis). The story includes overcoming prejudice to win. This morning, Jonathan observed that we also face prejudice, but ours is impossible to overcome. No one cares.

It's funny. I used to see our cause in everything—books, movies, news. Last night, I just saw a beautiful film. Jonathan saw a parallel to our cause. Interesting how we switch roles.

Now that Flora is at Camphill, I have more time to reflect on the damage done to her. I'm coming to terms with it as much as I can. And I still have hope that we can somehow unlock her, find a spark or two to blast open those brain pathways that are barricaded. A book, an activity, a movie that will bring joy and growth. Hope springs eternal. She's not a vegetable, she's a living being with likes and dislikes, joys and dreads, skills and desires. Onward!

June 16, 2020: Very disturbing news last night [...]. A Rasmussen poll shows that 62% of Americans have a favorable opinion of Black Lives Matter. Wait, WHAT? People who peddle that America is fundamentally racist, who want to defund police, who want to allow in all immigrants enjoy a 62% favorable rating?? Jonathan said some people may have said they have a favorable opinion out of fear [...].

Jonathan and I both planned on donating more this year to the Police Benevolent Association, even though police unions are supposedly part of the problem. Jonathan says, "There are no bad cops in Morris Township."

Six hundred plainclothes policemen were let go in NYC. How am I supposed to feel safe in a city that does not respect police? [...]

Research is falling into place. The results are strong and robust. Regardless of how I slice the data, the result remains: women who received the HPV shot are less likely to have ever been pregnant than those women who did not receive the shot. And birth rates keep falling in the United States.

I'm feeling better, though I'm sometimes lethargic. Allergies could be influencing my health. Twinge on left side still there, but not as intense as two weeks ago when it first appeared.

June 17, 2020: [...]. We watched a video of Flora doing Applied Behavior Analysis [...] in 2005. She was attentive, more or less alert, and somewhat talkative. Jonathan questioned whether we did the right thing with the treatments.

At first I said, no, no. But then I thought about it. Maybe we should have allowed the poisons to stay in her body; it appears they were encased to some degree. The biomedical treatments opened up the encasements and brought out the mercury and aluminum and yeast.

Still, there were so many days when she just sat. So sad. And ABA is so artificial. Plus, we did the ABA the school offered. We didn't stop it, we just did other treatments as well.

Jonathan later pointed out that maybe Flora needs the structure that, for example, ABA provides. Camphill also provides that structure.

And certainly some of the doctors were mistakes […] with the steroids they prescribed. Those are the only two medical professionals who did any real damage. The others were simply time-consuming and expensive. I don't think any of the others did any real harm.

And Jonathan didn't blame me. He said, "Maybe **WE** did the wrong thing." For that I am grateful.

June 18, 2020: The Last Straw. I was on a video call with Dr. Isaacs yesterday, and she asked me about my research. As I was describing my work, Jenny flew into a rage: screaming, hitting herself. When I ended the call, I told Jenny she couldn't do that, she couldn't disrupt my call. She then started physically attacking me. When Jonathan intervened, she physically attacked him […].

From now on, if she disrupts **anything**, I deduct $5 from her tab. If she calls any of my friends, I deduct $5 […].

I have tried, in vain, to instill a sense of respect in Jenny. Respect for other people, starting with the people closest to her. I one time asked her why she attacks me when she's upset. Her reply? Because you're the closest one.

How is Jenny ever going to raise children? Will she attack them?

The report from Dr. Isaacs was good. We're going to stay the course. While a conventional oncologist would prescribe a hormone blocker, she said we could continue to watch the situation.

I've hit my lifetime limit of doctors. I do not want to meet or work with one more doctor ever again. Not for the girls; not for me. Getting used to each of their different personalities, their idiosyncrasies.

Research is going well. I'm actually able to recreate my original findings!

And I was feeling so much better until Jenny's flare-up. My health is currently precarious, and I was too weak to go for a walk last night. I'm somewhat concerned about having Flora visit this weekend, but it's a risk worth taking. I am feeling better—as long as Jenny doesn't cross me—and neither Jonathan nor Jenny show any symptoms, so I don't appear to be horribly contagious. Plus I just don't know how we would explain it to Flora.

June 19, 2020: Juneteenth. A national holiday. The day in 1865 when slavery ended (I think).

What about April 12, 2028, the date autism ended?

In my dreams. That's more likely the date when half the children born in the United States develop autism […].

Yesterday morning was explosive, but Jenny is now back to her sweet self. It's always the same rants: "I can't live here any more!" "Speak more softly!" "We need to be more marketable!" "People are making fun of me!" (I wonder why.) […].

I just wish Jenny would realize how very, very lucky she is to have Jonathan and me as parents. Many parents would have given up long ago.

Flora comes to visit today. It will be nice to see her […] for two days. It's all so tragic.

June 20, 2020: My entire body aches—ah, symmetry! I guess it's mainly my back. I wonder why!

Flora came home yesterday […]. This morning, I woke to find the back sliding door open. It appears someone opened the door last night and perhaps went outside […].

We never get a break, Jonathan and I. If Jenny isn't having a sudden outburst, Flora is eloping. No wonder I feel so old.

June 21, 2020: Jenny had another horrible outburst last night. My muscles ache, and she attacked me. "Hugging my dolly!" She also attacked Flora by squeezing her wrist; Flora was on the verge of tears. She punched Jonathan. Then she called Terry [our neighbor] and said we didn't love her.

The sooner she understands that we are doing everything we can to help her live independently, that our motives are pure, the better off everyone will be. She is sending me to an early grave. Without me, she has only one cheerleader, and Jonathan doesn't know which pills she takes. [I didn't, but when the time came I greatly simplified her pill regimen.] When we're gone, there is no one standing between Jenny and the loony bin.

People ***do*** treat her differently, but it has nothing to do with our research. It has everything to do with her strange behavior. She needs to realize that before she can get better, before she can address her outbursts. I've tried everything to help her control these outbursts. Biomedical, supplements, psychologists, acupuncture, homeopathy. She needs to know what to do when the feeling comes.

Triggers such as "Dara Berger" [author of the book *How to Prevent Autism*, who was attacked online by neurodiversity activists] and talking about my

research, e.g. with Dr. Isaacs, sends her absolutely mad. The viruses flare up
[...].

June 22, 2020: We took Flora back yesterday. Thank God. She broke into
the fridge and ate a pound of yogurt and drank almost a pint of heavy cream.
Interestingly, that was all. But still [...] ugh!

I feel like crap. Last night, I went to bed around 7:30 pm. I read for a
while—*Loserthink* by Scott Adams; good book—but total shut-eye by 9:30. I
don't feel totally rested, but I do want to get up. I feel kinda gross. The pain on
my right side is not constant, but when I roll on it a certain way, it hurts. The
pain on my left side is subsiding. Growing old sucks [...].

Tragic to see Flora just being. Not growing, just existing.

So grateful we found Camphill. And that we should be able to afford to set
her up in a similar living arrangement for life.

Jenny is getting worse. Jonathan noted that we had based all our plans
on the assumption that Jenny would get better, that she would hold a job and
be able to live at least semi-independently. But her outbursts started becoming more vicious last year—I have the picture of my neck, which she tried to
strangle—to prove it. And now she is not just attacking me, but also Jonathan.
When I asked her why she attacks me, she said, "Because you are the closest
person."

Jenny cannot be trusted to raise a child. I'm almost ok with that. Bringing
children into today's world is almost a crime.

But not quite. And I'm sad about not having any grandchildren.

Scott Adams said he had a horrible childhood. He doesn't elaborate, but
does say that he replaces the thoughts of his childhood with good and positive
thoughts. That sounds like a good idea. Onward with my research!

June 23, 2020: I am in severe pain. Only when I move the right side of my
body without supporting my upper rib cage. As long as I have my hand on the
back of my upper rib cage, I'm fine. Trouble is, there are lots of things I want to
do that involve being able to use both hands so I can't always support my back.

The pain is intense, like a stabbing. I suppose anyway; I've never been
stabbed. It's difficult lying down and getting back up.

I toyed with the idea of going to the hospital, but I'm glad I didn't make that
choice. The arrogance of the ER doctors—they would probably tell me my
cancer treatments are all wrong. And then they would put me in with Covid
patients and I would die [...].

In fact, now that I'm up and around, it's not so bad. The area still hurts,
though, and I will get it checked into.

After a morning explosion—in public, during our morning walk—Jenny was as sweet as she could be. I think the Neuroprotek along with the homeopathic remedies, Dr. Turner's supplements, and the P5P and zinc are helping […]. I wish I could have more guidance, but I can't start with another doctor.

Now, I want to use my limited energy to work on my HPV vaccine & fertility revision. Last night, I felt close to death. I have a few more things—ok, a LOT more things—to accomplish before that time comes.

June 24, 2020: I'm healing […] without drugs! Dr. Weiss—via telemedicine—deduced I'm having muscle spasms. [Howard Weiss was our local family doctor.] He recommended Arnica and CBD oil. He's so into weed! Lyn recommended a homeopathic remedy (Biotium), Epsom salt bath, and Arnica cream. She also said she can offer a more intense hormone blocker if the need arises.

Self-reliance. That's what naturopaths offer.

The world continues to go to hell in a handbasket […]. Universal vaccination, more free stuff for less deserving people, more destruction—perhaps in the suburbs—fear, danger, corruption.

I thought the destruction of our civilization would take a little longer, as more and more kids got vaccinated. I thought we had until at least 2050. We may not make it.

So, I better speed up my research!

June 25, 2020: My body still aches. Much less than yesterday, but I hope more than tomorrow. ("I love you more today than yesterday, but not as much as tomorrow […]") Muscle spasm on right side is subsiding, though certain positions are still dicey. Cancer-scar area hurting again. Probably was hurting all the time, but I didn't notice, because the muscle spasms hurt so much more.

For all the joy mankind can gain, not in pleasure but in rest from pain. The plaque in Dr. Goldin's office. [Her family doctor when she was growing up in Lancaster.]

And I have a bump on my head. Of unknown origin. Actually, not really a bump. Just a sore spot. Still, of unknown origin. Brain tumor? Cracked skull? Broken blood vessel that leads to stroke? Who knows? […]

Jenny has been very good. More independent, more proactive about helping. I think the new remedy is really helping. Also, Neuroprotek four times a day.

Still working on my HPV vaccine and fertility revision. I better hurry up before my brain tumor sets in.

Jonathan is patiently waiting for my body to heal. I know he really, really likes sex (with me), but he's not pushing anything. How's that for a double entendre? He's the most wonderful man in the world.

June 26, 2020: Dad would have been 98 today. Except that "modern medicine" intervened. Screw modern medicine. Eighteen years without my protector. And see my standing in the family. I'm a nobody.

But, Dad, your spirit lives on in me. Your optimism—well, at least part of your optimism. Finding the good. Of course, you only faced getting bombed at and watching your comrades get eaten by sharks. You never had to face the "friendly fire" of the government telling you—highly recommending—that you poison your kids. There is zero good in this situation. Zero [...].

My muscle spasms appear to have subsided. The area is still a bit sore, as to be expected after such a workout. I'm sleeping better [...] and I'm better about to concentrate. I have had a taste of what it's like to be old, and it sucks.

So, back to research. And then maybe doing taxes this afternoon with Jonathan [...]. Dad would be so happy for us!

June 27, 2020: Will I ever feel good again? My body aches. The pain isn't as intense as earlier this week, but going for a walk hurts. I forge onward, but I'm exhausted afterwards.

Old age came on so suddenly.

I must be grinding my teeth at night, because I wake up with a sore jaw.

Jenny's stupid actions aren't helping. Yesterday, she discovered a $20 charge to her debit card. We saw that the charge came from "HealthSapiens." Jenny denied knowing the existence of this company. I asked whether I could look at her emails, and she reluctantly agreed (what choice did she have?). She had indeed signed up for a "free trial." So, she was charged $20 for the month and then another $40 cancellation fee.

I didn't bail her out this time. I'm not going forever to be around to bail her out. The way I feel now, I'm not going to be around much longer to bail her out.

Her lack of preparedness for living weighs upon me heavily. Flora is more or less set up. We need to find a permanent place for her, but we should be able to do that. A humane place.

But Jenny—caught between two worlds—attacks me when she's confused. Instead of dealing with the confusion and trying to figure out things, she attacks.

No wonder my stress levels are so high.

My body ached too much to make love with Jonathan yesterday. I hope we can make love soon. Today, maybe.

June 28, 2020: Jenny physically attacked me twice yesterday. The first time the morning when I was trying to guide her about proper use of the sauna. Also PNC Bank called, because Jenny is disputing the charge form HealthSapien, a "free trial" she signed up for. When I intervened with the call, Jenny got angry, but kept it together. Only when I told her how to use the sauna—that she needed to stay hydrated—did she lose it. She squeezed me. I yelled "Help!" or tried to, at least. My faint cries are nothing compared with Jenny's war screams. Lyn's drops. Apologies. "I'll never attack Mom again."

Then again last night, when we discovered she signed up for yet another "free trial" for makeup that costs $30 a month. She squeezed and punched my cancer area. Jonathan called the police.

Morris Township police are some of the finest people I've ever met […] and I've met many Morris Township police. They arrived—one officer, his boss, and back-up—and scared her straight. They asked whether we wanted to send her to the hospital. We declined. The officer offered to come out any time we needed them. We explained how their presence calms Jenny. He repeated we could call any time. Even if she was upset again in five minutes. I said I was sorry for everything they are going through, that I've only met only fine people in the Morris Township Police Department. The officer thanked me, and said it meant a lot […].

I spoke with Angela [a family friend and autism mother of Amy]. She said we needed to take care of ourselves. What would happen, she asked, if one of us gets severely injured; how would the other two feel? She told me about Amy's residence, Community Options. Angela is actually happy with the arrangement! The highest praise I have heard from Angela up to this point was she was "not unhappy" with services from an agency. We're calling Monday. I hope we can get Jenny out of the house soon. She's killing me.

My muscle spasms are back, this time on the left side. Excruciating pain. I can stand, sit, and lie down, but the act of lying down or getting up from lying down is very painful. I'm getting better at lying down, but rising is still an artform. I roll onto my left side, then hoist myself up while breathing out. That way, the pain isn't quite as excruciating. I'm taking Bryonium and rubbing Arnica on the area and I'm getting better.

June 29, 2020: I'm still in pain. The most intense pain is when I move from lying down to sitting up. But sleeping is difficult and not completely restful […].

We'll probably call Community Options today. I can't imagine that a placement will be easy, given the waiting lists.

I haven't been able to take care of Jonathan for the past three weeks. I feel so bad. He's so patient. I love him so much.

June 30, 2020: Muscle spasms continue. Pain on left side, right side, sometimes the back. During the day, life is more or less fine. Sleeping is difficult, knowing that I'll need to rise. It's the rising part that is so excruciating. I'll check the web to see what else I can do. Maybe I should see Dr. Weiss. It's interfering with my ability to take care of Jonathan. Yes, I should see Dr. Weiss [...].

The more I hear about hydroxychloroquine, the more I realize how much the elite really don't care about human life. The WHO and the UK designed studies to overdose patients with HCQ so they could say, see, the drug not only doesn't work, it kills [...].

I'll work on submitting my revised HPV paper to *Immunological Research* today.

July 1, 2020: The aches are subsiding somewhat. Yeah! Advil seems to help. For me, taking Advil is defeat, but sometimes I need to lose a battle to win a war.

Now my cancer area is hurting again. It probably hurt the entire time, but when other parts of my body were aching more, I didn't notice the cancer. There's a small blotch of goo from the cancer site on my t-shirt. Dr. Isaacs was always concerned about the integrity of the skin. But I don't want to call her. She'll say I need an oncologist. I just can't deal with another doctor. Lyn returns from what I assume is a vacation on July 7. I don't want to bother her before then, but I will if I have to. She said we could do homeopathy before resorting to prescription hormone blockers.

Jenny is being a true pain in the ass. Jonathan mentioned a slow recovery for the economy. She yelped. I agree that the observation is painful, but I don't yelp. And the trailer for *1986: The Act* [a film directed by Andrew Wakefield] has a two-second cameo of me, and Jenny went ballistic. Thanks, Jen, for respecting my work [...]. It's like walking on eggshells. And she forgot to take her evening pills. How is she ever going to live on her own? Answer: she can't.

Fortunately, things are moving at DDD [Division of Developmental Disabilities]. Jim Ruskin called yesterday to let us know that she has been approved [for housing] and they are expediting the case. Jim, the way, is furloughed. Yet he still called and even replied to my email. People need to work, even if they don't get paid [...].

Jonathan and I made love yesterday. Very pleasant. We should do it again sometime.

July 2, 2020: I am in intense pain. Yesterday, walking was difficult. Reaching hurts. My upper back, my middle back, my lower back, my right side, my left side. Everything strained.

Guess it's finally time to call the doctor.

Jonathan has been so sweet. He attends to my every request. I hate being such a burden, but Jonathan doesn't seem to mind.

I'm preparing two manuscripts for submission. Both very controversial. I can't stop now. I know too much, and I have too much to share.

Interestingly, I learned yesterday that the *Lancet* had an article already in 1966 linking premature ovarian failure to autoimmunity. That's fascinating.

So, how can I investigate the lowered SIDS rate during the pandemic as an economic question? That's my next challenge.

July 5, 2020: Dr. Weiss […] is testing me for Lyme. Good thing, because the pain is getting worse. Yesterday, I spent most of the day in bed […]. Dr. Weiss and I discussed the possibility that someone might be trying to poison me. I brought it up, only half in jest. We both immediately agreed the person was not Jonathan. But then I mentioned my paper on HPV vaccine and lowered fertility and the multibillion dollar industry I am challenging. Greater men have died for less, I'm sure.

Jonathan is so sweet. He's always sweet, but I notice it more when I'm weak. And weak I am.

Lately, flickers of depression are making themselves felt. In a couple of weeks, Flora will be coming home. While I'm dreading her six-week stay with us, I'm also terribly sad that it will probably be the last time she will have an extended time with us. I want more than anything in the world to find the spark to excite her, to make her happy, to help her find her way in the world.

Jonathan and I had fun last night watching the fireworks (after suffering through some Grand Ole Opry music). Macy's sponsored the TV show and kept interjecting sycophant acknowledgments that we must atone for our systemic racism […]. Jenny joined us to watch the fireworks, and then we all watched the Greg Gutfeld Show. Surprisingly to me, Jonathan really got into the show. I'm so glad, the show is amusing, and we all need a laugh right now […].

I'm going to […] submit the HPV vaccine and fertility paper today […]. The cover letter has the symbolic date of "July 4." It may be too late, but I'm going to keep going as though we still have freedom of speech, freedom of research, and freedom of thought. Otherwise, it's all over.

July 6, 2020: Horrible night. The pain. This morning, the stiffness. I'm walking like a 90-year-old, shuffling along. The molding on the walls provide support as I move from one room to the next. Fortunately, I was able to sleep, but getting up was very difficult.

And Jenny, Jenny, Jenny. She had a horrendous flare-up last night. Yes, I've been criticizing her lately—don't get water on the floor, put shoes away, lower the music. She's really been getting on my nerves lately. Probably because, even if I don't die from what I have now, I will someday not be here. She has to figure out things for herself, and she seems so incapable of doing so. Jonathan says it's because she doesn't like to be reminded of her disabilities. But how is she going to improve if she doesn't recognize her weaknesses? At first, she took my criticisms ok, but then—I think it was the music—she had had enough. "I can't live here anymore!" she screams. When Jonathan told her to blow out the candle, she went ballistic for a second and more intense time.

And she's not staying on topic anymore. It's so annoying. It's like living with a five-year-old who wants to enter the conversation. We indulge five-year-olds; it's more difficult to indulge 24-year-olds. And she keeps repeating the same stories and phrases […]. She's not growing, not able to talk about anything outside herself.

Jonathan is ready to call the police and have her taken to the pysch ward. I'm not quite ready for that. She didn't physically attack me last night […].

We never get a break, Jonathan and I […]. The people who did this to our children […]. How many children have they murdered, how many lives have they destroyed? How many children will not be born, because of their greed, their lust for power and money? And there's no end in sight.

July 7, 2020: I'm still in great pain. Rising after having lain for a while is difficult. The longer I lay, the more difficult to rise. Rising in the morning is the worst, and rising in the middle of the night to pee is the second worse. Sometimes I miss. I sense this is how old age feels, and IT SUCKS.

Dr. Weiss prescribed a homeopathic remedy, Rhus toxicodendron. Jonathan picked it up for me last night from Dr. Weiss' office. No man (or woman) is an island.

Jenny & I are getting along better. She seems genuinely concerned about me, as I am genuinely concerned about her […].

Jonathan seems to be holding up well. I feel so bad that I can't be a good wife. We've done taxes exactly one time in about a month. I'm focusing on getting better. For him. For us. I love him so much.

July 9, 2020: I.am.going.to.live! And I am never, ever going to take my health for granted again.

We're still waiting for the test results to see if I have a tick-borne disease, but Dr. Weiss prescribed antibiotics. It looks like a duck, walks like a duck, quacks like a duck: It's a DUCK!

I'm still moving slowly with a few kinks to work out. But I no longer need the cane I started using two days ago. I am able to think more clearly—funny, when you're not racked with pain how much more easily ideas flow [...].

And the depression has lifted. I kept thinking, "Is this how it ends?" I've spent the better of the past two decades caring for others, tending to the girls' needs, trying to help them to heal. And then, ironically, I'm the one who needed overwhelming support from others. I didn't want it to end that way.

I don't think I'll call Dr. Isaacs about noncancer things again. She said it didn't sound like metastatic bone cancer, but you never know [...]. I like her, I respect her, but I prefer to take one step at a time. Yes, try the antibiotics. If that path doesn't work, let me know. I know she was just being honest, and I guess I needed to know what other possibilities my symptoms suggested, but maybe just say if the antibiotics don't work, perhaps we need a CAT scan to see if anything else is going on.

1986: The Act came out yesterday. I was too sick to watch it.

When Dr. Weiss called yesterday, I needed to confirm the phone number of the pharmacy, so I asked Jonathan to find a medicine bottle. "He's such a peach," I reported to Dr. Weiss. "Just like all you Stuyvesant guys." [We both attended Stuyvesant High School in New York City.] Scott Adams says you should embarrass yourself often, so you know it's not the end of the world. I hope Dr. Weiss realizes the statement came from a foggy mind racked in pain.

July 10, 2020: I'm feeling better, though I still have many aches and twinges. No longer do I need a cane (!), and I wore padded underwear last night only as an insurance policy. I didn't need them. ☺ I'm able, with some difficulty, to roll around in bed. Yeah! Sex soon.

A couple of days ago, I noticed droplets of ooze from my cancer site on my t-shirt. Dr. Isaacs said to be careful of ooze. Ugh. I really don't want to call her again.

Yesterday morning, I gathered data on fertility rates; this morning, I'll gather data about HPV vaccine uptake. Then, I'll send it to Josh [Joshua Guetzkow, on the law faculty of the Hebrew University in Israel]. In case anything happens to me, he'll have the data.

Jenny got upset last night when Jonathan told her to put on more clothes. She still doesn't get it.

July 11, 2020: The pain continues, but seems to be dissipating. Slowly, very slowly. I'm never sure when a movement will result in a yelp of pain. But move I do. I do believe I'm feeling stronger every day.

Scott Adams says we all have movies in our heads. They filter the information around us. People can observe the same facts, but their movies interpret the facts very differently. If the filters we use to understand the world make us happy and help predict the future, they are good.

I don't see movies as much as hear music. I'm hearing the song by Chicago, "I do believe I'm feeling stronger every day."

But the words of Dr. Isaacs give me pause. "It doesn't sound like metastatic bone cancer, but you never know." Metastatic bone cancer, metastatic bone cancer. Not to add any stress, but metastatic bone cancer.

Scott Adams is a great persuader. I wish he could persuade Flora to talk and Jenny to be calm.

I have never felt so close to Jonathan. It's a culmination of our lives together. Tomorrow, I'll feel even closer, because we will have had one more day together. "I love you more today than yesterday, but not as much as tomorrow." It's also the idea that if the end is near for me, Jonathan and I don't have much more time together. That makes me sad. Not a good filter.

I do believe I'm feeling stronger every day.

July 13, 2020: Tick found! It was the black "pimple" that suddenly appeared in early May after biking. I was in the shower and felt the very odd growth. I tried washing it away for several days and the decided, oh, screw it, and just yanked it off. The growth was so weird that I decided to save it. Now, we might be able to use what I saved to determine what kind of tick is making me so miserable.

Part of the critter might still be in me. I'll ask Dr. Weiss whether it should be removed.

I'll ask Dr. Isaacs whether—with so much going on—I should do a juice fast right now.

I'm taking double doses of Advil. Otherwise, the pain is excruciating.

I love Jonathan so much.

Acadia powder seems to be helping Jenny. She's reading a book! About Malala. She's also less defensive when I ask her to turn down her music.

I, Gayle DeLong, will become healthy. Scott Adams is into affirmations. I think they're weird. But, hey, at this point, I'll try anything. It may have something to do with focusing energy.

I, Gayle DeLong, will become healthy […] with a little help from my doctors and my antibiotic and Advil and my husband.

I love Jonathan so much.

July 14, 2020: Pain still excruciating […]. I'm so sick & tired of being sick & tired.

Lyn's remedies seem to be helping—I think they are the reason I lasted until 3 am with no Advil fix. She'll be sending an arsenal.

Dr. Isaacs seems so tired. She's probably wearing her mask too long. She said I didn't need to do a juice fast this break.

I'm getting to know Dr. Weiss. He really is a Mensch, even if he's a Grumpy-Pants from time to time. He's a New Yorker, what do I expect?

I want to work on my letter to the editor pointing out the lack of evidence that masks prevent Covid […].

I love Jonathan so much. In sickness and in health. He's a man of his words […] and actions.

July 15, 2020: Thank God for adult diapers! For the past couple of nights, I've filled mine […] on the way to *going* to the bathroom! I'm so pathetic.

I so look forward to the pain subsiding. Jonathan sent off the tick on Monday (ticknetics.com, cute name). Yesterday, I went for blood work […].

Jonathan is so wonderful. I am not worthy. And yet he makes me feel as though I am.

July 16, 2020: Pain has decided to invade my lower back. Those muscles are so tight […] There is a joke in there somewhere, but I'll have to think about it […].

I don't remember my energy ever being this low. Pain reduces energy, and I've got lots of pain […].

Jonathan continues to be a peach.

Jenny is being ok, under the circumstances. Still demands wifi at a moment's notice, but is taking her supplements on her own (a BIG plus).

I will contact Lauren O'Toole to see if emergency respite exists.

July 17, 2020: Flora comes home today. For 50 days. Not that I'm counting. OK, I'm counting. The saddest part is that this will be the last time she is home for any stretch of time. No more chances to find the sparks that make her happy, that make her feel alive. I do hope we can find a place for her that continues to search for those sparks. I think we can....

I'll be accompanying Jonathan and Jenny on the trip to pick up Flora. I prefer to stay at home; I'm still in great pain. But I do worry about Jonathan driving the entire distance without someone checking to make sure he's awake. More than once, I've had to strongly encourage him to let me take over the wheel. Staying home today would be more difficult than going. Who knows? It may actually be good for me. In fact, it will probably be good for me. I haven't been out of the house, except for a doctor's visit and blood draws since early July.

I hope we do find out what's wrong with me [...].

July 19, 2020: Yesterday, I sat in the big comfy chair all day. Hence, no musing. The world is taking care of itself without me. The kids are eating and taking their supplements. OK, I'm helping when I can. But I'm still in much pain. My hips and lower back mainly. And my left knee. God, I hope this isn't metastatic bone cancer. I'll ask Lyn. I very much like and very much respect Dr. Isaacs, but I sense she has seen the worst and is geared toward that perspective.

[But what we thought was Lyme disease turned out to be much more serious. The diary resumed 20 days later.]

August 9, 2020: Dad always said not to worry about the bullets you dodged. I dodged a lot of bullets these past weeks. Here's what happened.

Was it July 22? I forget. Anyway, I was feeling lousy. Really dreadful. The doxycycline that was supposed to clear my supposed Lyme was not kicking in. I barfed some green liquid. Dr. Weiss called and said my calcium levels were high—they went from 10 to 12. My bones were rejecting calcium and spilling the mineral into my blood. Get to the ER. Now.

Metastatic bone cancer. So sudden. It was only since early July that I felt really awful. And the pain would come and go. First my right rib, then my left. Then my lower back.

The people at the hospital took excellent care of me. I needed surgery for an exploded fracture in my lumbar region (L5). God, that sounded awful. Not just a fracture, but an *exploded* fracture. More troubling perhaps was the lack of bone in my neck. The plate for my C5 was gone. If I understand correctly—which is dubious—any shock to the region, such as a mild car accident, could have left me paralyzed. Bullet dodged.

Very fortunately, the surgeon was able to surge relatively quickly. July 30. The operation went smoothly.

I met some of the most wonderful people during this adventure. Christina, Eric, Marybeth—it was her last day at MMC [Morristown Medical Center]—Paula [...], Aditi (who obviously loves her work), the nurse's assistant who introduced me to the Reggae performer Lucky Dube (I forget her name), Samantha who will be taking her nurse's exam this coming Saturday, Brianna who was very competent, but also a drug pusher ("I have to give *something*.")

The hospital did push drugs for pain management. Many people were shocked that I didn't press the patient-controlled pain button (for 0.2 ml of liquid morphine) even once. Lyn Farrugia gave me homeopathic options, and

Jenny delivered the goods ("So, I'm your dealer now, Mom?"). It was a "don't ask, don't tell" situation as I snuck the homeopathic remedies for pain.

Looking to the future, […] I'll most probably need radiation for the "innumerable" bone mets on my spine. You do what you have to do.

In other news, Jenny has been very good except for Friday night. She ran out of Valtrex and went ape shit. She's back on Valtrex and is no longer ape shit. Flora has been very sweet. Sometimes, we just hang out together in the living room.

And Jonathan, wonderful, wonderful Jonathan. So supportive, so caring, so calm. Where would I be without him? I would be so, so lost. But I'm found, and together, there's nothing we can't lick.

August 11, 2020: My current condition appears to be a taste of old age, and I want nothing to do with it. Mom is still very active, and that's the way I want to be. I suppose old-age decline is more gradual than the tsunami that hit me. Fortunately, I have the hope and great prospect of healing and getting back to "normal" life. Without that prospect, I don't know what I'd do.

Jonathan is being absolutely wonderful. It's so hard on him. Of course, *I'm* the easy one. Jenny spilled sangria all over the kitchen last night—probably did not tighten the spout. And she took no responsibility for her actions. "I wasn't doing anything." And, of course, she did a half-ass job of cleaning up the mess. When we try to guide her, she becomes defensive and aggressive. "Sorry I'm such a burden!" she'll wail. If she were so sorry, she would learn from her mistakes and not make them again.

We're looking into long-term placement for Flora. We can get assistance from New Jersey only if the placement is within the state. There is nothing like Camphill here. We will explore what's here, but Camphill (and similar arrangements) are perfect for several reasons. For "co-workers," Camphill is a way of life, not just a job. It is also a system. When one co-worker leaves, another enthusiastic and dedicated person arrives. The thought of Flora living in a group home, where staff have no mission and merely clock in, scares me. Let's see, let's see, let's see.

I will try to take the semester off from teaching. I just need a doctor's note […]. I look so forward to getting back to research. The HPV & fertility paper was rejected—at the editorial level!—at *Immunologic Research*. What a bunch of pussies! I'm thinking of *Journal of Economic Population*, also a Springer publication. The research is important, and the truth needs to be told.

August 12, 2020: Jenny has spun out of control. Last night, she slammed the front door so hard that it jammed. Now, we cannot use that door […].

Jonathan is so exhausted.

Last night, she admitted she had taken some propranolol she found in her room. She claims she took six pills. She's still alive and not showing any strange physical reactions, so we didn't call 911 (like last time, when she took a handful of her antidepressants "to get rid of the pain.").

She doesn't learn. She blames me and Jonathan, her most fervent supporters. She takes no responsibility and lashes out when we try to correct her uncivilized behavior (starting to eat before everyone is at the table) […]. She has twice physically touched me when she was angry. She's scary when she is in those moods. We thought it was the fact that she ran out of Valtrex, but then yesterday occurred.

She hasn't been taking her liquid supplements—why would they stop, just because I'm in the hospital?—and shows no responsibility when it comes to taking care of herself.

She felt that confessing to taking the propranolol absolved herself of the stupidity of doing so.

I need to focus on my health, my healing. I've given her everything I can […] and more. Helpless. Hopeless. Horrible.

August 13, 2020: Twenty-five years! Jonathan and I have been married 25 years. Today.

We've been through so much, yet we keep getting stronger. So much of who I am is because of Jonathan […].

How has our marriage "worked" when so many—especially under our circumstances—fail? Ok, true, we: (1) seek pleasure and avoid pain; (2) skipped our first marriage and went straight to our second, and (3) I asked Jonathan never to grow up, and he never did!

How did I get so lucky, though? Jonathan brings out the best in me, the very best. He says the same of me.

We both have the same desires in life—a healthy and happy family, work that is fulfilling, and great sex.

Yesterday was a much better day than Tuesday. Jenny was on an even keel, sweet even. If only she could always be that way. For her sake (and ours!).

I continue to heal, though this bone cancer has thrown me for a loop. Never a dull moment. Not in 25 years.

Last night I had a thought about Flora's long-term living arrangements. If she stays in New Jersey, she will be dependent upon the N.J. government to provide for her. What are the first programs to be cut when the budget tanks? People who don't vote. The thought scares the shit out of me. Private pay to a Camphill-like arrangement, here we come.

Speaking with Christy from Dr. Levitz's office was wonderful. She's so refreshingly upbeat. She says Dr. Levitz [an oncologist] will work with me. If she's correct, I think we found ourselves the right doctor. I already sense I can be more honest with him than with Dr. —.

Being able to be myself. That's a fulfilling life.

August 14, 2020: What a delightful day yesterday was! The occupational therapist came by to show me ways to make my life easier. Then the physical therapist came by to show me ways to make life stronger. Then Jonathan picked up the doctor's excuse from Dr. Gatto's office; Dr. Gatto says I should be out until January 2021. Perfect. I do hope my request for leave is approved. I'll be able to get back to my research.

Then Jonathan and I met Dr. Levitz. His patient in-take person, Christy, sang his praises, saying he would explain things to me and would listen to me and would work with me. I thought, that sounds ***great***, but I'll believe it when I see it. Christy is right—Dr. Levitz is very knowledgeable, yet listens and incorporates a patient's desires. We all had an instant rapport. He explained I have stage IV cancer, because any cancer that has metastasized is considered stage IV. That is the **dumbest** thing I've ever heard. My cancer is very slow growing (3%—whatever that means). Jonathan asked whether I could outlive my cancer. Dr. Levitz said probably not; that people with stage IV breast cancer typically live seven to ten years. Jonathan freaked (silently). First of all, I'm not just doing conventional medicine. I'm also doing Dr. Isaacs' protocol. Secondly, I don't have chemo or radiation crap already in my system. Dr. Levitz said I will most probably respond well to treatments. Thirdly, I'm married to my best friend.

Dr. Levitz has no problem with my continuing with Dr. Isaacs […].

Last evening was topped off by an enchanting dinner to celebrate our 25th wedding anniversary!

August 15, 2020: Yesterday, we figured out that the "propranolol" that Jenny took on Tuesday was actually my arimidex […]. The arimidex pills are the same size as the propranolol pills. The different color wouldn't matter to Jenny. She associated the two. After asking her for the bottle—which she claimed she recycled—and not finding it, Jenny finally confessed. She wanted the "pain to stop."

When are you going to learn, Jenny? You overdosed bigtime once before. Then you popped Valtrex when you were upset, but I made you spit them out. Now, ***my*** pills. Anything prescription, huh? […]

So, extra work for me. I had to call the doctor's office—the doctor whom I just started working with—and explain how my autistic daughter popped my pills. David at Dr. Levitz's office said we'll figure out something […]. [He] asked whether Jenny was ok to which I replied, "Yes, but *I want to kill her!*"

Flora's wandering at night concerns me. [She insisted on taking long evening walks by herself.] I wish she would come in before dark, but she steadfastly refuses […].

Jonathan continues to be a total peach. Life will get easier when Flora is back at school. And we can have sex again. My body just isn't cooperating.

August 16, 2020: Jenny is such a selfish bitch. I turned down the volume of her radio—the one we bought for her—explaining that I wanted to work. As soon as I had left the room, up goes the volume. Not too, too loud, but annoying that she can't honor a simple request with an explanation.

And her candles. She's into candles. Last night, two of them, even though she and Flora were running late for the outdoor movie. I noticed a candle in her room this morning. We need to explain to her that candles are dangerous. If we have a fire, we can't get out the front door because it is jammed. We could be trapped. Moreover, my mobility is limited, and I could more easily die […]. She accepts no responsibility when she does stupid things, and she does a lot a stupid things […].

I explored one of the medications Dr. Levitz suggests, Ibrance. Apparently, it kills bad cells, but good cells as well. Mmmmm. I'll discuss with Dr. Isaacs. I'll also ask her about mistletoe.

I know I have to relieve stress. Like not concentrating on what a selfish bitch Jenny is. Venting helps, as long as I don't dwell.

I'm tired a lot, and I guess my back does hurt. Not really hurt, more sore. Like I've just done a workout (when I haven't).

I love Jonathan so much. Lucky I'm in love with my best friend. That song was playing in the restaurant when we celebrated our 25th. How appropriate!

August 17, 2020: Jenny had another flare-up yesterday. I forget what set her off; it doesn't matter. She ranted, she raved, she hit Flora and herself. She said something about how some parents care about their children's self-esteem.

It's the ingratitude that gets to me. Jonathan and I have been working the past 20 years to get Jenny healthy so she can live a happy, independent life. We've tried everything, and yet she blames us for her shortcomings. She takes no responsibility for when she doesn't take her supplements or when she doesn't organize them correctly.

And then she plays that stupid song by Taylor Swift about "all you're ever going to be is mean." That hurts, cuts like a knife.

I was reading about survival rates of breast cancer with bone metastasis. It's somewhere between six months and over ten years. I should stop wasting my time reading that stuff.

What I do need to read about is Ibrance. Dr. Levitz recommended the drug for me, but I'm skeptical. It kills off cells that divide quickly, including but not limited to cancer cells. Hair thins. Who knows what other quickly-dividing cells are also attacked? I'll ask Dr. Isaacs. I'll also ask her about mistletoe, which to me looks promising.

I love Jonathan so much, who stays calm throughout it all. I know all of this is so hard on him; we have to take care of the caregiver. I look forward to taking care of the caregiver.

August 19, 2020: Got up late yesterday—8:20 am!—and had to get ready for a phone appointment with Andrew, the lawyer helping us with Flora's DDD application. Then Jenny had a flare-up, a big one. I was scared of her. Jonathan stood between her and me as Flora was throwing things in the living room. Jenny *is* a burden. She keeps saying she is, and she's right. So, why doesn't she do something about it? She says she doesn't want to be a burden. Really? […]

Oh, Jenny. You don't get it. When I say you won't ever hold a job, it's after you engage in self-destructive behavior. Notice, I always preface my observation with "If you continue to behave the way you are currently behaving, you will never hold a job."

She's so selective in her hearing, so self-centered, so **mean**.

Jonathan says the draft of her new book is dreadful. Whiney, complaining, no sparkle. I'm hoping he can pull out some nuggets and suggest she expand upon them.

What happened between her first book—where she sparkled—and now? The real world intervened. We've protected her for so long, getting her out of her scrapes, and when the real world of college greeted her, she was totally unprepared. We tried to help her negotiate around the mean-spirited people […] and gravitate toward those who are understanding […], but she fixates on the negative. What a sad, sad life she is leading. Always blaming others. Focusing on the negative. It's as though Doug [Gayle's penultimate boyfriend, before she met Jonathan] is my child! […]

I'm concerned about Jonathan. The whole situation is really wearing on him. I think he'll feel better when school starts, though it probably won't be in-person. He so very much misses the classroom. The **real** classroom. So do I.

August 20, 2020: Yesterday was a good day. Of course, when you have bone cancer, **every day** is a good day. Except that the radiology oncologist assured us that people with bone cancer can live years and years.

I like Dr. Wagman. She explains things and doesn't seem to want to radiate just because she can. The plan is just to radiate my lumbar area now and in a few months, after my neck has healed, to do my neck. Ten trips each time. Jonathan is a peach. No problem.

Dr. Isaacs had warned me about radiology oncologists, that they tend not to be people persons. That may be true for the males [...] but the females I've worked with—including Dr. Wagman and even the lady at Sloan Kettering—or heard about—including the ladies at Morristown Memorial—are great [...].

Jenny had no flare-ups. Yea! Jonathan recommended she turn her Manimal script into a book and then into a cartoon TV series. She took the advice well. Maybe this project will lighten her up so that she doesn't dwell on the past negatives of her life. [Manimal was a 1983 television series about a professor who can transform himself into an animal and fight crime with the assistance of a beautiful blonde police lieutenant. It was cancelled after 8 episodes, but it still has a tiny cult following, including Jennifer.]

Flora screamed in the middle of the night. Jonathan gave her two Advil, which seemed to calm her. Autism is such a Gift in the German sense of the word "Gift," which means "poison."

Jonathan has a busy day today. He's taking it all in stride. He noted the other day that I am the only person who has never let him down. His mother admitted—toward the end—that she was "a lousy wife and a lousy mother." Jonathan had to agree [silently]. Our kids—through little or no fault of their own—are not exactly bringing total joy to our lives. But we have each other, Jonathan and I. Our fathers didn't let us down. But everyone else—our mothers, our siblings, our children—have.

Dr. Weiss noticed—as have many people—that I must have a high tolerance for pain. Maybe it's the homeopathy that's helping, or maybe it's all relative. There is no greater pain than seeing your children drift away from you into seas that they cannot navigate and you can't help them. No greater pain.

August 23, 2020: One month since I went to the hospital. One month until my birthday. I wonder where I will be in a month.

I missed several musings. Jonathan and I have been getting up about the same time. Once I have breakfast—which I wouldn't miss for anything to have with Jonathan—a musing is difficult to write. Plus, I was having some pain in my left side. I think I overdid it on Thursday, when I tried to do an enema. For the first time in a while, I experienced pain. I was scared. Did I fracture something? Or was it just a pulled muscle? Was a pulled muscle bad?

I hate being so fragile. I'm so used to being **strong like bull**. Or at least *agile as butterfly*. Now, I have aches and pains—mainly aches—everywhere.

My central back, my lower back, my left rib (#7), my right ribs (#10 and 12, I think), my upper left arm. And let's not forget the neck brace. Ugh.

Still, I believe I was five minutes away—one slight case of whiplash—away from being paralyzed from the neck down. That does put things into perspective.

Anyway, I felt better this morning. Still a small twinge in my lower left back, but I seem to be mending. Bad things don't mend. They just get worse.

Jonathan starts "teaching" on Monday. Scare quotes, because this semester on online. Talk about fragile! Our democracy, our democratic rights have evaporated since mid-March. All it took was the fear of sickness to terrify the US—nay, the world!—population to cower. We can't gather, can't protest, we can't attend religious services. How did this happen? Fear. Lack of information.

We saw it with autism. If you don't vaccinate, your kid will **die** of a horrible disease and **it will be all your fault.** We saw it with cancer. Poison yourself to save yourself or something dreadful will happen **and it will be all your fault.** Well, something dreadful did happen to me—something that, given my daily stress, probably would have happened anyway—and, at least the attending physician at Morristown Hospital, blamed me. In fact, given my daily stress, something even more dreadful would probably have happened. Ovarian cancer, anyone? Brain cancer? Pancreatic cancer? I'm fortunate to have bone cancer as my wake-up call.

Jonathan is now about to have breakfast. So, I will go share precious moments with my best friend. Forever.

August 24, 2020: Jonathan starts teaching today, so I had to set an **alarm!** First time in forever. He wanted to be up by 7, so I set the alarm for 6:30 so I could have a few moments to myself. Those moments were taken away as Flora stumbled upstairs from her first-floor den and Jenny was already sitting downstairs with her cup of coffee. Not really a cup of coffee. More like coffee grounds mixed with water. She seems incapable of making a decent cup of coffee. But the swill does not seem to bother her, and she doesn't ask for a refresher course on how to make coffee.

Jenny is anxious about getting her period. I advised her to take her drops from Lyn. She did, and she's back to bed. Those drops are amazing. And Lyn sent some super-duper (1M, whatever that means) pellets for when Jenny is in a rage. We haven't needed the pellets yet, but I'm glad we have them [...].

Jonathan continues to be my absolute soulmate. An article in the *Wall Street Journal* described how a nonagenarian husband moved in with his slightly older wife at her nursing home when he was told he could not visit her. He continues to feed her and be there for her, even though the ravages of Alzheimer's have taken her faculties. The story was incredibly touching. Jonathan and I agreed we would do the same for each other. Since neither of us allows ourselves to receive flu shots, I sincerely hope we don't have to deal with Alzheimer's. But we will have—we **do have**—other ailments. And we are there for each other. Always and forever.

August 26, 2020: Jenny attacked me last night. Both Jonathan and me. We were having a peaceful dinner. Jonathan suggested that Jenny get hitched with Matt, that they complement each other. "Like your mom and me. I'm the words person and she's the numbers person." Jenny flew into a full-blown rage, ranting about how I should be a "real woman." She started cursing at Jonathan to "put me in my place." I left the room and removed her laptop from her desk. She lunged at me, putting her palms on my head.

Her rant continued for about 45 minutes. I gave her Lyn's pellets about 15 minutes into the rage.

Then, it was over. "I'm calming down now," Jenny noticed. And then she was fine. Apologetic to a degree.

Jenny's autism is literally killing me. And you don't seem to care, Jenny. You don't acknowledge the depth of your insanity. You blame others. After your rages, you want to live and let live. You desperately want to live independently, but you can't. You are unable. You spent $90 to talk with a former actress in *Manimal*. "But I have the money," you protest. That's not the point. You flushed $90 down the toilet.

And when was the last time you spent money on someone other than yourself? Matt created a lovely birthday celebration for you—balloons, donut holes, several very nice presents. Have you ever done anything like that for him?

You are a danger to yourself and others. True, 95% of the time you're ok. You make stupid—very stupid—financial decisions. You are disorganized with your schoolwork and your room is a mess. We could deal with that.

But your rages, your violence […].

I hope the people who did this to her—the executives at Merck and GlaxoSmithKline—all rot in hell.

August 27, 2020: I called Jim Rankin yesterday to tell him Jenny needs to be in a group home. Now. He has not yet returned my call. Jenny is not happy. I don't care. Neither does Jonathan. She needs this next step. It may not be forever. In fact, we hope it is not forever. But for right now, she needs daily supervision and care.

She shows such little respect for Jonathan and me. But I don't want to focus on negative thoughts again so early in the morning.

*** NEWS FLASH *** It appears Flora did not steal any food last night! No lamb chops, no cheese, no yogurt.

I'm getting further into the republication of my HPV and fertility article. Interesting analysis by Nathan Seltzer finds the fewer middle-class jobs, the lower the total fertility rate. The hollowing out of economic opportunity accounts for at least some of the lowered fertility rate. A one percent increase in "goods-producing" jobs is associated with a 0.02 increase in TFR. But the TFR changed by more than 0.02 between 2006 and 2014. Seltzer could be correct, but something else may also be happening.

I love thinking.

I love Jonathan more. Especially when I'm not thinking. Like when I'm moaning and making monosyllabic grunts.

August 28, 2020: Yesterday, I was to have begun classes. In a normal world, I would be healthy. My kids would be out of the house—one at college, one starting her career.

But I shouldn't go there. It's far, far too painful.

So, I deal with what I have. Bones wracked with cancer. A daughter who couldn't write a paragraph to save her life. Another daughter who is so selfish and self-centered that she can't learn, she can't grow. No one can tell **her** what to do. That trait is fine, up to a point. When a person can't function in society, s/he needs to deal with reality and figure out what's going wrong.

Jenny has no respect for others, especially the ones trying to help her the most. She pushes us aside—both figuratively and literally. She's furious that she won't be able to live on her own. She's furious at us, because it is our fault that she can't live on her own. True, her current rages are directed solely at Jonathan and me. But we're the only people in her orbit right now. When she had other people in her orbit—at Drew, at St. E's, at the bank—who told her she needed to do something or she couldn't have something (a bank card), she went ballistic at them.

I look so forward to using my brain again. This morning, I need to focus on keeping Jenny calm so that Jonathan can teach. Yesterday, she blew up while Jonathan was on the phone with a student. He was able to take a break and call back the student. He can't do that to an entire class. [I was teaching remotely from my home computer.] So, I have to suck it up and keep Jenny calm. I can feel my cancer cells laughing with excitement at the stress this morning will bring. They are partying hardy at my increased levels of cortisol. Ugh.

August 29, 2020: Jenny was good yesterday, and I was much better able to concentrate. Reworking my HPV & fertility paper for *Demography* will be interesting. Seltzer makes a compelling case that the drop in fertility is associated with—oh, what's the term?—labor readjustment. No, that's not it. The United States has lowered its demand for goods-producing jobs (GPJ)—manufacturing, mining, construction. Blue-collar workers who used to be able to make a good living with those types of jobs now need to take lower-paying service jobs. So, they have fewer children. He regresses total fertility rates by metropolitan statistical area (MSA) on percentage of GPJs and other independent variables and finds a statistically significant relationship between MSA and GPJs.

However, Seltzer's model does not appear to explain the entire change in fertility. OK for white women, but only a small fraction of change for blacks, Asians, and Hispanics.

Also, Selzer's analysis does not explain the dramatic drop in teen pregnancy.

Internationally, we see birth rates falling in some countries, but not all.

So, something else seems to be going on. Make my case.

Seltzer's explanation and my explanation are not mutually exclusive. HPV vaccine covered under Vaccines for Children so even unemployed have access [...].

Also, I need to explore converting to Judaism. Converting would bring me even closer to Jonathan. [My initial response was, "Now this is going too far." And I wasn't entirely joking.]

August 30, 2020: Yesterday, we learned that Jenny may not receive her certificate [in school librarianship because her grades are low]. Jenny has known for about a week. Perhaps that is one reason she's been so volatile. Still, she's scary when she's volatile. And it shows that her volatility is not just a function of Jonathan making an off-hand remark that he "is the words person and Mom is the numbers person."

Jonathan and I did everything we could—in our own ways—to help Jenny lead a full, productive, and happy life. I with the biomedical interventions to get her body healthy; Jonathan with the education—first Drew, then St. Elizabeth's, then the librarian certificate. Neither of our strategies was successful.

SO WHAT? NOW WHAT? [This was the theme of the commencement speech delivered by professional footballer David Clowney when Jenny graduated from the College of St. Elizabeth. That is, when you run up against adversity, what is your Plan B?]

The "so what?" part Jonathan and I answer with our own work. So what? An entire generation has been poisoned. Some are less affected than others; a few escaped by not getting vaccinated. But for the most part, the entire population starting in 1988 has been poisoned.

But it's the "now what?" part that we have to deal with. I'll call Mike O'Brien [the son of our neighbor] today. He works for the Jewish Family Services in his area. I'll pick his brain. And we'll call the case manager at Division of Vocational and Rehabilitation Services.

Jonathan noted that it's odd that Flora is more employable than Jenny [...].

We watched *I Love You Again* with William Powell and Myrna Loy. It was cute. A fun-loving scoundrel develops amnesia and turns into a mousey penny-pincher. A knock on the head wakens him, and his wife likes the scoundrel more than the penny-pincher. The ending is precious. 1940. Escapism.

2020. Escapism sorely needed. The only truth I know is Jonathan.

August 31, 2020: Akeem's birthday. The young man who transported [me] from the MRI back to my room when I was in the hospital. Everyone— including Akeem—kept asking me my birthday, so I asked him his. August 31, 1996. I assured him he was more mature than my daughter born the same month in the same year.

She's never had a job, I thought. And if her rages continue, she never will.

When I say that to Jenny—*If your rages continue,* you will never have a job—she accuses me of not believing in her. That's why she's so messed up; I don't believe in her.

No, Jenny, you're messed up, because you were poisoned. Deliberately and methodically poisoned. I do hope the perpetrators of these crimes against humanity are brought to justice. Paul Offit, Bill Gates, Anthony Fauci, Francis Collins, the CEOs of Merck, GlaxoSmithKline and Astra-Zeneca [...].

With my time left on this earth, I will continue to shine light on their crimes. I will get the HPV & fertility paper republished as well as work with Josh on health outcomes of school mandates.

And I will continue to love and worship Jonathan. He is an amazing human being and an unbelievable best friend. How did I get so lucky?

September 1, 2020: First of the month and I paid the major bills [...]. Our AmEx bills are about $2,000 less per month than before the lockdown.

The lockdown, the riots, the vaccine-injured [...]. And Jonathan and I are some of the lucky ones. Our lives have touched by only one of three scourges. One is enough.

Already today is shaping up better than yesterday. This morning, I entered a kitchen that Flora did not heavily use. The dirty dishes suggest she had a couple of eggs last night. Unlike Sunday night, when she ate about 1½ pounds of meat. Jonathan was furious. Just at the end of his rope. Flora got upset at his yelling and threw a tantrum. She backed into the bookcase and it collapsed.

She's ok, and I guess learned her lesson about eating food she is not supposed to eat.

So, we have a jammed door thanks to Jenny's outburst and a collapsed bookcase thanks to Flora's tantrum.

Good news about Jenny's living arrangements. According to our ICM—intensive case manager—Jenny could live in an apartment complex where a supervisor is always on-call. The supervisor could check-up on Jenny once a day and also be there if Jenny flips out. But the person would not live with Jenny. Jenny might have a housemate. Jenny will probably thrive in such an environment. I need to call the Support Coordinators to see if they can help arrange such a situation. We also need to gather documentation of Jenny's violence (police records). We are an emergency case. There's hope for us all […].

I'm excited about converting to Judaism. The process will bring me closer to Jonathan. Should I reconsider B'nai Or [a Reform Temple]? Can I stomach their "How to be an antiracist" baloney? Or is the Conservative [synagogue] the better route? We might have to eat kosher. Ugh. This is a little more complicated than I can ponder right now.

Jonathan continues to be an angel.

September 2, 2020: Yesterday was pretty good. Flora didn't eat us out of house and home (unlike Monday). Jenny was on a pretty good keel until later at night. She got pissy when I bristled after Sean Hannity promoted the testing for the BRCA gene for breast cancer and the subsequent protocol of prophylactic double mastectomy. I can't think of anything dumber than a prophylactic double mastectomy. It's like the joke where an executive is having an affair with his secretary on the couch in his office. Get rid of the secretary! Is the first response. No, she's too good; we need her. Get rid of the executive! No, he's essential. Get rid of the couch!

Women with the BRCA gene are susceptible to cancer, which has a strong affinity for breast tissue. Take away the breast tissue, and—I assume, but, of course, I'm no doctor—the cancer will find other tissue to thrive.

I didn't argue with Jenny, though I wanted to. It's no use discussing my ideas with her, especially if she disagrees.

I started radiation on Monday. I'm not sure whether it is making me more tired or if I'm just more tired in general. But I am more tired. So, I take naps […].

Jonathan continues to be my saving grace. I do like our excursions—getting away from Jenny & Flora. At first, I was concerned we had to drive half an hour each way for the radiation […]. But I like spending time with just Jonathan. Ah, just Jonathan. So richly deserved by us both.

September 3, 2020: I've been complaining about Jenny a lot lately. It's time to focus on other things.

I wish I could express my love for Jonathan more physically. My body hurts; I feel so fragile; I'm afraid I'll break. But I love him so much.

September 4, 2020: Paperwork sent for Jenny's new living arrangements. We are an emergency case—partly thanks to my cancer, I assume. Let's hope things move quickly and well.

Flora returns on Sunday. I'm so out of it that she doesn't bother me much. Still, I know she creates tension for Jonathan and Jenny (although she is also Jenny's gravy train in that Jenny earns money by taking care of her). Also, I don't often feel a stress until it is lifted.

Stress is literally the air that we breathe, Jonathan and I. For a brief moment, we had it all. Right after we were married, we had everything. We had each other, we had great jobs, we had high hopes. I finally felt I was becoming a solid part of my extended family. Up to that point, I had always felt like an outsider. An accepted outsider, but not quite part of the family. Dad did his best to make me feel part of the family, but he himself was a bit of an outsider. Then I got married and started a family of my own. I could share pregnancy stories and baby stories. I could relate to my, uh, relatives.

Then autism ruined everything. I could no longer relate to the people with whom I share a last name. They pushed me and my family away […]. Family gatherings were a chore, and then they no longer occurred. Or at least we were no longer invited to them. No living member of my extended family gets it about the struggles my immediate family faces. And most—with the exception of Mom—don't bother to try. Mom tries, but still doesn't get it.

Enough bitching and moaning. They will never change […].

Jonathan was very touched by what I wrote about him yesterday. I'm a little surprised that he was so touched; that he didn't already know how much I want to take care of him physically. [Of course I knew, but to see it in writing was deeply affecting.] I don't tell him often enough how much I love him. The punctuation of the following sentence is obvious to me: A woman without her man, is nothing.

September 5, 2020: My brain feels as though it's going to mush. I'm so tired, lethargic. Ugh. I don't like this feeling. It could be the radiation. It could be Flora. It could be that my brain *is* going to mush.

Flora goes back to Camphill tomorrow. Yes! For everyone. Especially Flora. I have three-day hiatus from radiation. Hiatus. Good. I can remember multisyllabic words. Multisyllabic is also good.

And only five more radiation treatments for this round. I'm somewhat concerned about radiation to my throat area—so close to the brain. I'll ask questions. I'll be in the pain in the neck [...].

Our new door will cost over $2200. Twenty-two hundred dollars. Autism is expensive.

Dr. Stu has found a new product—stem cell patches. It sounds far-fetched, but who knows? I guess I never give up.

Jonathan continues to be wonderful. He laughs at the stupid jokes I read on *Babylon Bee*. The arrest of the Antifa guy who shot the Trump supporter in Portland? Mostly peaceful (the Antifa guy was shot dead). Why didn't Nancy Pelosi melt when they got water on her in the hair salon?

September 6, 2020: Flora goes back to Camphill today. The farm is a much better environment for her than our house. She thrives at the farm. Eats well, sleeps well, learns.

Last night, I tossed and turned about Jenny. She isn't doing her reading assignments. She doesn't know what her written assignment is. She doesn't seem to understand the importance of doing well in this class or she doesn't know how to do well in a class or both. She is more or less capable. But she bristles at reminders. Not just bristles, she becomes outright hostile.

If I were in the early days of this autism journey, I would try to find ways to convince Jenny to do her work. OK, I guess I didn't do that in the early days. When she didn't understand an assignment back then—I'm thinking of a French project in 7th grade—I yelled. But she didn't seem to get it back then either. Sometimes you have to do work just because. And you do your best. Or else you won't pass. Life has many tasks you do just because. You try to figure out a way to make those tasks enjoyable. If you can't find a way, you just do them and then reward yourself by doing tasks that are enjoyable.

I am reminded of when Simi told me she never had to help her twins with homework. They did it, and they did it well. When I think of the time and energy I've spent on both my children, yes, I feel a sense of resentment. I could have been a contender.

Contender for what? Why, if I could have spent my time focused on bank mergers—who knows?—I could be deputy chair of the Fed in Philadelphia by now. I'd certainly be a full professor. I'd be presenting research in at fine conferences and working with grad students on their research.

And what would it matter? I don't know. I'll never know. Like I'll never know what it's like to [...] watch a child grow into a fine young lady and then an independent woman. Those pleasures have been denied to me and Jonathan.

For what? For the profit of a few greedy bastards who don't give a damn about destroying people's lives. So, I must continue the fight. I have to get the word out […].

Life will get easier when Flora is back at Camphill. Jonathan will have to take care of only two demanding women instead of three. He says I'm easy. He's hardened by his upbringing—trying to please his mother and keeping his sister at bay. He's such a good person. He deserves all the good that is possible.

September 7, 2020: Flora is back at Camphill. When we dropped her off yesterday, she scampered up the steps to her house. No tears, no regrets. She seemed excited to be home.

My brain is working better already. I'm not going to water down my HPV & fertility paper, but rather *temper* it. "Watering down" and "tempering" might amount to the same thing, but I want to get the paper past the censors. Just like Vaclav Havel in Czechoslovakia. Get it past the pharma censors.

Jenny continues to be a pain in the ass. Yesterday in the car, I wanted Jonathan to slow down in front of a car, but all I could do was squeak. When I observed, "Sorry, I couldn't find the words," Jenny flew into a rage. "Be a *real* woman!" she demanded. To keep the calm, I sucked it up and felt my cancer cells just laughing in glee as they multiplied.

I talk with Dr. Johnson today about mistletoe. [Dr. Steven Johnson, an oncologist based in a Camphill community in Chatham, NY]. Can't wait! I am getting better—slowly—by the day. Walking better, not peeing at night (!), sleeping better. Ugh. I do hope my life does not revolve around the care and feeding of this bag of bones. My brain needs to function, too.

Jonathan continues to be a great support. Maybe someday—soon!—I can express my appreciation *physically!*

September 8, 2020: Mike O'Brien called and we talked about agencies that can help Jenny. When—after having talked with Mike for almost an hour and being very tired—I couldn't quickly find the words to relay the conversation, Jenny blew up. I wasn't a **real** woman, because I needed to grope for words. She wants me to stop taking the estrogen blocker. In other words, she wants me to die.

Then Jenny called Liz [the mother of Jenny's boyfriend Matt], who then spoke with me. Liz thinks Jenny has a mood disorder that might be remedied with prescription lithium. Whatever it takes. We'll ask Dr. Feingold.

If Dr. Feingold prescribes lithium, Jenny will still need to take it. Therein lies a great problem. She knows what's good for her, but she doesn't follow through with action. During her blow up last night, I suggested she drink some of the water with her "pissy pills" (pellets Lyn gave her). She snorted that she drank it all. So, instead of refilling it when she finished the bottle—or asking how to refill it—she allowed it to remain empty.

That's how Jenny and I are so different. If I have a problem, I do everything in my power to address and alleviate it. Working on a PhD was a struggle, but I faced the challenge head-on and succeeded. Publishing articles is a challenge, but I keep going. The girls have autism, but I keep searching for ways to heal them. Even today, I'm talking with Dr. Stu about patches. Who knows? Maybe it will help.

After a drink or two, Jenny was so lovey-dovey. It's just so hard to respond to someone who scares me.

Jonathan remains rock solid. He was about to commit Jenny last night, but now looks forward to taking her to see Dr. Feingold. As soon as possible. I'll make the appointment today. Jonathan has had much more experience with neurotic women than I. I can learn from him. Like so many things, I can learn from him.

I'll also contact the B'nai Or rabbi today.

September 9, 2020: Yesterday, I drafted an email to Rabbi Satz [of Temple B'nai Or] inquiring about converting […]. This is a nice adventure.

Jonathan continues to be an angel. This morning, he had his hands on me (again!). "I love touching you," he whispered. It reminds me of when we were in the used bookstore in the town across the river from New Hope […] and he slipped his hand into mine and whispered, "I love holding your hand." That's when I knew I was going to say yes.

September 10, 2020: Jonathan said he got a hard-on when I mentioned one of the reasons I wanted to convert was to get closer to him. He's so adorable! […]

Jenny's been good lately. ***That's*** the real Jenny.

September 11, 2020: 9-11. Nineteen years ago, I thought the worst travesty ever had hit the United States. Five years later, I learned that the worst travesty ever was an internal blow—the National Childhood Vaccine Injury Act. In both cases, the elite showed how little they care.

Flora was a baby, and still healthy. We bought the CD of patriotic songs, and Flora stood up in her crib and belted out, "God bless America!"

I still have hope that we can recover more of her. She's not obsessing as much about, for example, the clogs that need repair. She ***is*** obsessing about when we will pick her up. Maybe the patches will help; maybe the homeopathy will help.

[…]. Jenny's so good lately, perhaps because she is taking her pills. Maybe the patches will help her be even more better. Homeopathy seems to help […].

Jonathan was very tired yesterday. I wonder **why?** He's better this morning. I look forward to helping him release tension [...] Lately, my stirrings have been increasing.

September 12, 2020: Nothing much going on [...]. These are quiet moments, full of quiet potential.

These are also the moments I am able to share more fully with Jonathan. Not rushing around. Just quiet, peaceful moments. They are the best moments.

September 13, 2020: We watched *Back to the Future* last night. Absolutely adorable! [...]

Jonathan remains healthy. He was on the verge of illness on Thursday, but overcame it. There's nothing we can't lick!

September 14, 2020: Lately, Jenny has been wonderful. She wants to learn to cook, and Jonathan is patiently obliging. Maybe the thought of getting free is enough to keep her in equilibrium. Also motivating her to learn to cook. Still, we should check for mood disorders [...].

I need projects to keep me happy. I don't think I'm unique. The idea of guaranteed income is insane. People need work, a purpose, a reason to bitch.

One reason **not** to bitch: Jonathan. He is everything good and right in my life. Yesterday, he put together his bookshelf (to replace the one Flora slammed into during one of her few tantrums; it was a piece of shit anyway and Flora did not hurt herself). When the two pieces didn't stack properly, I recommended placing the bottom piece on top. My suggestion worked! I like being able to help Jonathan. He does so much for me.

September 15, 2020: First, a thought of thanks to Jonathan. When the surgeon's statement reflecting a charge of $300,000 arrived, Jonathan said (without hesitation) I was worth $300,000. Wow. I didn't marry Doug. [That morning she sent me a dirty email with a photo of a radiantly naked beauty from *Women's Health* magazine, and wrote the caption: "It's wonderful, feeling healthy again!"]

September 16, 2020: Another awful day with Jenny yesterday. She was rude and infantile when we met with [the director of a group home]. She pulled out her cell phone even after Jonathan told her to put it away. She chewed on her mask and put her hand to her throat several times.

Quite frankly, she's not a good candidate for The Group Home [the fictitious name of a local group home]. Her screaming and rantings would be enough to cause grave concern. If she were to be violent there, it would be all over [...].

We always thought a change in environment would help Jenny to grow. Live on campus, get away from her parents, become more independent. It didn't work at Drew. It worked somewhat at St. E's, but she still had rantings. And she was only there for four months.

Four months. That's the length of the break Jonathan and I have had since the girls were born. Even then, I had to field calls and concerns from Lisa [the Disability Coordinator at the College of St. Elizabeth].

Back to the present. I thought Jenny could step up to the plate and understand that I am very fragile and sick. But instead, she attacks. Touching my head, pinching my foot, wanting a "hug." And the screaming and ranting.

No wonder my cancer cells are just living it up. With Jenny creating unbelievable stress, my cancer cells are partying all day and night.

You'd think she'd rise to the occasion. That she would maturely understand that I need rest, peace, and quiet to heal. You'd be wrong.

She needs to leave.

Jonathan teaches three classes today. I need to suck it up and keep Jenny as calm as possible.

Jonathan keeps saying he wanted to give me a happy family and he is so sad that he didn't. I have him. That's **ALL** I have, but he's enough. He's more than enough. Dayanu!

September 17, 2020: After a rough morning yesterday, Jenny is back to her sweet self. Still somewhat immature, but at least sweet. In her good moments, she's stuck at 14. She wants independence, but no responsibility [...].

But my back is feeling better and my ribs. I can even rest on my left side; until recently sleeping on my left side was irritating due to the cracked ribs.

I'll call Suzanne this Sunday. She's always calling us; it's my turn this time [...].

And, as always, give thanks to Jonathan [...] for being Jonathan.

September 18, 2020: Ugh. Dr. Levitz is pushing Ibrance. I thought he was ok with my "waiting." He's saying in his experience it prolongs disease-free progression. He's had some people on it for five years, some for two years. The FDA approved the drug in 2015, so if he has had a patient on it for five years, he jumped on the bandwagon when Ibrance first emerged.

I trust Dr. Levitz in that I believe he is sincere. He sincerely wants me to live the longest, most happy life possible. He is convinced Ibrance can help me. However, he signed on to the drug early on; it is very difficult to say, "Oops. I was wrong. This drug isn't really prolonging life or preventing cancer progression." It's very difficult for him to admit that, both professionally—all his colleagues say what a wonderful drug this is—and personally.

I've seen it myself with the protocols I've tried for the girls. I couldn't fathom that a protocol—GFCF diet, the listening programs, any number of drugs [...] suggested for the girls—didn't help. Sometimes the interventions made them worse. But I couldn't see that. Since my ***only*** motive is to get my girls well, it's easier for me to admit a treatment isn't working than anyone else. Even I had difficulty admitting the time and effort (and money!) I spent on a protocol was making them worse.

So, I recognize Dr. Levitz's conflict of interest. But Ibrance could still be good for me. However, there are risks to the medication. White blood cell counts go down, which could increase the likelihood of infection. Dr. Levitz says the WBC is just a number and that none of his 50 patients have experienced major infections. I saw that video, too. The video where the guy trying to sell the drug says "WBC is just a number." He was obviously a stooge for Pfizer, noting only the good side of the drug.

Other common side effects include nausea, something that sounds similar to leukemia, loss of appetite, vomiting. Delightful! And I would have to suspend turmeric. Also, a large percentage of women in one of the studies stopped taking the drug due to side effects. Even the FDA—one of the most captured industries in the Swamp—admits that there are "rare, but serious lung infections" that appear to be affecting women who take Ibrance. Just like the "rare, but serious side effects" from the HPV vaccine.

And for what? Studies ***sponsored by Pfizer*** couldn't find a statistically significant difference between those who took the drug and those who didn't in terms of disease-free progression or life expectancy. What?? Not even studies sponsored by Pfizer could find solid evidence of improvement. Those who took the drug had disease-free progression of seven months longer than those who didn't but the result was not stat sig. Life expectancy was similar. "But life expectancy wasn't the goal," pointed out Pfizer's marketing guy. Oh.

And the people in the study have all kinds of metastatic cancer, most of them visceral. I'm assuming non-visceral is bone cancer. How does the drug help people with bone cancer?

I think I'll play the Covid card for as long as I can. Covid—and now the flu!—are out there. I don't want to lower my immune system. Which is true, actually [...].

Jonathan is very concerned about this whole Ibrance thing. He loves me and wants me around as long and as healthy as possible. Me, too.

September 19, 2020: Yesterday was eventful. Ruth Bader Ginsberg died, throwing a chaotic election into more chaos [...].

I'm feeling better. I can roll on my right side with no rib pain! [...]

Best news from this morning: Jonathan and I can cuddle again. Dayenu!

September 20, 2020: [...]. People are threatening to burn down Congress if there is a vote for new Supreme Court justice. Does at least a majority of Americans see what Looney Tunes these people are? I hope so [...].

Having a date with Jonathan yesterday was so much fun! We picked up sandwiches and green beans prepared with garlic (fresh!) and parmesan cheese at a deli and enjoyed them at a picnic table. The weather was gorgeous: there was a slight nip in the autumn air, and the sun shone through the leaves. Those are some of the most real moments in life.

September 21, 2020: Jenny pissy again yesterday during dinner. We can't have a regular conversation without worrying she will blow up [...].

My neck brace is beginning to be, well, a pain in the neck. I can wear the other, less intrusive brace either during the day or during the night (I forget which) [...].

I stayed in bed until 7 am this morning. Normally, I get up at 6:30 to have a few moments to myself. Anyway, it was fun bantering with Jonathan. I threatened to take advantage of him in his semi-somnolescent state. Except I couldn't quite pronounce "somnolescent" being myself also in that state. Jonathan understood what I meant and said "please do"

September 22, 2020: Damn! Upper left groin hurts like heck. Not like hell, but like heck. Last night, during our walk, it hurt like hell. My recovery was supposed to be linear! Each day, I was supposed to get better and better [...].

Interesting conversation among Lyn, Jenny, and me. Mainly between Jenny and Lyn [...]. Jenny said Jonathan was gay, because I'm so masculine.

Jonathan continues to be an absolute sweetheart. He's very concerned about my new ache. He was brilliant yesterday when he gave his lecture to the English-Speaking Union [in Florida via Zoom] [...]. The people in Florida are praying for me. They are so nice.

How did I get so lucky to find my soulmate?

September 23, 2020: Happy birthday to me, happy birthday to me!

Mom sent me a card, but I think I accidentally threw it out. Rats! See, this is what happens when I take chemo!

For the past several days, I've been taking 40 mg of melatonin. Finally, I remember my dream from last night. I was walking through people's homes, just the front parts, to get to my home. Along the way, I was collecting information about the health of the children living in the home. One family, a very large, multi-generational family, asked me what I was doing. I tried to explain, but I had difficulty describing the information I was collecting. So, I winged it. They were absolutely fine with my explanation. When I first saw them, they were disheveled because they had just gotten up. Later, they were much more presentable […].

OK, Dr. Freud. So, I'm working on this project with Josh, looking at health outcomes of children by state. One independent variable is the number of vaccine mandates. So, maybe I couldn't explain what I was doing in the dream, because I didn't want to explain. Or maybe I just had trouble explaining difficult concepts, and I should take a Dale Carnegie course, as Scott Adams suggests. But the family was ok with what I was doing. Who wouldn't want to know about the health of their children? […]

Jenny screamed once last night and banged her bed against the wall a few times. I screamed at her to get the "happy water." When will she learn that screaming is not ok? That banging her bed is destructive? Of course, if I call her out on it, she'll scream more.

After telling Lyn that I am not a warm or nurturing mother on Monday evening, Jenny on Tuesday morning asked, "Are we friends?" I answered unemotionally, "Yes, but what you said really hurt." Jenny seemed pleased with herself. How sick.

Jonathan cut short his shower when he heard me scream. I feel bad about that. He does so much for me, for us.

September 24, 2020: Nothing much new. I'm twisting and turning more in bed; I can even sleep on my side for a while!

Police called yesterday about Jenny. Someone saw her chewing on her phone and seeming disoriented. A concerned citizen. Thank you, concerned citizen. I do appreciate your looking after my daughter. She needs looking after. I wish she didn't, but she does.

Jenny interrupted my writing.

I love Jonathan.

September 25, 2020: Three months to Christmas. Oh, joy.

Last night, I didn't sleep well. Having Jenny here is so nagging. Either she's interrupting with stupid stuff or she's enraged. For me to heal, she needs to go.

But I'll still have to take care of her supplements and her doctors' visits and DVRS and housing not to mention miscellaneous tricks to help her—e.g. chewing gum instead of chewing clothes. And I'll still get the phone calls. In the past, the calls were from the school […]. Now they are from […] the police. I'm so tired of the phone calls. **When** is Jenny going to grow up?

And she's so mean to me. How much longer am I supposed to take this?

I'm so tired. My body aches and my brain is mushy. I'm not half-dead, but I'm only half-alive. My sex drive is low. It could just be the achiness or it could be a side effect from the arimidex.

So what? Now what? Wise words. I'm in the process of organizing my desk area. Slowly, but surely. I'll do that while Jonathan teaches. I learn so much when he teaches.

What if the guy from DVRS doesn't ever call back? We keep calling (ugh). What if Jenny never grows up? Too overwhelming to contemplate.

I love Jonathan so much. He keeps me going, but I hate being such a burden. PS I just had a massive bowel movement, and I feel better. But that's what it's all boiling down to. I've been fighting for health for the past 20 years. First for my kids—and I failed—and now for me.

September 26, 2020: Jenny read my musings yesterday, even after I told her not to. Now she knows what I think, but I sense she knew most of the stuff already. I need to heal. She needs to live (semi) on her own. We all want that. Stress for all of us will be eased […].

Jonathan & I had a nice quiet dinner last night while Jenny & Matt had fun in Morristown. I'm glad they have each other; I hope they can both grow to enjoy life to its fullest. Matt has such an amazing flair for clothes. He needs to work in that area; he would be phenomenal.

Jonathan and I have found professions we love. And each other. Who could ask for more? Well, healthy kids, but we're working on that.

September 27, 2020: Judge Amy Coney Barrett has seven children, and she is able to have a profession. I have two children, and I can't even make it to full professor. Yeah, I could have been a contender. Thanks, Pfizer; thanks, Merck.

Jenny screamed last night while we were watching *Cast a Dark Shadow*. I turned my head quickly. Fortunately, I had on my neck brace, so I'm not paralyzed.

September 28, 2020: Dare I write? Jenny might, as she did yesterday, read my musings and explode. Then all day she was on an emotional roller coaster. Twice during the day she exploded, once after reading my musing and once at dinner. Jonathan reported she also went berserk in the grocery store; people stared. Then the screaming at night and the banging of the bed. With no comprehension of how her behavior is so odd.

We are held hostage by Jenny's mood swings. She's so right—she can't live here anymore. But where can she live?

Our children are both monsters. Born of us, but not us. They are possessed. And I can't help them. God knows I've tried.

I would not be able to survive without Jonathan.

September 29, 2020: On Sunday, I wrote that the reason I'm not a full professor is that I needed to tend to the girls. That's not completely correct. The main reason I'm not a full professor is that I changed course in my research […]. And that's fine with me. Just *fine*. No, really. The research I'm doing now is so much more important than bank mergers. And people—for better or worse—actually read the research I'm now doing. Except the paper on the decrease in vaccine safety that deserves more credit than it is getting. The papers on HPV & fertility as well as on the HPV vaccine & increased HPVs are vital. Deirdre Little emailed me that some people owe their existence to my research. Now *that's* important research.

Amy Coney Barrett learned that adoption had gone through on the same day that she found out "Jessica was on her way." (Notice she doesn't say, "I was pregnant.") She took a walk and ended in a graveyard. "Life is difficult," she thought. "But at least it's short." Now *that's* inspiring. "And what is more important than raising children" […]

Jonathan and I agree there is nothing more important than raising children. For us, the experience has been very different from most people's journeys. We didn't have the joy of watching our children grow, because they didn't. And yet we are a family. We love and care about each other. It is tragic that Flora will never experience raising children. If we can free Jenny of her demons, she might be able to raise children, but that's an if.

The journey of raising children has brought Jonathan & I closer (though we would have been fine—just *fine*—without autism). He is an incredible husband, father, and human being.

October 1, 2020: Jenny's been great lately. Glutathione patches? She's coming up with clever ideas […].

Jonathan continues to be an angel. Unfortunately, that's all we can do these days. I so look forward to bringing out the devil in him!

October 2, 2020: Yesterday, October 1, I spoke with the rabbi. Converting to Judaiasm, er Judiaiism involves learning how to spell "Judaism" which I consistently misspell. Thank God (ha, ha) for spellcheck. Some formal study, some one-on-one conversations with the rabbi, a comprehensive exam in front of three rabbis and a mikvah. But I'm postmenopausal, I wanted to tell Rabbi Satz. But I didn't. We'll figure out whether I need a mikvah as we proceed.

We also saw Dr. Levitz yesterday. He keeps pushing Ibrance, and I keep telling him no, because I'm concerned about side effects. He keeps saying a low white blood count doesn't matter, and I keep wondering how it could not matter. Even the package insert says that infection was more likely in the test group taking Ibrance than the control group. Ugh. Then I blurted out the girls' autism came from vaccines. Jonathan was taken aback. OK, OK. I won't dwell on it, but now Dr. Levitz knows where I am coming from. I don't trust pharmaceutical companies. They are willing to poison babies. How can one possibly think that they are truthful about medications for cancer patients? Pharmaceutical companies lie to regulators; they lie to doctors. Doctors then unwittingly pass on incorrect or incomplete information to patients. And the patient is the one that lives with the consequences. Every day.

I'm sure Dr. Levitz is sincere in his hopes that I take Ibrance; he truly believes it will prolong my healthy life, the time I have before I need to go on chemo. He started prescribing Ibrance when it first appeared five years ago, and it would be very difficult for him to admit that he made a mistake.

Interestingly, at the beginning of our discussion, we all agreed that pharmaceutical companies might be cutting corners in the development of the Covid vaccine. What prevents them from cutting corners for other vaccines? Regulators? But government agencies regulate the Covid vaccine. So regulators do a perfect job with all medications except the Covid vaccine?

Dr. Levitz asked what other treatments I was using to address my cancer. I mentioned mistletoe, supplements, diet. I look forward to doing coffee enemas again, but currently I don't bend well enough to do so. As soon as I can do coffee enemas again, I'll restart pancreatic enzymes. I forgot to mention homeopathy, and I purposely did not mention the patches […].

So, I'll close with a word of thanks, as always, to Jonathan. He would not have mentioned the vaccine-autism link to Dr. Levitz, but he did not chastise me for doing so. Jonathan seems positively delighted that I'm converting to Judaism. (NB: I spelled it correctly *on the first try*.) I'm happy he's delighted.

October 3, 2020: I spent yesterday morning looking at cancer sites. Kinda depressing. They all say Stage IV is really serious. But I don't feel horribly sick. When I heard that any cancer that has metastasized is considered Stage IV, I remember thinking that was one of the dumbest things I had ever heard. There's a huge difference between bone mets and pancreatic cancer. But nobody asked me. I'm just a patient.

So, I'll stop wasting time reading depressing stuff. At least for now […].

Jenny got a little pissy yesterday at the dinner table when I struggled for words to describe *On Becoming a Jew*. I became a little agitated and calmly explained that I need peace & quiet or my cancer will get worse. Jenny got herself another drink, and she was fine. A true DeLong woman!

Jonathan and I are able to cuddle more. Last night, while watching television; also in bed. It's so wonderful to cuddle. I missed it more than I knew.

October 4, 2020: I finally figured it out. I did everything correct concerning the physical aspects of cancer—the diet, the supplements, the coffee enemas. I threw in HBOT and sauna for good measure. The vital piece missing is the emotional healing. I'm very angry and I'm very sad. So much has been denied my children; so much has been denied my husband; and so much has been denied me. I hate the people who did this to us. The people who ruined Flora's life, took a large chunk of Jenny's, and created a permanent hole in my soul.

But I need to heal emotionally in order to live. I have Jonathan and he has me.

Jenny seems to be learning. This morning, she played her Sunday morning "acoustic sunrise," but did not blare it as in Sundays past. That's progress! She couldn't find her glutathione patches, which seem to help, and she panicked. She eventually did find them, and, I think, felt proud to have done so. That's some progress. She still doesn't seem to know what's important and what isn't. She throws out important things while hoarding junk.

We watched *H.M. Pulham, Esq.* with Robert Young last night. The film is about the unfulfilled lives that WASPs lead. The ending was happy—as I suppose films about WASPs need to be—if a bit rushed and not quite believable.

But what of the undeniable sorrow in our lives, Jonathan's, Jenny's, Flora's & mine? How do we resolve it?

Now that I've figured out the missing piece, I have to figure out how to address it. Jonathan will help—he already is—but he has his own private hell. A hell we share.

October 5, 2020: I know what my dreams are—health, for me, for my children; continued health for Jonathan. And happiness for all of us. There are a few people outside my immediate orbit for whom I also wish health and happiness [...]. But the most important people are the ones closest to me.

But first a word of praise for Jonathan. Did I ever mention the raunchy emails he sends me ***every day***? He's amazing.

October 6, 2020: Nice conversation with Dr. Johnson last night. I am reacting to the mistletoe BIG TIME [...].

Jenny continues to be very good. A couple of hiccups, but no fierce blow ups. Yeah!

Jonathan continues to be amazing. Yesterday, he taught two classes, drove Jenny and me to see Dr. Feingold, fought with [a colleague] over some of [her] stupid ideas, drove Jenny to and from her yoga class, and remained a perfect angel (except when he was zooming with his department). A true mensch.

October 7, 2020: [...]. I'm working on my HPV vaccine & fertility paper. Polishing the paper for *Environmental Research*. Why? I'm not sure it will ever be republished. And if it is, it may be pulled again. Jonathan says I'm doing it for Humanity. What has Humanity ever done for me?

Jenny is up and down again. It really is like living with a drug addict. Her violent moods, her stealing of money. I cleared my throat, and she screamed I wasn't being a "real woman." I gave her $40 for her haircut, telling her I wanted the change. She lied that Nino [her hairdresser] had increased the price to $30 and she gave him a $10 tip.

And she has no concept of how much her behavior negatively affects both Jonathan and me. I have metastatic breast cancer; Jonathan has high blood pressure. She's killing us. Her autism is killing us.

Jonathan is getting his blood pressure checked into […]. I'm glad he's going to see Dr. Weiss. When Tina confirmed his appointment yesterday, she suggested I consider CBD. We'll see. I get loopy on CBD ("And what is the problem?" asks Jonathan.)

I'm loopy in love with Jonathan.

October 8, 2020: […]. Jenny blew up at my flannel shirt yesterday. I locked *myself* in my room, and she calmed down […]. Jenny needs to be more appreciative. I overheard her saying to the person who drives her to Writers' Group, "Are you picking me up tonight?" A little more gratitude will go a long way.

Jonathan continues to be a saint. He's steady and calm. And a great lay, which we will do again sometime, I'm sure.

October 9, 2020: I wonder what great and wonderful things will happen today. While lying in bed this morning, that's the thought I had. My second thought was, woah! where did *that* come from? From Dad, where else? […]

I so cherish my early morning moments. Quiet. Alone. Not for ever, not for long. But a few, very quiet moments. To collect my thoughts.

A bone mass is accumulating on my chest, I think the result of the neck brace. So, I switched the "daisy" neck brace—the yellow dot in the middle makes the apparatus look like a yellow flower with petals—for the oatmeal cloth neck brace. The new brace is less confining, but also less supportive. Oh, what to do?!?

I slept well, so today I'm raring to go. I'll polish up the HPV vaccine & fertility paper; maybe even send it off […].

This morning, after my 6:30 am alarm went off, I rolled over and cuddled with Jonathan until his 7 am alarm sounded. Ah, bliss!

October 10, 2020: […]. Jenny's been good. Continued messing around with candle after Jonathan told her to stop. Candle then broke. Natural consequences. She apologized, but didn't get all pissy and blame us. That's progress.

Jonathan […] [is] helping with the Amish project […]. I very much respect him and his ideas […] not to mention his great bod!

October 11, 2020: "Good morning, Mom!" Jenny greeted me. No, no; Jenny, I just need a few moments of silence when I first get up. The pitter patter of little feet used to be a joy; now it's a drudgery. And it's not exactly a pitter patter; more of a clump clump clump.

And we never really had the joy of the pitter patter. Oh, no. The kids are up. I need to get them their supplements on an empty stomach. And then keep them away from food, which I need to prepare because they are on a special diet. Sometimes, a super special diet.

No, the good old days were awful. The pictures of the kids are cute, but life with two young children with autism was not easy or fun. Now life with two older children with autism is neither easy nor fun.

Fortunately, we found a place for Flora. For now. But she ages out soon. What then? […]

And then there's Jenny. We need to find a place for her that is NOT with us. Soon. It has to be soon.

And the bastards who did this to our children live in mansions and look down on the "little people." Those bastards are evil.

Jonathan was a wonderful chauffeur on our trip to see Flora yesterday. He complimented my coffee! I'm so glad I can make him happy.

October 16, 2020: Wake up America! The coronavirus is way overblown. Dana Freed [a neighbor] talking about how college students—***college students,*** the ones who are ***least*** susceptible to *anything*—need to sign up to use the shower and the commode. Imagine that, timing your bowels so that your urges match your allotted schedule! INSANE.

And yesterday, Jenny fell apart again under the strain. We learned that one of the possibilities for Flora is $8,000 a month, which we do not have. When Jenny got upset and I suggested to her that the best thing she could do to help would be to take care of herself, she utterly freaked out. She bopped me on the head and then punched me on the arm before I could escape to my room. Apparently, she took some swings at Jonathan and then hit herself and banged her head against the powder room door.

October 17, 2020: Seven months since the lockdown began. St. Patrick's Day (actually, a few days before, but St. Pat's Day is easy to remember) […].

Jenny becomes very agitated whenever I work on Flora's permanent placement. Yesterday, when I was on the phone with a possible home, I could hear Jenny hitting herself. ***That's not helping!*** She did get her period, but ***that's no excuse***. Yes, it's stressful. *Life* is stressful. The thing with kids—unlike any other relationship—is that you can't move on. You can't say, "It's over between us!" and start a new life.

That goes for Jenny and Flora. I think that's what my family doesn't understand. They don't understand—they can't understand—the heartache and the fear Jonathan & I live with constantly. The sad part for him and me is that my family doesn't even try. It's too much work; it's too sad. So they ignore the problems we're dealing with; they blame us for not "letting go." As though it is possible to "let go" of your kids. Maybe they could have done that—maybe they already do. I can't. Jonathan can't. And that's why the girls are so fortunate to have us as parents. I hate to be one of *those* parents, but, damn, I wish they would appreciate what we've done, what we're trying to do. Especially Jenny. A little appreciation would make all the work we're doing easier. And, of course, not getting literally beaten up [...].

I forgot to send Jonathan a raunchy email yesterday. Everything he does for me, the least I can do is send him a raunchy email. He sends me one *every day.* What a guy!

October 18, 2020: Last night, I had trouble sleeping [...]. Jenny [lied] to us about going to an event this morning [...]. She's going to be upset when we ask her about it. I hope she doesn't hurt me.

And Jonathan. Sweet, wonderful Jonathan. All we have is each other, and that's enough. Dayenu!

October 19, 2020: The [Introduction to Judaism] class is rather boring, but it's fun with Jonathan. The instructor appears young and relatively new. Judaism is a *family*, a very large, **dysfunctional family**. But they also wanted to know our pronouns ☹ and how to make the learning environment a "safe space." To the first inquiry, I wanted to respond "I/me/mine" and to the second, "I want an *unsafe* space; an environment that challenges me and my preconceived thoughts and biases." One woman brought up politics. Uh, oh. ***Don't go there*** unless you are prepared to hear what ***I really think!*** [...]

Jonathan is so incredibly dear. We voted on Saturday and bought a toaster oven on Sunday. These small, domestic chores are so much fun with him. We'll hang pictures soon. He hangs so well (as in, yes, he is well-hung).

October 20, 2020: Ruth [Jonathan's mother] would have been 98 today. I'm glad we were friends in the end.

Corruption—what country do you think of? China, India, Burkina Faso? No, folks. Right here in River City. The millions the Biden family amassed over the lives of U.S. citizens. Promoting China's entry into the World Trade Organization costs millions of American jobs. Allowing China to become more assertive in the China Sea gave China a sense the United States would do nothing to curb China's aggression. Being instrumental in the firing of a Ukrainian prosecutor allowed Ukraine to become more corrupt.

[…]. The information on Hunter Biden's laptop is not the main story. The manner in which Big Tech and the media responded is terrifying. Twitter blocked the laptop story. Facebook did something also to downplay the story. The sole reporter who attempted to ask a question was mocked and ridiculed.

We in the vaccine hesitancy community know the tactics. First they ignore you […]. But eventually you win […].

The only people remaining are the voters. The workers. The people who care about their families […].

Jonathan continues to be my everything. Actually, my only thing. He's the only thing in my life that makes sense.

October 21, 2020: The Biden Family corruption scandal is disgusting. The lack of coverage in the lamestream media is even worse. The *Wall Street Journal* is so disappointing. Not a peep. Of course, *WSJ* doesn't cover our story—and the few times it does, it is horribly biased—so I should be used to it. Still, I expected more.

I did read some great jokes. The Barrett Family recently adopted a new troubled youth named Hunter […]. The best place to practice social distancing is a Biden rally […] Joe Biden is promising to anyone who votes for him a seat on the Supreme Court […].

Jonathan continues to be my everything. It's fun teaching him Judaic minutia. On Sabbath, you light the candles first and then say the prayer since after you say the prayer Sabbath has begun. Normally, you say the prayer first and then do the action, but you're not supposed to do work on the Sabbath. So, you light the candles first, *close your eyes*, then say the prayer Leonard Nemoy was Jewish, right?

October 22, 2020: So nice this morning lying in Jonathan's arms. He has this wonderful masculine aroma that is so comforting. So protective, like nothing can hurt me when I'm in his arms.

October 23, 2020: […]. Lying in Jonathan's arms this very early morning. He is all that is true and real and pure. Except when he's dirty; then he's impure. ☺

October 24, 2020: […]. Jonathan & I were so cute yesterday at the ophthalmologist. Kissing through our masks. Love in the age of covid. Love in the age of anything.

October 25, 2020: […]. Jenny & I watched *Madea's Big Happy Family* about a woman trying to get her family together to tell them she is dying of cancer. Squabbles ensue; hidden secrets are revealed. It was heavier than the other Madea films I've seen; it had great messages. Be thankful for the days on this earth and the ones I have remaining. I can do that, even if I don't necessarily believe in God. Forgive others for my sake, not theirs. (I'm not there yet with Dave and his family.) Sit up straight, show respect, take responsibility. Amen [...].

I have to go. The family is having breakfast, and I have not yet read the raunchy email that Jonathan me *every day*. What a guy!

October 26, 2020: Jenny went on a hike yesterday. Jonathan is getting tired of driving her everywhere. Lyn is right—we need to plan out driving requests at the beginning of the week. Perhaps on Saturdays.

Our "Introduction to Judaism" course is going slowly. Jonathan is beside himself in how boring the instructor is making such a lively subject. Just like Prof. Weaver [one of Gayle's teachers at American University] saying it is so difficult to make economics boring, but some people work really hard at it [...] and succeed! It's fun taking the course with Jonathan. No one with whom I'd rather take it.

October 27, 2020: Radiation to my neck started yesterday. One treatment down; nine to go. People amazingly nice [...].

It looks as though we may have to pay $2,000 for the anesthesia I received during my surgery. Bummer [...]. See, both New York and New Jersey have very strong "surprise bill" laws, but only for the insurance plans and hospitals in their respective states. If, like me, you have an insurance plan issued in one state (NY) and a hospital in another state (NJ), you're screwed.

Speaking of being screwed, Jonathan & I haven't in almost—what is it?— four months. Yikes! I'm glad we can be physically close; we couldn't even do that for two months. He's so patient as I mend.

October 28, 2020: Jenny & I seem to be entering a new phase. She seems more in control, and I am more accepting of her limitations. Thank you, Lyn!

Radiation treatments continue. Two down; eight to go. I could feel the vibration on my neck this time [...]. Jonathan & I kissed through our masks yesterday at St. Barnabas Hospital before I went into the treatment room. The woman who greets us and takes our temperature (to confirm we don't have Covid ☹) smiled. I confirmed, "Love in the age of covid!"

October 29, 2020: Radiation treatments continue. They put a mask on me so I don't move my head. I feel as though I'm in an Edgar Allen Poe novel, except that I am able to breathe [...]. The people [...] are very patient-oriented. They tell me what they are doing and try to make me as comfortable as possible [...].

It's so odd that everyone except doctors in the medical field are supposed to make the patient as comfortable as possible. Many—not all—doctors are so arrogant and condescending. Male doctors especially. Though the Bitch on Wheels […] from Sloan Kettering was female. I think […].

I think if I were a doctor, I would be so humbled by my knowledge and my abilities. We know so much about the human body and yet we know so little. Why do some treatments work for some people, but make other people worse? How can we decide who should get what? Why is it our tests tell us a treatment should work for a person, but it doesn't? Or it works for a while and then stops?

It's possible that humans are not machines. That so many variables are involved with whether a treatment works that generalizations are nearly impossible. That's why patients must be involved. And that's why doctors hate patients—like me—who ask too many questions. Some doctors, not all. Mainly male doctors. Yes, I *do* want to be sexist about it.

Yesterday was Jonathan's long day—three classes. He's so easygoing while he's teaching, but exhausted afterwards. He gives everything his all. Including me.

October 30, 2020: Fifth radiation treatment to my neck today. Amazing, the stuff I'm doing that I never thought I would do. Radiation, pharmaceuticals […] are conventional treatments I never thought I would do […] or need.

I do wish people in the conventional world […] would let me know how I'm doing compared to other patients. Am I bouncing back better than most? I sense I am. Yesterday, Dr. Wagman asked about my energy level and seemed surprised when I reported that I'm bouncing back. Maybe my vitamins help?

I still feel some soreness—not pain really, just soreness—in my upper left arm and a quarter way down my spine. As though I've just completed a 10-mile bike ride, but I haven't. I guess I'll always be a little nervous that any ache or pain portends something worse. But I need to live. Or else I die. And I refuse to die while I am living.

Dr. Wagman and I got into a conversation about masks. She [said] emphatically; masks are unequivocally good. I shrugged that I haven't seen any studies confirming that masks are useful. Oh, but they are. Oh, ok, I replied, not wanting to get someone who aims a radiation beam at my throat to be pissed off at me. For example, she persisted, one study found teachers can transmit the disease by speaking to a class. Maybe my facial expression of doubt betrayed my words; I did my best to convey it's ok. We disagree, but it doesn't matter for my radiation treatments; in fact, let's drop it. She persisted a bit longer, and then dropped it. Whew. I don't think she changed my protocol to instruct the technologists to aim the beam at my head to knock some sense into me. But you never know […].

It was so great cuddling with Jonathan this morning. Quarter to seven, raining outside. No place I'd rather be than in his arms.

October 31, 2020: Hope for the best; prepare for the worst. Stay busy. That's my mantra these days [...]. But I'm afraid to have hope. That's sad, isn't it? So often with the girls, I had hope. This therapy will work; a new location with help Flora to blossom.

But the hope was shattered. And that is so painful. Now we're in the process of finding living arrangements for Flora. A humane setting where she can feel comfortable. As though she is a patient in a hospital. Which in some senses she is.

Regardless of the outcome of the election, Flora won't be getting better [...]. And the stats from Belfast. One in 15 boys [diagnosed with autism]. Dear God. How did this happen? Is man so greedy?

Hope for the best; prepare for the worst. Stay busy.

Jonathan is also feeling sad, numb, helpless. We're propping each other up. That's what we need to do in times like these.

November 1, 2020: I slept *very* late this morning, even though we just got off of Daylight Savings Time. Jonathan pointed out that my body is repairing itself. Go, body!

I'm writing a tribute to my father, lessons I learned from him. The exercise is quite fun. I wonder what Dad would have thought about the current state of affairs in the United States. He would find something good. Like him, America is always "Great & getting better!"

Hope for the best, prepare for the worst is still my mantra. Deep breaths. Laugh whenever I can; *Babylon Bee* helps, so does Scott Adams. Even gallows humor makes me laugh [...].

Jenny went to three Halloween parties yesterday, with one of them albeit online. She's so happy getting out. I'm happy she's getting out.

Jonathan & I watched *The Best Man* last night. It's so much fun watching movies with my boyfriend on Saturday nights. I love Jonathan so much. We will survive.

November 2, 2020: [...]. Jenny's been her delightful self lately. Quick, funny, enjoyable. She worked a phone bank yesterday. She's drinking a bit, but she seems to be calmer when she drinks. And it's sangria, if you can call that drinking.

I love travelling through this crazy life with Jonathan. He's the only balanced person remaining on this earth (OK, a few exceptions).

November 3, 2020: [...]. I sense Jonathan & I will be making love soon. Hallelujah!

November 4, 2020: Jenny was very good, even though she was nervous. She poured herself a glass of wine and helped herself to a big bowl of ice cream. That's my girl! The food and drink seemed to calm her [...].

I love Jonathan so much. Last night, I held his hand most of the evening. This world is absolutely crazy, and I'm absolutely crazy in love with Jonathan.

November 5, 2020: Fortunately, I'm feeling stronger every day.

Jenny has been very good lately. She can identify her feelings and ask for a hug.

Jonathan has a busy day yesterday, and we were all exhausted. I made him some iced coffee that he sipped all day. I so love when I can do little things to make his life better. He does so much for me and the girls.

November 6, 2020: [...]. Last day of radiation! Yeah.

Dr. Levitz said my tumor markers (C27/29) have fallen from 9,000 to 4,000 to 3,200 to 2,300. Yeah me. I must be doing something right.

Jenny has been handling the stress of the uncertainty well [...].

Jonathan continues to be wonderful. He's all I need; he's all I want. The rest of the world can—and is!—go to hell. Jonathan & I have each other.

November 7, 2020: Concerning my health: Dr. Gatto said I may wean myself off my brace! Ah, how ***liberating***. The yoke—and I do mean *yoke*—of oppression is lifted! It's funny; I had gotten so used to the brace that I sometimes forgot I was wearing it. Now that I may remove it for stretches of time, I didn't realize how confining it was. There's a metaphor in there somewhere [...]

Jonathan & I are both excited about the prospect of sex. ☺

November 8, 2020: Trump's loss will be ok. Anything he could have done for autism would be too late for our girls anyway. It's just sad to see more families suffer the ways ours does. For no reason except greed and fear. The greedy people who have a conscience are afraid to speak out. Non-greedy people who know the truth are also afraid to let their insights known. Lisa Fidler could lose her job if she told the mothers what she knows about the cause of their kids' distress.

Scott Adams is quite cavalier about politics. I would like to emulate that, but my kids have been poisoned because of the government. It is very difficult to be objective, but I must. Objectivity allows for a calmer response, for finding a way out [...].

I am concerned about the power of the internet to funnel news. Still, Americans did seem to vote against identity politics and open borders [...].

Also today we'll have sex, if we remember how [...]

November 9, 2020: Jonathan and I tried sex yesterday. Fortunately, we remembered how. Unfortunately, I have a herpes outbreak ☹ so we had to stick to handy tools around the house.

November 11, 2020: Veterans Day. Dad, thanks for your service. I know it was just a great adventure for you, but you helped save the United States from external tyranny.

Now, I'm trying to help save the United States from internal tyranny. Just doing the best I can, but the forces are mighty against us. We are not permitted to discuss vaccine safety, unless the Orange Man puts forth a vaccine. Then even Kamala Harris wants vaccine choice […].

Jenny continues on an even keel. Housing may be coming soon. She's too high-functioning for emergency aid, but she does qualify for a housing voucher. All this shit that I have to figure out, thanks to the greed of the pharmaceutical executives. Not a single one of them stood up and said, "This is wrong." […].

Jonathan continues to be my great pal (inter alia). Ever and always.

November 13, 2020: Kim [another autism mom] called last night. Jenny arranged for one of the "Real Housewives of New Jersey" to send Kim a video with birthday wishes. How clever! How creative! Jenny had asked me for an advance on her allowance […]. She wanted to raise money to purchase a birthday greeting. I said, NO. But she figured out a way. Clever.

Kim will be coming over today to bring me soup and lollipops. We'll socially distance, because she's about to see her 67-year-old aunt. Sixty-seven sounds so old, until I realize, I'm 62. How DID that happen? Kim is also concerned about my health. I am, too, but I'm not concerned about covid. We are shutting ourselves off from what makes us human—contact, family gatherings (see below), visits to the elderly. But the elite are able to visit their families. Just us peons are not.

Yesterday, Jenny and Jonathan went for Jenny's intake into the job training program. Jen was very nervous and bopped me on the head […]. She's so dense when she's nervous. When she returned home, she was quite proud of herself for having done a great job […].

Flora may not be able to come home for Thanksgiving. If she were to come home, Camphill—probably under the directive of PA—says she would have to quarantine for two weeks. Then she would have to quarantine for two weeks in PA. Dear God, what are we doing to ourselves?? […] Thanksgiving without Flora. Goddamn them! Goddamn […] the elites who are drunk with power […].

I want to reply to the stupid-ass critique of my HPV vaccine & fertility paper. The reviewer just doesn't like it. S/he's just not convinced. No specifics.

No arguments. Just no. I hope the journal accepts my rebuttal, which will be polite—even though this review really is garbage. Of course, I think most reviews are garbage until I reread them and find they actually have some valid points. This review has no valid points, because it has no points.

I may venture to Lord & Taylor's today. Shopping. What a concept! And a haircut. I desperately need a haircut.

Jonathan continues to be my everything. I can't imagine going through this crazy, crazy life in this crazy, crazy world without him.

November 14, 2020: America so desperately needs what Google and Twitter and Facebook promised when they were founded. An open exchange of ideas […].

Thursday evening, we learned Flora could not come home for Thanksgiving unless she quarantined for two weeks when she returned to Pennsylvania. Friday morning, we learned she could indeed come home. Friday evening, I think we learned she would have to quarantine. This is what happens when government dictates your life. Bureaucracies can't anticipate every eventuality. They are not flexible. They are riddled with corruption and conflicts of interest […].

November 15, 2020: Great seeing girlfriends yesterday. The only commonality we have is a special-needs child. I guess that's enough, because otherwise I don't have much in common with any of them. All wore masks and socially-distanced. All are afraid of Covid. All want the best for each other.

I guess in a different world, I'd hang out with more people. But the mercury poisoning that crippled my early social life put a kibosh on that. [Gayle felt that as an adolescent she had been adversely affected by mercury in her braces.] Very fortunately, through a stroke of complete and utter luck, I found my soulmate. The first roommate I ever got along with […].

Mom says she's not sure whether she wants us to visit. At first, I thought she was joking; she had followed the statement with a laugh. But the laugh was actually a nervous one, and she is really afraid that we might infect her with wretched New Jersey germs.

The reaction to Covid is absolute nuts. True, at the beginning we didn't know much about it. Now, much truth is being hidden. Asymptomatic people do not appear to spread the virus. That's great news that no one is sharing. We have therapeutics for people who become infected; witness the President.

But the morons who have gained power as a result of the fear are loathe to relinquish their one and only chance to control lives. So, control they do! Thanksgiving gatherings must be outside! No more than three families! No longer than two hours! Underwear to be worn on the outside!

I have a busy, but pleasant day ahead [...].

And the Judaism course.

And wonderful, sweet, non-herpes lovemaking with Jonathan.

November 16, 2021: Jenny is doing well. Talking quite a bit and sometimes annoyingly. But I just say, "uh huh" and move on. I don't point out how a comment does not fit into the conversation, but I don't reward the comment either. She seems to be picking up when a comment is not exactly appropriate.

Jonathan & I made love yesterday. Ah, so nice (except I still have remnants of a herpes outbreak). Still, I'm glad we haven't forgotten how to do it.

November 17, 2020: The ampersand is such a delightful character. There's a difference between "Jonathan and I" and "Jonathan & I." In the latter, we're closer, happier. The ampersand also allowed Dad to be remembered for his essence. Military regulations permitted only 22 characters on a gravestone. "Great and getting better" is 24, while "Great & getting better" works! I have a huge debt of gratitude to the ampersand.

Ugh. Housing for Jenny is going to be more work, more research, more decisions. I'm just so fucking tired of arranging my children's lives. We were all set to hold our breath and have Jenny live on her own. Of course, it would be a disaster. There are programs that can help her manage time and money; programs where she can learn to cook and plan meals. We thought the programs were all out of state, but there is one in South Orange, right up the street. Jespy House [a residence for special-needs young adults] seems good for Jenny. But we'll look into the other programs in CT and MA. Cause that's what we do. And why, exactly? Not sure. Jenny got pissy again last night, ragging on me for rolling up the sleeves of my flannel shirt. "I'm feeling better now," she announced. "That's nice," I replied sarcastically. From now on when she gets pissy, she needs to offer a sincere apology—acknowledge that her behavior is incorrect—and hand over the remote.

[...] The world has gone completely mad over this virus. Mom is afraid for us to visit. People are afraid to hug. Politicians say we can't be with our families, we can't attend religious services, we can't eat at restaurants. Protests against the lockdowns are forbidden, while Black Lives Matter and Joe Biden victory celebrations are encouraged. Slimy hypocrites.

I'm back doing research. First replying to snarky and vague review of HPV vaccine & fertility paper. I have to stay professional and not reveal what I think about the jerk who wrote the review [...].

Jonathan let me vent twice yesterday about Jenny. I love him so much. For his patience [...] and his cock (inter alia).

November 18, 2020: *NEJM* rejected my commentary on the very flawed article they published that found a lower incidence of cervical cancer among women (under the age of 30!) who received the HPV vaccine. The journal does not want to hear any arguments. Shut up & obey.

Jespy House seems great for Jenny, and Stanton Home [a residence in western Massachusetts] seems great for Flora. There, we're done.

If only.

Jonathan was so great when I was losing it on Monday. He is great all the time.

November 19, 2020: I feel as though I'm witnessing the end of civilization as we know it. In fact, I have a front-row seat. Everyone is afraid of everyone else. Mom does not want us to visit […]. To be fair, I've always said we need to protect the elderly. But Mom does not have any respiratory issues. And, honestly, this is how she wants to live the remaining years of her life? Isolated from her children and grandchildren? It's certainly her call, but I would make a different decision […].

Jonathan has only one more busy Wednesday in this semester. It's difficult for me to work when he's teaching, because his [Zoomed] lectures are so damn interesting.

November 20, 2020: The CDC and state governors are attempting to cancel Thanksgiving. Interstate travel is extremely difficult. For Flora to return to Beaver Farm, she needs to have a PCR test taken within 72 hours of her arrival in PA. The problem is, it takes about 72 hours to receive the results of the PCR test. And that's assuming we can find a place that will give Flora the test. Insane! […]

Jenny's acquaintance at Writers Group [a circle of aspiring young authors who met weekly at a local restaurant] said Jenny's hygiene stinks (I'm paraphrasing). Ugh. I'm so tired of hearing about Jenny's shortcomings. I'm always the one who hears from the school, from the other school, from the college (actually, Jonathan fielded most of the complaints from Drew), from the other college, and now Writers Group. I explained to Jenny that we don't make the rules, but are trying to offer her guidance in surviving in this world. She took it relatively well. And then forgot to turn on the toaster oven to cook dinner. And got water on her bathroom floor. I'm at wit's end.

Jonathan is adamant that we be a family at Thanksgiving. I love him more & more each day.

November 21, 2020: So much shit going on. And I do mean scheisse! Drawn-out conversation with Dana yesterday really got on my nerves. She started out by telling me how horribly the school district failed Jenny, that

Jenny needs "Social conversation skills" to express herself so that she doesn't have these rages. Then, painstaking detail about different (expensive) programs Jenny could enroll in. Some of the information is useful, but I'm tired. I'm utterly exhausted from all the consultants who tell us, "Oh, I can help your child. In fact, I'm the *only* one who can help your child. All those other people who tried to help your child, they were awful. Too bad you didn't find me earlier; you've wasted so much time. But now *finally* someone is able to do a good job."

Ugh. And then we talked about the Covid lockdowns. I knew I should not have, because my nerves were already frayed [...]. I was rude. In the future, I need to talk as an economist looking for balance. We're destroying our kids' lives to keep them safe [...].

Jonathan is having a rough time. He's reflecting about the girls and how unfair life is to them. Jenny threw out a match yesterday and set the trash on fire. She doesn't get it. It's scary. I want to help Jonathan as best I can.

November 22, 2020: All this hysteria over a disease that kills fewer people under the age of 70 than the flu! The Dark Side of the lockdowns is costing millions—18.7 million to be exact—of life years lost. And that's just deaths. What about the abuse, the alcoholism, the drug use, the depression? [...].

Jenny got herself to a movie and a way home last night! ***That's*** responsibility. Hallelujah! [...]

Jonathan is so wonderful as I navigate the Covid testing infrastructure. Maybe we can have it all! We do deserve a break.

November 24, 2020: Jenny had another bender last night [...]. I left the room. She exploded; hit Jonathan twice. She pounded herself and the wall several times. I had to remind her not to break another door. What a pain in the ass she can be.

And I'm supposed to say, "What can I do to make you feel better right now?" while she taking swipes at me. I don't think so.

The stress of finding a place for Flora to receive a Covid test is not helping. For two nights in a row, I get up when I take my 1:30 am pills to come to the computer to sign her up [for a test] on a fresh new day. I know I'm overstressing, but I don't know where I can cut back the stress. If I believed in God, I would say, "Everything will be all right." But it's not all right.

[...] Supposedly, Covid is very contagious. But we don't really know, because the tests are so inaccurate. Elon Musk—for whom I am gathering more respect—took four tests and received two that were positive and two that were negative. Or so he says. It would be great if he provided pictures of his results. Of course, the pictures could also be faked.

Everything could be faked. "Is this the real world; is this just fantasy"? Of course, if it's fantasy, I sure as hell would make it a better dream. It's a nightmare. The powers that be have poisoned our kids and now put half the country in a complete state of panic and the other half in a complete state of anger. Guess which half I'm in? [...]

Jonathan and I might work together on a special issue of *Vaccines*. An interdisciplinary issue on autism prevalence and vaccine uptake. It would be so much fun to work with Jonathan.

Jonathan is the only thread to life that keeps me hanging on. He's the only thread that makes sense.

November 25, 2020: We did it. We picked up Flora. We made it to the State Line without getting caught. I feel so *criminal!* Of course, these arbitrary and senseless rulings will backfire. Now that I've committed a small sin, I'm empowered to commit ever greater sins. Next, I'll host a party and invite more than six people!

And the lockdowns have no effect on reducing overall morbidity. One or two lives might be saved from not transmitting the disease now, but the disease will transmit. That's what diseases do. And other lives are lost from loneliness and despair [...]

I'm up early to have a few minutes of peace & quiet. The HPV vaccine and fertility revision is shaping up nicely. Deirdre's extraordinarily kind words about how some people owe their existence to my research sustains and encourages me.

We're all calmer now that Flora made it home. Jenny needs to stay on top of her supplements. I need to stay on top of Jenny to stay on top of her supplements. Ugh. I do get tired of having to be the grown up *all the time*.

It was delicious getting an almost entirely uninterrupted sleep. For three nights in a row, I got up to set up Flora's Covid test. Walgreens opened a new day of appointments at midnight, so I dragged my arse down to the computer to sign her up. The first night, I misjudged the days they made available (only until Tuesday); the second night, I signed her up but never received a confirmation; the third night, I was successful [...].

This is what I'm reduced to thinking about. I could be thinking great thinks, but *no*, I need to plot out my daughter's escape.

The story of my life. Except that I'm plotting out both daughters' escapes.

I do treat Flora differently from Jenny. I'm nicer to Flora, indeed more caring. Flora doesn't try to choke me; she doesn't hit me when she is frustrated.

Jonathan continues to be incredibly sweet. Last night, I realized we needed bagels for Flora's breakfast. Although he was dead tired, he went to the kitchen and started defrosting some frozen bagels. He takes such good care of all his chicks.

November 26, 2020: Thanksgiving 2020. Actually, Thanksgiving is cancelled. So, it's just November 26, 2020.

But we're celebrating Thanksgiving in the Rose-DeLong household. We're together as a family, despite what the tyrants decree. We snuck into Pennsylvania, whisked our hostage, and made it to the state line. Getting Flora back is an ordeal, but we'll do it. We are a family [...].

[...] it wasn't the CCP that poisoned our kids. It was good old Capitalistic greed and American ingenuity. Of course, you mix American ingenuity with CCP greed for power and you get the totalitarian society we are headed for. We're losing our democracy so quickly. In many ways, we've already lost it. Those of us who have lost our kids to vaccine injury saw the Covid [hysteria] for what it is—a desperate power grab from the elite losing their collective grip. Since it was based on health and fear, they are getting away with it. People are ever so slowly, but surely, awakening to the loss of our rights. I hope it's not too late. I'll do everything I can to make sure it isn't [...].

Jenny got upset last night over something. I was lying in bed when I heard her wails. Flora got upset. I figured I would just make things worse if I intervened. Of course, if Jenny had physically hurt Flora, I would have called the police. The kerfuffle ended without major incident. Jenny seems to have no awareness of how she affects those around her. If she is aware, she doesn't seem to care.

Jonathan continues to write raunchy emails *every day*. Honestly, who could ask for more?

November 27, 2020: This morning, the musing is the second thing I did on the computer. First, I wanted to find a nice—and by "nice" I mean *raunchy*—meme for Jonathan. Mission accomplished!

We zoomed with Suzanne & Mark, Doron & Michelle [Jonathan's nephew and his girlfriend], & Mom. Suzanne asked why I was converting. I said family. Did you hear that, Mom? *FAMILY.* Family is important to me. By adopting a new family, maybe I'll feel less anger toward the people with whom I share a last name. I hope. I don't want to feel too angry, but I do. Angry and hurt.

Jenny bashed a hole in her bathroom wall. She needs to get out of this environment.

Flora & I went for her Covid test. All the planning in the world—getting up at 1:30 am when I take my pills to sign up for the test—meant nothing. We found a place that didn't have a line and just did it [...].

I'm glad I was able to find a nice raunchy meme for Jonathan. Actually, I found several and stockpiled. He deserves the best!

November 28, 2020: You wake up one morning and realize your entire country is a fraud. The elite control the resources and throw you crumbs if you obey.

You thought the corruption you discovered 16 years ago was a fluke, a small corner carved out by slick mobsters. Then you realize that all major decisions—not just vaccine policy—are determined by people who have major conflicts of interest; by people who don't care about the consequences for others. Just the benefit they reap.

The corruption reveals itself in the hypocrisy. Enjoying dinner with family and friends—22 people all together—while mandating others hunker down and "socially distance." An oxymoron, proposed by morons. Or you get your hair done, Kardashian-like, while you prohibit others from the same luxury. Or you greet your married lover across town in your apartment while you, in your expert opinion, recommend a total and complete lockdown of society. OK, the last example is from Great Britain, but the British informed our institutions and even our current Covid policies.

And people follow. We wear our masks, we socially distance, we cower in our homes. Intelligent, reasonable, rational people do this. Of course, a celebration that involves Black Lives Matter or a Biden "victory" is allowed, even promoted. Protests against lockdowns or even religious gatherings are illegal.

You wake up one morning and you realize you're living in a Third World country.

You saw inklings. The crumbling infrastructure, the petty bribes, the nonsensical vaccine policy. But you didn't think it could go this far so quickly […].

It's disgusting. And the ramifications are huge. Mandated Covid vaccines; more lockdowns; greater misery.

And yet you fight on. You've fought for 15 years, no sense—not even the ability—to stop now.

Jonathan helps me to hang on. He—and helping the girls find their places in this horrid world—are the reasons I'm living.

November 29, 2020: We watched *Yesterday* last night. Such a sweet movie. Flora would not watch with us, perhaps because she had seen it several times already since she's been home. Jenny—quite astutely—vowed next time not to show Flora a film we would like to watch as a family.

Flora goes back today. She is talking more. But still watching the same lame video of the guy singing Beatles songs out of tune. Ugh. And she's still fat. But she did manage to open the freezer one night, ***and only took two ice***

cream treats. There were two gallons of ice cream along with another full box of treats, but she didn't touch those. I think she only eats things from packages that are open. And fruit. She'll eat any piece of fruit she can find.

Jonathan & I danced last night to the Beatles music. Jonathan kept singing "My Girl." Right era, wrong group. Sometimes I feel as though he & I are in the right group, but wrong era. We belong more in the radical '60s. Actually, no. We're ***ahead*** of our times.

November 30, 2020: We took Flora back to Beaver Farm yesterday. I so profoundly miss the person she was supposed to be. I'll bet she would have been excited about life and intelligent. Very, very smart. And fun. Clever, for sure (that she is even under her horrid circumstances).

I don't know about Jenny. She might have been mean. I just don't know. I do know Jenny is awfully mean to me. My looks, my work, how I try to guide her. She is less mean about my looks lately, but she still has no respect for the work I do and certainly wants no guidance (except in a few brief moments).

Jenny & I watched *Madea's Christmas* last night. It's a cute movie, and it was fun watching with Jenny. I do hope Jenny gets into her own place soon. I think our relationship will improve. Seeing her might become a treat, a pleasure [...].

And I worry that the Covid vaccine will be mandatory. We'll cross that bridge when we get to it.

Jonathan continues to be my anchor. So strong, so sweet.

December 1, 2020: Last night, I had trouble going back to sleep after waking to take my 1:30 am pills. Flora, Flora, Flora. How can I find you? You were supposed to be a little bit of Dad of and a little bit of me. That's how it was supposed to be. But we don't know who you are.

Maybe stem cells will help; maybe Dr. Johnson can help.

I reached over to Jonathan when I couldn't sleep. He said we have to move on. He's right. And I would certainly do that, if I were able.

December 2, 2020: Dikshit. Someone actually has the last name of Dikshit. Stumbling upon his name yesterday provided immense comic relief. Jenny was on the verge of getting pissy, and I just started cracking up. So, are you a Dik or are you shit? This guy is ***both!***

These days, I do my best to ignore Jenny. She gets on my nerves, but when I ignore her, she gets on my nerves to a lesser degree. She needs to be out of the house. Yesterday [...].

Jonathan outdid himself yesterday with the raunchy meme he sent. "Your pussy is like the weather: when it's wet it's time to get inside." How deliciously raunchy is that??

December 3, 2020: Flora is officially obese. OK. From now on, when she visits home, sauna every other day. Sit-ups twice a day. Low-carb as much as possible […]. If her mind can't be the smart & clever person she was supposed to be, at least her body can be the athletic person in there.

Memories of Purim as I prepare for the Judaism class. The girls were quite cute in their Indian garb.

As long as I am alive, I will strive for their health […].

Jenny & I are in equilibrium. I do my best to ignore her. If she would be nicer to me—no, if she just wouldn't be so mean—I could care more. But I can't.

Jonathan is almost finished with classes. Next semester, he'll be on campus. Concentrating is difficult when he's teaching; I just want to listen to what he says. Maybe next semester, we'll become empty nesters; 'tis a consummation devoutly to be wished!

December 4, 2020: Jenny blew up again last night. Wailing, screaming, yelling. After banging something against the wall (her bed? Her head?), she proclaimed she was upset because of what happened last night. She had signed up to attend a gym session at the YMCA. We said ok, but it was strange that they didn't require membership. She insisted they didn't. Then we read the fine print, and indeed one needed to be a member. Of course, Jenny got mad at us. She was calm when she went to bed, but around 3:30 am, she started screaming and banging. Jonathan gave her two Advil. After about half an hour, she was calm.

I have tried everything. How many doctors? How many protocols? How many suggestions? **She** needs to know when Advil would help. She needs to figure out what works for her. I don't understand her, and I am not her.

I noticed this morning that she cut her Valtrex in half in the evening. That could have influenced her behavior.

Her autism is killing me. My back is bothering me. It actually started bothering me yesterday while trying to get out of HBOT. Not bad, just annoying. The kind of ache you get after a ten-mile bike ride, except that I didn't just complete a ten-mile bike ride. Dr. Levitz is still pushing Ibrance. My tumor markers are going down: from 9,000 to 4,500 to 3,200 to 2,300 to 1,818 (or 1,880). He says the cancer will start growing again after ten months, but that Ibrance retards the growth until 20 months. But it will grow, he seemed to promise. Except he doesn't know about the protocols I'm using. Why is it my Ki-something, which indicates the speed at which cancer grows, was 10% in 2015 and down to 3% now? Could it be the pancreatic enzymes or something else I'm doing? Also, he has not once spoken to me about diet or supplements or anything except pharmaceuticals. He is well-meaning—very concerned and caring—but ignorant about alternatives.

What I really need is to lower my stress […].

Jonathan is such a peach.

December 5, 2020: Jenny's hissy fit from Thursday night spilled over into Friday morning. By mid-afternoon, she was ok. She doesn't seem to realize that such behavior is not acceptable. Ever. We have some more indentations in the wall, this time near our family photos.

I'll have her write actions she can take when she wants to hit, to bite, to scream. Get a system in place […].

I forgot to send Jonathan a raunchy email yesterday. Rats! And he does so much for me. I'll get back on track today.

December 6, 2020: Slept late this morning (until 7:30 am). Had trouble going back to sleep after taking 1:30 am pills. Worried about being forced to take Covid vaccine. Worried about Flora gaining 25 pounds since starting Camphill. How did that happen? Much of the weight probably gained when she was home. I tried. We tried. Now, we're going to try harder […].

Seeing Dr. Johnson tomorrow! And Lyn & Mary [Coyle, a homeopath specializing in autism]! I'm not sure whom I am more excited about seeing and spending time with. **This** is what life is made of. Friends, road trips, exchanging ideas. **This** is what the Dark Side (Bill Gates, Anthony Fauci, Phil Murphy, George Soros, Mark Zuckerberg, Jeff Bezos, Twitter guy etc., etc.) want to destroy. When people gather, they share ideas; when they share ideas, they learn; when they learn, they see the hypocrisy of their leaders.

I've been mean to Jenny lately. The meaner I am to her, the nicer she is to me. OK. We'll keep it that way.

Jonathan continues to be incredibly sweet. We tried making love yesterday, but I'm still having pain with my lady parts (only when we have sex ☹). I'll see a doctor. I loathe doctors, but this cause is so important.

Pearl Harbor Day, 2020: Seventy-nine years ago. Wow.

Amazing what a good night's sleep will do for the spirit! The night before, I tossed and turned about being forced to get a Covid shot—both for me and my family—as well as Flora's weight and her life in general. Yesterday morning, I was crabby to Jenny—she deserved some of it—and just felt sad.

This morning, I'm feeling better. Fauci claims there won't be federal mandates, but employers might require the vaccine. What bullshit.

And we'll help Flora with her weight. She probably packed it on over the summers she was home. Now, she'll unpack while she's home. Patches, locked food, sauna, exercise.

Jenny was up and down yesterday. Mad at me when I called her out on things. If not me, then who? If not now, then when?

Today is my road trip with Lyn. We'll meet Mary in NY. I can't wait! […]. Jonathan doesn't get to do road trips with guy friends. That's a shame. Guys are lucky in that they are not expected to call or take care of the sick; they aren't expected to come over for coffee, so they don't feel bad when they don't. On the other hand, they also don't have road trips.

December 8, 2020: Jenny & I are getting along better. I really needed the break from her.

Where would I be without Jonathan? I love him so much.

December 9, 2020: Another alternative medicine person murdered […]. And Paul Thomas lost his license. [Thomas was an Oregon physician who authored *The Vaccine-Friendly Plan*, which offered flexible and individualized vaccination schedules for children. His license to practice medicine was suspended in December 2020 and restored the following July.] Tragic on some many levels. For the people themselves and their families, but also for the families they directly serve and society in general.

This time, a woman's young son found her. That suggests the murder took place in her home, not, as is usual, in a desolate hotel room.

I sense I'll be murdered before any cancer has a chance to knock me off. Not that I expect cancer to kill me. I still see me living to a ripe old, crotchety age.

So, I better stop being a bitch now to Jenny. There's plenty of time for that. Having a day off with the girls was heavenly. And things are happening for Jenny: […] Jespy House, job training. Things are **really** happening. She deserves good things […].

I do hope I get my lady parts in working order […]. Jonathan deserves pure, unadulterated sex.

December 11, 2020: Flora comes home in a week. The penultimate time she will be home for any stretch of time. I need to order a book about clouds. Something she & I can read together […].

The Group Home is coming through! OMG. Jenny is very cool with the idea. I'm so glad. She's not freaking out about a huge change. She's looking very forward to it. She's been good with changes. We thought she'd figure stuff out once she was on her own. I still believe that, but she needs guidance sometimes to help her figure stuff out […].

I love Jonathan so much. What more can I say? He is my everything.

December 12, 2020: Jenny insisted upon going to an outing at Jockey Hollow this morning at 8:30. When we said we wouldn't drive her, she called someone after 10 pm last night. Ugh. You can't do that, Jenny. It's disrespectful and rude [...].

Sadly, as a result of the pandemic [...] the rest of the United States is now experiencing what we in the autism community have faced for decades. Whenever we questioned vaccine safety, we were told to "shut up and listen to the experts." Debate ceased, and open questions were never resolved. The legal system offered no relief, because we never had our day in court.

We can hope—yes, and pray—that more people push back against the draconian measures taken by the power-hungry and non-scientific tyrants who run our state governments [...]. We've seen too much to go back and pretend.

Jonathan is such a wonderful father. He got up & drove Jenny to Jockey Hollow this morning. He is now picking her up. Soon—I hope & pray!— she will be on her own. Then Jonathan & I can be together. The two of us. In peace.

December 13, 2020: I had lunch with Louise Habakus [the coauthor of *Vaccine Epidemic*] yesterday. She reached out to me to provide suggestions for my spiritual life. Quite frankly—and I was honest with her—when I dwell on my negative thoughts, it only makes them worse. So many people told Jenny to "talk about her issues." She talked all right. And talked and talked. To absolutely no avail except to have her focus on the negative instead of emphasizing the good and growth [...].

Jonathan continues to be my everything. The one & only thing that matters. He & the girls. Now, I have to run & see what kind of raunchy email he sent me today [...]

December 14, 2020: Jenny is getting nervous about The Group Home and taking it out on us. She "hears voices in my head." She banged her bed against the wall and screamed. Ugh. She needs to find better ways of dealing with excitement [...].

December 15, 2020: [...] Jonathan continues to be my everything. He's very excited about Jenny's next step and hoping she can start moving out before January 15. It will be grand spending time with just him!

December 16, 2020: Jenny humming a lot lately. She's nervous about The Group Home, but at least she could identify what is bothering her. I assured her the transition will be gradual. I think all she needed was for us to remain calm [...] as she puts dents in the refrigerator and her bathroom door [...].

Jonathan shakes his head about Jenny. Moving out is everything she wanted. I explained that the excitement part of her brain is right next to the anxiety part. It's difficult for our kids to express unadulterated excitement without anxiety. And I'm just the opposite. Unless I'm excited about life, I'm anxious. That is, I become anxious when I'm not excited.

Jonathan always makes me excited. ☺

December 17, 2020: Flora comes home tomorrow. Jonathan & I are going to give it the old college try today. I hope for a Hannukah miracle!

December 18, 2020: Jenny's going to The Group Home! What a relief. For everyone. Especially Jenny. Jespy House is a fall back, but I very much hope [this] works out. For everyone's sake. Especially Jenny's.

Flora comes home today. There goes life as we know it. That's ok. I have several projects, none of which is pressing […].

Jonathan & I made love sweet, sweet love yesterday. Ahhhhhhhhh. It's so wonderful being married to my best friend.

December 19, 2020: Flora is home. She very diligently put together the puzzle we got her for Hannukah. We need to find more puzzles for her!

She also broke into the refrigerator and ate the candy from Camphill as well as the cream.

I put a Lifewave sticker on her that is supposed to reduce cravings and addictions. I hope something works! Her obesity is unhealthy.

Of course, what does it matter? Her life is ruined. Vaccines poisoned her and destroyed her life. We'll maintain hospice […] for the rest of her life.

But we do keep trying. Maybe Dr. Johnson can help. Or stem cells.

I'm tired; I'm old. But I still have breath in me. And I'm a warrior. Warriors fight as long as they breathe […].

Both Yehuda Shoenfeld and Chris Exley have quoted my work. Deirdre Little says some people owe their existence to my research. Warriors fight as long as they breathe.

I told Jonathan I was a failure at everything—teaching, research, parenting—but somehow I don't feel like a failure. He pointed out that I have not failed, but rather, I have been failed. By our authorities and experts. We trust people, Jonathan & I, to be professional and honest. In the case of medical authorities and experts, the trust was very much misplaced.

But we're going through this together, Jonathan & I. There is no one—***no one!***—I could go through this with other than Jonathan.

December 20, 2020: A ***bitch*** of a night last night. Jenny went to a party a half an hour away, which meant we had to drive her a total of two hours. Except that Jonathan got lost and spent two and a half hours on the road. I was in a grouchy mood when I picked her up, which spoiled her good mood.

Then, Jenny couldn't find her key so she started perseverating. Then Flora started perseverating about the Beaver Farm yearbook from 2017 to 2018.

Eventually, both found each but not before screaming and wailing and punching (Jenny on me).

Jonathan instructed me to go to bed. Wise man.

At 1:30 am, when I got awake to take my pills, Flora was still up. She was on Jenny's computer and making soup. With scallions. Not a bad snack. I turned off Jenny's computer, and Flora said she would go to bed.

At 3:30 am, Flora was still up. Jenny's computer was on again. Flora realized we had forgotten "to ask." "What's something good that happened to you today?" she inquired. "Nothing," I responded. "What are you looking forward to tomorrow?" I provided the same response. What else can you say when you have two daughters with autism who don't seem to be getting better?

While drudging myself back to bed, I noticed my hand. My fingers were slightly spread in curved positions, almost as though I was about to play the piano. My pinky was bent as though about to pick up a teacup. My hand seemed separate from my body, almost angelic. Flora won't be with us much longer. I want her to think of me fondly. So, I got up again and said I thought of something that was good today ("Finding a journal for my article") and what I was looking forward to tomorrow ("Working on my article").

This morning, Jenny asked whether I had seen her note. She had written an understanding that her behavior was wrong and she apologized. She also provided ideas on how to handle the situation in the future. We are getting through to her. Hallelujah!

Jonathan continues to be my rock.

December 21, 2020: Much better day yesterday than the day before. Jenny wrote me the sweetest apology note. Are we (finally!) getting through to her? We love her; we want the best for her; we are trying to help her navigate this world.

Flora is more animated. She's talking more. Still not a ton, but there seems to be progress.

I'm going to work on getting my article on HPV vaccine & lowered fertility paper republished. *Fertility Research and Practice* might be interested. I'll toss the dice.

Yesterday, I gathered information about the girls for Dr. Johnson. Damn. We have tried so many different protocols over the years. Most of them did more harm than good [...]. So many drugs, all of which made the girls worse.

We'll be having our Solstice celebration tonight. Jonathan bought brisket, in honoring of my conversion to Judaism. We're having fun with the Judaism course, even if the instructor is making one of the most interesting subjects as boring as possible.

December 22, 2020: Another evening of frustration and incredulity. In the afternoon, Flora insisted upon buying glue. Jenny, to her great credit, took Flora first to the local gas station and then to RiteAid. But I'm sure it took a toll on Jenny. In the evening [...] Jenny insisted upon using the sauna. No regard for how much she inconvenienced us (Jonathan wanted to get ready for bed) and no understanding that the sauna takes a while to heat up for it to do any good. She sat in the sauna at 80 degrees Fahrenheit. That's a warm Spring day. And then she wanted water, which she had not procured before entering the hot place. So inconsiderate. So selfish.

I have a herpes outbreak. I wonder why [...].

Jonathan is such an adorable absent-minded professor! Yesterday, he drove to the liquor store. When he went to open his car, the electronic system didn't work. He & Flora walked home (Jenny's phone, of course, was not working.) I suggested he use the key to **manually** open the door on the driver's side. It worked! I feel so needed. And so loved.

December 23, 2020: Ugh. Jenny dragged me to Boonton to deliver a Christmas present to some unknown organization. I should not have bitched & moaned the way I did. Jenny is very sweet to want to deliver presents to the less fortunate. What bothers me is that Jenny does not seem to realize that "Charity begins at home ... and more or less stays there." See, Dad, some of us still remember you. Every day. Well, I try anyway. Sometimes the challenges are too great for me to remember that I'm "great & getting better."

But the fight to "take care of those two little girls, those two beautiful little girls" continues. That's always & forever. We'll be seeing a new doctor next week. And stem cell. Three doses for Flora. Wouldn't it be grand if the stem cells help?

Flora *is* more animated. And is talking a bit more. She's still very hung up on glue, but now that she is broke she needs to earn money to buy glue. That's where encouraging her to do things comes in. She listened to *Help!* one time last night, and then went to bed. OK, she gets a dollar for that. And reading; we pay for reading.

Jenny lent Flora $5 yesterday, so maybe Jenny realizes charity *does* begin at home [...].

Jonathan continues to be my everything. We laugh together [...] about the absurdities of the girls. We're in this together. Forever & always.

December 24, 2020: Jenny had another hissy fit last night. As hissy fits go, it wasn't too bad. No hitting, only some chewing & head banging. She expects us to drive her around to all her events. And she doesn't tell us much in advance. When we push back, she expects others to drive her places. I'm trying to help her understand that if she lives on the way, it's fine to ask for a ride. "But I'm only ten minutes away from her house." Yes, but if the ten minutes are in the opposite direction you are asking her to go out of her way.

And the laws of physics are all my fault [...].

Jonathan & I continue to be on the same page with the everything [...]. We're definitely going to the protest at Pfizer global headquarters on January 13. Why do all the best protests have to be in the winter? Like the Trenton protests of 2019. Was that only a year ago? It seems ages ago. We raised our voices, and we won that round. [Those protests defeated efforts to end religious exemptions for vaccinating schoolchildren in New Jersey. The protests were entirely peaceful but extremely loud.] I hope we can do it again this year.

December 25, 2020: Jenny went to a Christmas Eve service last night in Liberty Corner. I drove one way, and she brought an Uber home. Fine. That worked.

She & Flora are so cute together.

Flora is getting to bed at least by 1:30 am. The lights are out at that time. I'm paying her, but the $1 is well worth her change in behavior. I'll also pay her a dollar not to play the sound on her Beatles video. She may play the video, just no sound. Now that she's broke, she's much more compliant.

That's what the elites are doing to us. Hollowing out that wretched, independent middle-class. Those deplorables who value more in life than just a paycheck. Family, faith, enjoyment. Choke them, say the elite. So they bow to our demands.

People seem to be rising up. Let's pray this tyranny ends soon.

[...]. Jonathan pointed out that most people throughout history have not been free. Freedom is a relatively new construct. That's such an odd thought [...].

I love the walks Jonathan & I take. He's so smart [...] and such a great lay. He's the whole package!

December 26, 2020: A very nice Christmas. Jenny had three great ideas—sort of a reverse Scrooge. We zoomed with the DeLong Family [...], saw *Wonder Woman 1984*, and watched *Madea's Halloween*.

Flora acted up a little during the movie, and one patron complained. I was shocked when he accepted my explanation—that Flora has autism. I'm surprised he didn't say something like, "You shouldn't bring her out in public if she is going to be so disruptive." I could have also explained that we thought the movie would be loud enough to cover the funny sounds she makes. I did suggest he inform us if Flora's behavior was bothering him. I would have removed her. The movie was incredibly stupid, and Jonathan joked that the guy felt he must have been missing out on the "scintillating dialogue" or something to that effect.

Joking with Jonathan makes this life bearable.

December 27, 2020: Mistletoe seems to be working for me. I feel the poison course through my veins, killing the cancer, but not the healthy cells. I do look forward to IV mistletoe, regardless of who administers it.

Jenny played her acoustic sunrise music quite loudly again this morning. I stormed into her room and turned it down. Jenny apologized! Not in a frantic, hissy-fit kind of way. But rather an "oops, I forgot" kind of way.

Jonathan was touched by *Ben-Hur* last night, which Jonathan suggested needs to be called *Ben-Them* in today's Woke World. Said it would give him nightmares. I'm finding the movie (we're watching it over two nights) a bit hokey. The constant music makes it artificial. The film probably has a different effect on the Big Screen.

December 28, 2020: Today's the big day. First Dr. Johnson, then Stanton Home. Or, as Flora puts it, first we eat out for lunch then we go to Massachusetts, then we eat out for dinner. Does that girl think about anything other than food?!? [...].

Tomorrow stem cells. And every day with Jonathan. WhAAAat a journey. What a soulmate.

December 29, 2020: Good heavens! The 29th already. The year is quickly coming to an end. Thank goodness.

Yesterday went well. Dr. Johnson had some wonderful—and doable!—suggestions for the girls. His approach to each was quite different and different from his approach to me. A true healer.

Today is stem cells for the girls (are stem cells?). Dr. Johnson said he didn't have much success with stem cells & couldn't continue to charge so much for a protocol that didn't produce enough results. Wow. A healer AND a mensch!

Stanton Home is nice, but not work $8K a month. Glad we visited.

Jonathan is so wonderful about driving the girls to all these appointments. As he pointed out, it was great to get out of the house!

December 30, 2020: I had trouble falling to sleep last night. Every sound was so LOUD. The boom box outside, Flora's clanking in the kitchen, Jenny's vocalizations, Jonathan's snoring [...].

And I need to survive. Which I'm doing ok with. My breast area hurts a little. Sometimes it hurts, and then feels much better. The healing process? Maybe we should zap this area with mistletoe prophylactically?

Jonathan continues to send raunchy emails. He's such a joy!

January 1, 2021: Whew. The first thing Flora did in the new year was elope. The police found her quickly, but, jeez, here we go again! Jenny unlocked the front door and Flora followed shortly thereafter.

Yesterday, I didn't get a chance to write a musing. Feels as though I dropped December 31, like a reverse leap year. Flora's computer died, and I was trying—in vain—to resuscitate it. Also, I slept very late yesterday—until 9 am!

Getting up early—defined as at least an hour before everyone else—is the way to live. The earth is peaceful, the time is quiet.

We went out for dinner at the Morristown Diner last evening. Jenny's brilliant suggestion. Hardly anyone there. The waitress told us about how her 85-year-old father is never scared of anything, but he was scared of Covid. The family stayed apart for Thanksgiving, but by Christmas said screw it (I'm paraphrasing). Twenty-seven people got together, including two policemen who are married to nurses and the waitress, all of whom are exposed to many people everyday. We all touched wood that no one got Covid. I pointed out that even if someone did, it wasn't the end of the world. That we need to protect the older people, but we also have to live. The waitress heartily agreed.

Glad I'm facing this year with Jonathan. I couldn't face it with anyone else.

January 2, 2021: 1/2/21—an auspicious day? We'll see.

Is America past the point of no return? Have the Chinese so thoroughly infiltrated our institutions, even our psyches, that we can no longer return to the fearless, rugged individualism that built and maintained this country for over two hundred years? "Toxic masculinity" removed the fathers— God, the Father; the Fatherland; and Dad. Now, "toxic individualism" will remove the remnants of personal agency.

But it didn't begin with "toxic masculinity." It began with the greed that capitalism can so easily sow. In our case, greed of the pharmaceutical companies to make money. That destruction was entirely home-grown. The institutions that were supposed to protect us—the regulators (appointed by the politicians), the media, the law, the nonprofits—have all been neutered.

The CCP is smart. Why can't they use the intelligence for good instead of conquering?

But the CCP saw the model of how we were destroying ourselves—neuter the institutions—and anything is possible.

How to fight back? Let them use their own weight against them. They way they did with us. Our weight—people's trust in the institutions we so carefully established—is destroying us.

The next book I read will be Gordon Chang's *The Coming Collapse of China*. Perhaps the book will provide insights on how to fight back.

Jonathan is also concerned. I brought up American's possible demise on our New Year's Day walk yesterday. He said we're in for a rough ride, and then Jenny wanted to know what we were talking about. I said mud, we were concerned the mud would make things messy.

There's no one I'd rather go through a rough ride with than Jonathan. Of course, we already are.

January 3, 2021: Something happened with Flora's handwriting—it improved! She wrote a thank-you note to Mom: Dear Jeanne Jeanne, [Their affectionate name for Gayle's mother] Thank you for the money! Love, Flora!! She wrote it on her own; all I did was mention she should write a note [...].

Jonathan & I are getting closer & closer. Just the thought of both girls being out of the house makes us mushy.

January 4, 2021: Jenny & Flora are interacting more. It's cute, even if it is LOUD [...].

Jonathan is so incredibly sweet. Both of us are looking so forward to having just the two of us. The very thought is making us so mushy.

January 5, 2021: Jonathan was on TV last night! He was a talking head in a documentary called *Churchill and the Movie Mogul*. The film analyzed Churchill's relationship with movie mogul Alexander Korda. Earlier in the evening, Jonathan was depressed about the state of the world—and he had much reason to be down—but the fame & glory lifted his spirits. Jonathan confided in me that as a talking head, you don't just want to talk. You want to create visualizations that the producer can then run as you speak. He alone among the talking heads in the film accomplished that. We saw glimpses of Jonathan, but for the most part when he spoke, we saw battles or relationships Jonathan was describing. Jonathan is so smart.

He has much reason to be concerned about the sorry state of the world [...].

Jenny had a hissy fit [...]. She banged her head against my bathroom wall. It's amazing she doesn't hurt herself.

Fascinating talk with Dr. Johnson yesterday. I'm on the road to IV mistletoe. The rest of the journey is simply mechanics. I so enjoy living, & mistletoe can help me overcome cancer. Let's do this! [...].

I love my life with Jonathan.

January 6, 2021: [...]. My cancer rash has worsened, and the area is very tender. I texted Dr. Johnson, and I hope he has some suggestions. I don't trust Dr. Levitz to have enough knowledge to really. Dr. L knows only pharmaceuticals. Drugs won't heal the stress [...].

Jonathan said it's going to be ok. We'll figure it out. I want to be here for him. I want to live.

January 7, 2021: Oh, Dear God. What a day was yesterday. Jenny & Flora went for a walk. Got lost. Police called. We picked them up. Later, Flora's DVD stopped playing. She became frantic, uncontrollable. At one point, around 11 pm, I had had it. I stormed, "Flora, just the f--- up!" Jenny freaked out—tension had been building. She called suicide hotline. Jonathan spoke to the person on the other end. Eventually everyone collapsed in exhaustion.

And the rest of the United States is falling apart, too. Angry Trump protesters stormed the Capitol. Smashed windows. Ran amuck […]. Tragically, a woman was killed. Tragedy for the woman & her family; tragedy for the person who killed her; tragedy for the United States. The hypocrisy is beyond reproach. BLM protesters are violent because they have a cause, says CNN; Trump supporters are just crazy […].

Jonathan held me & protected me from Jenny yesterday. We'll get through this.

January 8, 2021: Jonathan was sad yesterday, but I think I helped cheer him up. I'm glad. He's my BFF&E (best friend forever & ever). He emails me a raunchy meme every day, which I will go read now.

January 9, 2021: The rest of the United States is now experiencing what we in the vaccine safety community have known for over a decade. Our speech is blocked, our thoughts ridiculed, our issues ignored. But despite the blocking, the ridiculing, the ignoring, the lack of safety has not gone away. It has gotten worse, much worse […].

So what now? The situation is so unnatural—so against Nature—that it cannot hold. But how will it revert? Will it revert? Will it become the new normal? Like the garbled speech of our children; Lisa [Fidler] saw that a young child was not speaking appropriately, but her young colleague—who did not know what normal was—observed the child spoke just fine.

I love this country. My father and father-in-law fought proudly to preserve democracy and our way of life. It is up to us to continue their tradition. But how? […].

Flora goes back to Beaver Farm tomorrow. I'm always a little sad when she goes back. This time, however, I feel we made some progress. She *is* more interactive, happier. Is it stem cells? Anthroposophic interventions? Who knows? We'll keep doing what we're doing […].

Jenny is more in tune with my feelings. She noticed I was exhausted, but couldn't figure out exactly why […].

Jonathan & I are in this together. We are both disgusted and more than a little scared. But our world doesn't change much. It's just we have more people joining us.

January 10, 2021: Flora returns to Beaver Farm today. Not a day too soon. We worked through some things this break. Now that she understands the concept of money, we bribe her not to eat us out of house & home at night. Best $2 investment ***ever***! Stem cells seem to be helping—Flora describes requests in more detail. "Jenny, where are the stickers you gave me when we came home earlier?" […].

Flora, Jenny & I went shopping yesterday. It was fun, but I'm glad it's the last time for a while. In another reality, we'd be shopping for clothes; but this is the reality we have—glue sticks & keto bread. Still, we had fun.

Last night, we celebrated Flora's birthday at the Famished Frog. She was quite well behaved. Ahhhh […].

With Jonathan, we will survive. He's right though; we'd be so much farther along in autism research & treatments if the powers that be allowed Truth to emerge. It's up to us.

January 11, 2021: […]. Jenny has a much greater sense of family than I do. At least, toward my side of the family. That's Judaism for you.

We took Flora back to Beaver Farm yesterday. She OCD'ed about the thumb drive with family videos. Fortunately, Jenny found it (in her purse!). I'm glad I'm able to make a copy before sending it back to Flora. I'm also glad Flora likes it. Maybe we can pick up where we left off, when Flora was still with us. Before the second MMR shot sent her over the cliff. That would be a miracle. And something the State did not bring about; but rather prayer & hard work on all our parts, especially Flora. I hope—yes, pray!—we can help make her journey successful.

We all decompressed last night […].

I thought about writing a story about, what if our leaders cared about us, ***really*** cared? We'd have a cure—or at least a prevention—for autism. Probably cancer as well. At any rate, we'd be further along in research. But when voices of reason are stifled—Dr. Thomas losing his license, my article being retracted—the struggle is much more difficult. But Nature will prevail; it always does. I just hope—& pray!—to see it in my lifetime […].

I love Jonathan so much. He's my everything.

January 12, 2021: […] Democracy is dead. Authoritarianism is the modus operandi of the day. A small group of monsters—Jeff Bezos, Bill Gates, George Soros, Mark Zuckerberg, the Clintons, Jack Demsey, the CEO of Google—are taking over the world. Why? What are they going to do with the power? What's the point?

Jenny is freaking out these days.

We're on our own. There's no one I'd rather be on my own with than Jonathan.

January 13, 2021: Yesterday was quite pleasant. The drive to Dr. Johnson's office for the IV mistletoe is long, but once there, life is good [...]. Barbara, the IV nurse, said the doctor would be very interested in my work on HPV vaccine & vaccine safety in general. I'll send them my papers.

I had such a feeling of peace & calm during the IV. I see a once-a-week trip in my future. It's good when the doctor who coordinates the treatment is closely associated with the doctor who administers the treatment. Plus, these guys know what is normal—e.g. my puffy eye—and what is not right. The only hitch is the long drive after the treatment. If I ever have a really bad reaction, I can always stay at a hotel to recover.

I have hope again. Hope for the girls (Dr. Johnson & stem cells); hope for me. We will survive.

Jonathan is my perfect mate. We will survive. Too bad we can't do more than that; but in these times, surviving is good.

January 14, 2021: Today is Flora's birthday. Happy Birthday, Flora! I'm so, so sorry life has turned out the way it has for you. Dad keeps telling me it's not my fault, but I can't help but feel guilty for not protecting you. You must believe me that I didn't know. I didn't know—I couldn't even entertain the thought—that doctors would order me to poison you. The doctors themselves don't know, or else Steven [a local autistic boy] would not be sick. But the pharma execs know & the regulators know & the politicians don't think about it, lest a large flow of revenue dries up.

But I didn't know. And now, I—we—are doing everything we can for you to have as happy & productive a life as possible. That is my promise to you [...].

The gynecologist yesterday pointed out I'm getting old. Jonathan is concerned we'll never have sex again. I do wonder whether the Anastrozole is having a negative effect on my sex drive. Ugh. I love Jonathan so much; I will make him happy.

January 15, 2021: Flora seemed positively happy last night when we zoomed. She talked longer than ever before, more with us. Please come back to us, Flora; come home.

Iscador for the first time yesterday. I feel kind of achy, especially my joints. And my left eye is still a little puffy from IV on Tuesday. If these were conventional treatments, I'd be screaming from the rafters. Since they are natural, I say, "OK. That's part of the process." I'm funny that way [...].

Jonathan is so looking forward to sex again. Me, too. I do hope my body cooperates.

January 16, 2021: My hands hurt. I suspect this is how arthritis feels, and I don't like it […]. A body can be fun, but it can also be a pain in the ass […].

Jenny was so funny last night. She wondered aloud what Mrs.—excuse me, DR.—Biden's cause will be. Jenny suggested helping kids get over status anxiety.

It's late (8:40 am!). I need to get to work while my hands still let me.

Jonathan is so soothing. We discussed my hands this morning in bed, and he suggested it's probably not my spine. Maybe the mistletoe. Just hearing his voice was so soothing.

January 17, 2021: My hands & now my upper arms hurt. Could this be a pinched nerve? Dr. Johnson says it could be a reaction to the mistletoe, but that it would be temporary if it is. I'm getting a little fed up with this body of mine.

Last night, we watched *The Searchers* with John Wayne. It was quite good (a LOT to be said for low expectations!) […]. John Wayne & companion search for a girl kidnapped by Indians. Innocence was not rewarded in the Wild West, but neither was revenge. John Wayne was an almost total bigot against the Indians. Almost, because he thought about killing the girl once they found she had adopted the Indian ways, but he didn't.

The time for the search—over five years—the perseverance. I can relate. Only we've been searching for Flora for 15—no, 16—years. At least, we've been on a trail (biomedical) for 16 years. And when do we stop? ***Never!***

When Flora is home, I want to play school with her. We'll have spelling tests, like the word purple. I think she'll do well. Or she can be the teacher. I hope she wants to play […].

Jonathan continues to be my everything. Period. Now, I need to go read the raunchy meme I know he sent last night. I love him so much.

January 18, 2021: Jenny & I watched *Madea Goes to Prison* last night. The film inspired me to teach in a prison. Let me get a semester of teaching Personal Finance under my belt. Then I'll offer my services […].

Jonathan seems less sad. Still sad, but less so. I wish I could help more. He's my everything.

January 19, 2021: Dammit. My circulating tumor cells have increased. From either 2,300 or 2,800 to 3,200. I'm not sure what it means, but it can't be good. I haven't told Jonathan yet; no need to upset him until I have more information. Dr. Johnson might have some insights; I talk with him tomorrow.

My body continues to ache, especially my upper arms and especially at night. I sense the aches are a reaction to the Iscador, not the Pini. Again, Dr. Johnson may have some insights.

Oddly, I do not feel as though I am dying.

Right now, I need to focus on what's important. My husband, my family. A few research projects. Sadly, I don't have much of a research legacy. No students follow my inquiries.

So, as Phil Ochs sang, I guess I have to do it while I'm here.

January 20, 2021: […]. I told Jenny yesterday about my rising number. I'll tell Jonathan today, after I speak with Dr. Johnson. My hands & upper arms still feel a little funky, but nothing unbearable […].

Jonathan starts teaching today, another reason not to needlessly worry him. I love him so much. He's about my only reason for living—certainly my most important.

January 21, 2021: 1/21/21—auspicious? We'll see.

Conversation with Dr. Johnson so helpful yesterday […]. Tumor marker cells are up—since it's an exponential occurrence, rising from 10 to 30 is worse than rising from 2,300 to 3,400 (which mine did). Dr. J suggested if I would ever consider doing conventional medicine, I should do it now. So, I will. Dr. Levitz will be so happy. I wonder if he'll be as happy when things get under control & I decide to go off Ibrance. We'll see […].

Sorry, Jenny just interrupted me with a very intelligent & fun conversation. She promised we will survive. Thanks, Jenny […].

Jonathan took the news about my tumor marker cells well. He's concerned, but he didn't get all serious or depressed. I pointed out, it's not over by any stretch of imagination. It's just I have to be a bit more aggressive with getting rid of those pesky cancer cells.

January 22, 2021: Yikes. My CA 25.27 numbers went down in September, October & November, but started to increase in December & January. Yes, time for more aggressive interventions.

The odd thing is, I feel fine. A little achy, but nothing major. Of course, that's how it was in June. A little achy. Then more achy. Then pings of pain. Then full-blown pain. Then I couldn't walk.

I'm only achy in my upper arms—not my joints.

Anyway, let's move forward […].

So, what do I want to accomplish in life? Knock out a few more articles. Teach in a prison. Get my children well. Not necessarily in that order. Make sure Jonathan is ok if I go first. In fact, I've listed my goals in reverse order.

Jonathan is very concerned. I have to keep his spirits up. So often, the caregiver suffers to point of illness & early death. We're not there & we're not going to get there.

January 23, 2021: Jonathan & I will make love today. Ah, bliss! And then dinner out. Marriage is the reverse of dating—with dating, it's dinner first &

then sex; with marriage, it's sex first & then dinner. Marriage (to the right person) is so much better than dating!

January 24, 2021: According to my numbers, I'm half-dead. Odd, I don't feel half-dead. Still, I should probably get more aggressive with treatment. OK, some conventional drug (Ibrance?). I'll restart carrot juice. And stress, I'll aggressively try to reduce my stress […]

Jonathan & I had a delightful evening out last night. It almost felt normal. As though we had had a normal life with kids growing as they should & our growing older in grace. It's fun to pretend sometimes […].

Jenny is still a pain. She whined about coming with me to exchange the remote. Then she whined about not being able to have candles lit while we were gone. I told her she was causing me stress, but she didn't seem to care. Or if she did care, she was unable to do anything to prevent herself. My daughter with no discipline. Me, for whom discipline comes naturally, gave birth to a hopelessly impulsive id. No, I didn't give birth to an id; I gave birth to a healthy, happy baby. The vaccines blew up several parts of her brain. Worse for Flora, for whom vaccines blew up much more of her brain […].

I love Jonathan so much. I was looking forward to growing old with him. Maybe we still can.

January 25, 2021: Jenny is spinning out of control. Drinking coffee from a trash can—what were you thinking?? Signing up for a modelling school, at $55 per month (recurring). Then she explodes when I tell my friends how she hit me. During the summer, while I was wearing a body brace and a neck brace, she bopped me on the head. She's sick. Very, very sick. [At that point a sharp blow to the head could have left Gayle paralyzed. The *New York Times* reports the case of an autistic adolescent who subjected her mother to five concussions.][7]

Now, she has alerted my friends that my cancer is back, as though she had no influence. The best thing you can do for me, Jenny, is to 1) stop hitting me and 2) become responsible. OK, that's two things. For the love of God, GROW UP.

Jonathan & I suffered through the Judaism course last night. So glad I'm doing the course with him […].

And try to survive. With Jonathan by my side, I will. At least today.

---

7 Joseph Goldstein, "Sabrina's Parents Love Her. But Her Meltdowns Are Too Much," *New York Times,* June 1, 2022.

January 26, 2021: There's a strong possibility I'm not half-dead. Dr. Isaacs explained that CA 27.29 is a protein that cancer cells excrete. Live cancer cells excrete a little, so a higher CA 27.29 count could indicate more live cancer cells. **However,** *dead* cancer cells excrete even more of the protein in the process of dying. The higher number could be an indication that mistletoe is working. The CT scan (I assume) will be more helpful in determining how many active cancer cells I have than the CD 27.29.

I'm so glad I'm not half-dead. The fact that I don't feel half-dead—and that Dr. Isaacs's tests actually show improvement—suggest my cancer cells are the entities who should be getting their affairs in order […].

I started reading a short story by Jenny. It's quite good. I hope we can help her get rid of the garbage so that the real Jenny—and only the real Jenny—shines through.

Jonathan is greatly relieved that I'm probably not half-dead. Marrying him was the smartest thing I've ever done—and I've done a lot of smart things!

January 27, 2021: Jenny is a frickin' genius. Her short story is gripping & animated. I feel so bad for not recognizing her talent earlier. I see Jenny in such a different light now that I've read her short story from 2018. So creative! So vivid! Jonathan is better able to help her develop her talents than I, and he is quite eager to do so […].

Jonathan is excited about Jenny's prospects. I'm so glad he knows how to help her develop her creativity.

January 28, 2021: Jenny & I continue to be friends. It's great!

Jonathan & I also continue to be friends. BFFs as a matter of fact. On my trip up to [Dr. Johnson], I listen to classical music but on the way back I listen to historic pop. Tammy Wynette sang "Stand By Your Man." Yes! Always.

January 29, 2021: I'll call Mom either today or this weekend about the course. She so enjoys coming to my classes. I'm glad, even though my positive feelings for her have faded over time. My feelings are neutral now, I guess. She's limited & weak. I have asked one thing—*one thing!*—of my family (to get together for Christmas) and they couldn't do it. So much for Democrats being inclusive.

Anyway, to work!

I love being Jonathan's wake-up call. And his booty call. I guess you could say I'm his Call Girl!

January 30, 2021: I'm having serious qualms about converting to Judaism. The wokeness of Temple B'nai Or is something I'm not sure I can stay quiet about […]. Jonathan said he & his family have always decided they determine what it means to be Jewish. Rabbis don't tell them what to think.

Jenny overspent her account again yesterday. She signed up for several recurring expenses—including $55 for a modelling course. When she canceled the course, they charged her $55. It's most likely in the contract. We have to close her account entirely. It's a shame, but she needs to learn. So for the foreseeable future, she needs to use cash. If she wants something from the internet, she needs to ask us. Victor's granddaughter, stupid with money! […]. [Victor was a CPA.]

I'm so glad I'm married to Jonathan. I so look forward to our time together. Jenny should be moving into The Group Home on April 1 (no joke!). Let's pray (☺) everything goes smoothly.

January 31, 2021: 7 o'clock Sunday morning. A pleasant time. It's still quiet.

In these quiet moments, I always feel a profound sadness about Flora. And then I turn to the matters at hand, the tasks that I will do today. But I always pause first, and let the feeling come & then go […].

We watched *The Ipcress File* last night. Jonathan said we saw it before, but I have only a very vague recollection. Jonathan wanted to watch *Lord of the Flies*, but I just couldn't. Not last night. Maybe next Saturday. In fact, yes, next Saturday. Jonathan wanted me to be happy, so he didn't push for *Lord of the Flies*.

That's all he wants in life—for me to be happy. And that's all I want in life—for him to be happy. That's all that matters.

February 1, 2021: The first of the month, and all the bills are paid. We even have some money in the bank.

We're getting walloped with snow right now. It is lovely. Except I think of the homeless, who are hungry & now cold. And the children who are suffering with parents who are at the end of their ropes due to the lockdown. And the young man from Drew who went into New York City one Saturday evening a couple of weeks ago & has not been seen since. I wish there was something I could do. [The Drew student, Ajay Sah, apparently jumped from the Brooklyn Bridge; his body was later found downstream.]

Fighting the tyranny that is plaguing our country—our world!—is all I can do. In the most humble of ways.

But let me return to the good in the world. For my Judaism class, I need to write a passage about the ritual of a wedding. Here goes: The first Jewish wedding I attended was my own. It was lovely. The chuppah was adorned with simple, white flowers. I vividly remember how enthusiastically my husband smashed the glass. He explained that the glass symbolizes how fragile life is. Things break, but a strong marriage can overcome all obstacles. Fast forward twenty-five years to find us raising two children with autism and sorting through my metastatic breast cancer, just to mention a few of the curveballs life has sent our way. Jonathan is right—life is fragile, things break, but a strong marriage overcomes those challenges to find good and create in this world.

Yes, that's good enough […].

This morning, I semi-woke Jonathan with a pre-wakeup call. I love being his wakeup call (& his booty call)!

February 2, 2021: Next year will be 2-2-22. Auspicious dates indeed do lie ahead; I thought they ended with 11-12-13 […].

Last night, I had the strangest dream. Not a **teaching** anxiety dream, but rather a **research** anxiety dream. I dreamt I was at an academic institution—unclear whether NYU or Baruch—& I was caught cheating somehow, plagiarism maybe. But I wasn't going to achieve the goal I wanted—the PhD or tenure. But I have much to offer, I kept thinking. So very, very much. Interestingly, I wasn't much bothered at first by not achieving the goal. I'll figure it out, I kept thinking […].

When I related my dream to Jonathan, he held me & promised I was safe. Yes, with him, I'm safe. He keeps me warm & safe & dry & loved. Especially loved.

February 3, 2021: Class was ok yesterday. It's all so artificial. I hope we don't forget what it's like to be in a real classroom. Or have real offices. Or real get-togethers with neighbors. That, of course, is what the Dark Side wants—that we forget what it's like to be human. That our every movement is recorded, documented & archived. That we can be called to task for any misstep or any grievance we have with the elite. 1984 came so quickly.

But we're fighting back. We're finding other ways to communicate. Companies that don't track our every move. And Governor DeSantis is pushing for legislation to allow Florida's citizens to sue Big Tech for cancelling them.

I always saw the endgame. I knew my research would not make much of an impact now, but I looked forward to a time after the blockade had lifted. When we could talk about vaccines openly. But we're headed in the exact wrong direction. Censorship is growing & becoming more insidious.

But that worry is for another day […].

Jonathan & I snuggled this morning. So warm, so safe, so loving.

February 5, 2021: Ugh. Dr. Levitz doesn't agree with Dr. Isaacs that the increase in CA 27.29 could be the result of cancer cells dying off. "Dead cancer cells don't excrete any CA 27.29," he stated. Sometimes, he would see a spike in CA 27.29 after beginning a new treatment, but not a decrease and then an increase.

And yet, I found the following statement on the internet (so it **must** be true):

https://www.verywellhealth.com/cancer-antigen-2729-430607

"CA 27.29 levels will almost invariably rise during the first 30 to 90 days of cancer treatment for some patients as the disruption of the tumor releases CA 27.29 antigens into the bloodstream. Because of this, your oncologist may need to wait two to three months after the start of *each new treatment* to get an accurate test result [...]."

Still, they—Dr. Levitz & Jonathan—have convinced me to take Ibrance. I am **not** thrilled. In a perfect world, Dr. Levitz would have more tools in his toolbox besides drugs and Dr. Isaacs & Dr. Johnson would have more tools than pancreatic enzymes & mistletoe, respectively.

But I'm the cog in the wheel. I need to piece together the information from each of these very bright, very dedicated healers.

I'd love to do a study comparing cancer outcomes in Germany, where mistletoe is widespread, & the United States, where almost no one has heard of mistletoe. Prevalence of cancer, survival rates, quality of life.

Flora will be coming home for President's Day weekend under the following conditions: 1) no snow, 2) she reads a book about clouds with me, & 3) we watch *Phineas & Ferb* together. Flora agreed, and we're good to go.

Jenny continues to mature. It is so beautiful to watch her unfold into a lovely lady. Quirky, but lovely.

Jonathan said he's glad I'm taking Ibrance. I'm not. But I'm glad he's glad. For both our sakes, I want to live.

February 6, 2021: Angela & Mark are getting married today. I'm so happy for them! They are both wonderful people & they deserve happiness [...].

CT scan was quite pleasant yesterday (!) [...]. So, we'll find out in a week whether I'm half-dead. I don't **feel** half-dead. I feel very much alive. Healthy & vibrant. Whatever the results, we'll deal with them [...].

Jenny continues to mature!

Jonathan continues to be perfect, absolutely perfect. We picked out a very nice restaurant to celebrate Valentine's Day/our half-anniversary. I'd marry Jonathan again in an instant. Faster, in fact, than the first I time I said yes.

February 7, 2021: Angela & Mark's wedding was touching. They are both so happy. I wish I could believe in their God, the One who makes everything alright. [They were a Christian couple.] But I've seen too much.

It's snowing. So beautiful. So peaceful [...].

We watched *Lord of the Flies* last night. I think I saw it before. It reminds me of the Democratic party […]. When will the grown-ups in white shoes appear?

I told Jonathan that Mark looked like the Happiest Man on Earth yesterday. Jonathan said *he* was the Happiest Man on Earth. Debate ensued about whether there could be two Happiest Men, but it was decided that there can be only one superlative. That's Jonathan; he's superlative.

February 8, 2021: Yesterday, preparation for classes went nicely. The students are so cute! One admitted that the only way she survived last semester was by cheating. *I didn't hear that!* I thought to myself. Life is rough for them right now. All the uncertainty. How do you deal with that? How did Jonathan & I deal with the uncertainty of our girls' illness? A strong foundation. Figuring out how to enjoy life whenever & wherever possible.

The profound sadness of Flora's condition is constantly with me. I wrote as much on the paperwork for Dr. Ling. [Dr. Yuklin Ling practiced palliative cancer therapy.] Emotions as strong as these are bound to affect my health.

But I'm married to my best friend. Emotions as strong as those are also bound to affect my health […] positively!

February 9, 2021: Jenny continues to mature. One small hiccup on Sunday (head-banging), but she worked through it. Without attacking me. ☺

Jonathan is so wonderful. On my long trips to doctors, I listen to music from the '60s and '70s. When I was lonely, and looking forward to meeting someone like Jonathan. Not really sure that I ever would. But I did. I'm so glad I said, "I do."

February 10, 2021: Rats! I think I forgot to send Jonathan a raunchy meme yesterday. I'm more loyal to my Musing than to my husband. *That* has to change. The memes he sends me are so raunchy & delicious. The ones I send him pale in comparison. But he doesn't compare. He accepts my lame offerings with grace. What a guy, huh? […].

Jenny had a semi-hissy fit yesterday before dinner. During dinner, she promised, "I'll never wait to the last minute to make the salad again." Live & learn. That's how it works.

I had the most adorable conversation with Tracy at Uriel [Homeopathic] Pharmacy […]. Her dog died recently (they put him down), and yesterday she picked up his ashes. She was very sad, but also uneasy about her raw emotions. I suggested she just go with her feelings, not fight them. They are perfectly normal, because the loss of a dog means her everyday life changes. He's not there anymore to greet her. I then related my diagnosis, and Tracy said she would pray for me. Thank you, Tracy. That means a lot […].

Jonathan & I lay in bed for a couple of minutes before the 6:30 alarm. I feel so calm in his arms, warm & loved. Now, let me find a good meme for him!

February 11, 2021: I wonder what great & wonderful things will happen today. Yes, Dad, you're still with me!

Except—ugh—we get the results from the CT scan today. Whatever the results, we'll deal with them, Jonathan & I. Perhaps I'm disrupting the tumors & therefore allowing more cancer cells to be exposed. They were there the whole time, we just didn't see them […].

But I need to focus on what's important. My family, my husband, my kids. And my research & teaching […].

Jonathan & I snuggled for a while this morning. I hope for his sake—and mine!—the news isn't too awful this afternoon.

February 12, 2021: Abraham Lincoln's birthday. Happy Birthday, Mr. Lincoln!

I didn't sleep well last night. Dr. Levitz is ***really pushing*** Ibrance. I know he is sincere in his desire that I survive as long as possible. However, he is limited in his approach. He wants to keep the inevitable—in his mind—growth of the cancer at bay. In his mind, we need to suppress the immune system to do so. The only reason he is suggesting Ibrance is that my CA 27.29 keeps increasing. It went down for a while—which he totally credits the anastrozole—but then started to rise. For three months in a row. He said the tumor markers tend to be harbingers of future cancer. Although the scans showed improvement— yeah!—he suggested that the increase in the tumor markers predicts growth of cancer in the future. He does not agree at all with Dr. Isaacs that the increase in CA 27.29 could be cancer cells dying and excreting the protein.

I pointed out the FDA's Black Box warning that Ibrance could cause lung inflammation. He said he has never seen that clinically. So, we're supposed to believe the FDA when it suits our purposes, but ignore them when it doesn't fit the narrative.

Am I being courageous or stupid? I have a profound mistrust of pharmaceutical companies. And why shouldn't I? They have dramatically altered the lives of my children and by extension the lives of my husband and me. The information they provide is completely biased and self-serving. They are not able or willing to admit mistakes.

I came into this world as an ***oops!*** and I don't want to leave as an ***oops!*** (In that, "Oops! We shouldn't have given her a drug that can cause severe lung inflammation when a deadly virus is circulating.") [Gayle was the result of an unplanned pregnancy.]

I'll ask Dr. Isaacs for her opinion on Ibrance as soon as I receive the reports from Dr. Levitz.

Jonathan gets upset when I talk about all this. I'll talk with Lyn today.

February 13, 2021: Jeez, Louise. My CT scan report is very positive. The includes the words "healing" ***three times!*** Why on earth would we want to change anything we are doing? Why add a harsh drug that could throw my immune system into complete disarray—we don't know why white blood cells go down, but it doesn't ***really*** matter.

The issue, of course, is the CA 27.29. That's the only measure that's out of whack. Lyn had some good suggestions. Ask Dr. Levitz whether he's ever seen a scan that diverges so profoundly with the CA 27.29. Also, what should a person with these CA 27.29 numbers look like? Should they appear healthy & energetic like me? Would you expect these CA 27.29 numbers given the scans & how I feel? Have you ever seen scans showing improvements and CA 27.29 suggesting tumor growth? Could we look at other indications to determine whether Ibrance is really necessary? How long before we would see a difference in CA 27.29 on Ibrance?

Also, have any of his patients needed white blood cell infusions? What about the observations from Drugs.com where recipients (or their surviving relatives) report that Ibrance destroyed their immune systems? Dr. Levitz says markers are ahead of scans, but Dr. Isaacs says markers could be showing that cancer cells are dying off, that healing is occurring. I'll double-check with Dr. Isaacs. I'll also check with Lyn that I understood her correctly: doctors are recommending that many people take Ibrance. Have the people she knows indeed taken Ibrance? If so, what were their experiences?

Lyn totally agreed that Dr. Levitz's approach to disease is diametrically opposed to the holistic approach. Dr. Levitz wants to stop the symptoms, but can't even conceive of the idea of ***healing***.

Jenny became quite agitated when Lyn & I discussed cancer. She still doesn't realize how negatively she can influence the people around her. I need peace & calm. Jenny had about four episodes of pissiness on yesterday's trip. Ugh. Six weeks & she is out of here. Not a minute too soon, for everyone!!

Flora is home for a day & a half. She was pretty good until she couldn't get into her computer last night. She wailed & wailed. What a gift is autism! Finally, she figured out she could use Jenny's computer. Fine. It shut her up.

Jonathan is concerned about the stress on me of having Flora home. Of course, the next time she is home, Jenny should be at The Group Home. That will relieve some of the stress. Jonathan is also questioning Ibrance. "Everything we do is a battle," he noted. There is no one I'd rather fight beside.

February 14, 2021: Happy Valentine's Day!

I hate the medical establishment! Not the frontline workers—especially the nurses & nurses' aides—but the ***establishment***. The ones who make the rules. Yesterday, we tried to obtain a rapid covid test for Flora. Oh, no, they said. The rapid test is only for people with symptoms. And, besides, it's not very accurate. We couldn't ***possibly*** allow her to return to her residence with just a rapid test, said the nurse. Fortunately, the doctor said the turnaround time for the more accurate test (PCR) is less than 24 hours. I hope he's right. Otherwise, we have to lie to Camphill—that we sent the results to the central office—and I don't want to have to do that. Totalitarianism makes liars of us all.

Also, I'm not proud of ***my*** behavior yesterday. I had a hissy fit when the receptionist told me they ***couldn't*** do rapid tests. Then again when the nurse told me they ***wouldn't*** do the test. And then when I was overly happy with the doctor who indicated they ***could*** (and—I suppose—***would***) do the test, but advised against it since the turnaround time was so fast. He gave me hope. False hope, perhaps, but hope nonetheless.

The stress of having Flora home is big. The major stress yesterday was the covid test, so that won't be a problem when she comes home for Spring Break. But Friday night, she howled because she couldn't get into the internet. Interestingly, when I told her to go to bed, she said, "Sure, Mom," and actually started getting ready to go to bed!

And Jenny should be at The Group Home the next time Flora comes home. That's good & bad.

My extended family talked about getting the vaccine yesterday. Ugh […].

Jonathan insists upon taking Flora back today. He sees the toll it takes on me to have her here. He so wants me to be happy & healthy. I feel so loved. I love him so.

February 15, 2021: Whew! Flora's covid test came back in time. Of course, it was negative. The most stressful part of her being here was getting the covid test. Thanks, Medical Establishment, for making our lives even ***more*** complicated. When are you ever going to be happy enough to stop going out of your way to make our lives miserable? […].

They're calling for a wintry mix today. Rats […]. Jonathan & I had a date scheduled for tonight. Well, he knows where to find me, if he wants to postpone our date (I so hope he wants to!) […].

Jonathan is the best! Nothing new, just he is always the best!

February 16, 2021: Enchanting evening with Jonathan. We went to Bistro 46 on Elm Street […]. Jonathan & I talked about his *Playboy* project—it's so wonderful to see him so excited about his work!—and the fact that I'm not half dead (at least, according to Dr. Isaacs). [I was researching a history of *Playboy's* female readers.] I prattled on about my Subotnick Financial Services Center project that I am presenting today and how Andy Ngo's book on Antifa is devastating.

So, yes, according to Dr. Isaacs, I'm not half dead. I'm not even half half-dead. CA 27.29 protein excretion is not reliable, according to Dr. I, especially in light of the treatments I am doing. I have some follow-up questions. Like, she is correct—Dr. Levitz warns that the CA 27.29 elevation is a precursor to increased cancer. Is that a possibility? What could be causing the delayed reaction (better to ask Dr. L that question, perhaps)? [...].

While going out with Jonathan is fun, snuggling with him is even more so!

February 17, 2021: Thought about Ibrance. Pros & cons. I'll present analysis to Dr. Levitz to show why I will not (yet) take Ibrance. He's pushing Ibrance as the great savior. In his world, Ibrance staves off the inevitable for a few months by suppressing the immune system. No, thanks [...].

Jenny had a **huge** hissy fit yesterday after the computer went down. She has to get a grip. I've done everything I know; I don't know how to help her any more. She's on her own.

Same with the overdrawn account. She's on her own [...].

Woke up with Jonathan this morning. I murmured something about his beauty sleep. He said he's sleeping with a beauty. I replied how much I appreciate the beast in him. I love being married to Johnny.

February 18, 2021: This morning, I woke up with a peaceful, easy feeling. Just like the Eagles song. Lying next to Jonathan & then in his arms, a peaceful, easy feeling.

Today, I teach [...]. I hope the electricity stays on long enough for me to get through class. A frickin' Third World country, that's the United States [...]. God help us!

According to Jenny, she straightened things out with the bank. But I keep getting emails saying she owes the bank money. Victor's granddaughter, bad with money; yikes!

But everything's ok when I'm Johnny's arms. A peaceful, easy feeling.

February 19, 2021: Class is going ok. Difficult to tell, when you can't see students. This online teaching is for the birds. However, I don't miss the commute!

I think I've decided not to take Ibrance. Why should I? I'm feeling fine. My scans show vast improvement. Covid is still raging. Why interfere with what appears to be working?

Jonathan's leg was bent in bed this morning. "Oh, it's your knee!" I said. He laughed. I'm glad I can make him laugh.

February 20, 2021: Almost in accident. Service truck with arrow indicating lane closed was moving, then slowed. I almost hit it. Fortunately, the car behind me gave me space. Don't worry about the bullet you dodged. Of course, my brain can't comprehend "don't." All I hear is "worry about the bullet you dodged." Therefore, I'll stop thinking about the incident (***don't*** think about the incident) [...].

And I need to prepare for Judaism class tomorrow. I think I'll talk about the middah of "Sharp discussion with students" & how it's missing in today's society. [Middah: In Jewish biblical reading, a rule or method to explain the meaning of passages to address new situations.]

Jonathan & I will probably make love this afternoon. Ahhhhhhhhh.

February 21, 2021: Sunday mornings are pleasant. A little quieter than most mornings. No one has to work (outside the home ☺). Of course, these days ***no one*** works outside the home. Except for one of Jonathan's classes, everything is online. Life is online. So glad this isn't a growth period for me. Like the first year of college or eighth grade.

We watched *Lilies of the Field* last night. Sidney Poitier. He was excellent. The film was a little slow for my taste. Three stars, not $3\frac{1}{2}$.

Is the ridge where my breast used to be getting larger or did it always extend a little down the sternum? I suppose it doesn't matter. I still have cancer. I'm rereading Suzanne Somers's book and becoming more convinced that I do not want to take Ibrance [...].

I carefully kissed Jonathan this morning. I did rouse him a bit, but he went right back to sleep. I didn't want to rouse him; I just needed to kiss him.

February 22, 2021: Yesterday, I felt tired & slightly nauseous. Either I'm fighting a cold or [...] it's ***CANCER!***

Living in fear is a sucky way to live, and I refuse [...].

This morning in bed, Jonathan & I talked about how senile Joe Biden is. Kinda scary. The leader of the free world *non compos mentis*. I guess the rest of us must keep our wits about us.

February 23, 2021: Survival mode. Yesterday was horrendous. Jenny freaked out when Jonathan asked her to start the potatoes. She went & stayed totally psycho for several hours. There were periods of calm punctuated by violent outbursts. It's like living with a terrorist.

She banged her head on so many surfaces that it's amazing her skull is in one piece. She's destroying everything: our house, my health, Jonathan's shins (where he had an infection several years ago), her future.

I have her computer & her cell phone. She needs to write an essay explaining how her behavior is destructive. She needs to understand how she is destroying everything.

I keep thinking of Josh, whose son was playing cello in the background. The cello! The only background noises you hear from my kids are wails & screams & head banging. It's amazing I've survived this long.

But what's the point of survival? The world is crumbling around us. The government hates us […]. We are not permitted to assemble or to protest. Big Tech silences our voices.

And it all happened so quickly. In the name of a "health emergency." Programs of childhood vaccines were just a dry run for the big event.

Jonathan is the only person in the world I can trust. We will survive.

February 24, 2021: Much better day yesterday. Household walked on egg shells for a while, then warmed up again.

I hate those bad moods of Jenny. Or should I say "Lucifer"? There's Jennifer, and there's Lucifer […].

Lockdown not great for us, but what about people who are just starting out in life? They need to be with other people. Children, young adults, people figuring out who they are. And the elderly. Trying to provide meaning with their last gasps of life.

Jonathan & I make a great team. A dream team. We're the only two people looking out for each other. (I'm sure other people are looking out for each other, but not for us!)

February 25, 2021: Very touching email from Brian Martin [a friend]. His wife (!) has lung cancer. She's taking the conventional route & seems to be doing well. I look forward to responding this morning. I learn things about myself when I write. I guess that's the point […].

February 27, 2021: Dr. Levitz is sad that I'm not doing Ibrance now, but the phone call was short—less than two minutes. We'll still see each other. That's important to him. I guess they teach that in Oncology 101, keep communication with obstinate patients open. He will never admit that Ibrance is not for me. That's ok.

Jenny is going on a walk this morning. I said I would drive her there. We start out at 7:30 to get there by 8am. Yes, Jenny, I love you very much.

Stacy from Temple B'nai Or called to complain about Jenny's behavior yesterday [on a temple hike]. Actually, she was only the conduit for the complaints. Apparently, Jenny was interfering with the others' abilities to get the most out of their "contemplative walk." Helping Jenny was, well, too much of a bother. She wasn't dressed properly; she was afraid of dogs; she kept going in the wrong direction. They want us to hire someone to accompany Jenny. Jonathan is ticked. Where's the tikkun olam? Anyway, he's playing phone tag with Stacy. What a relief that I don't have to deal with this all by myself. I always got the brunt of the complaints when the kids were growing up. "Are you ***the mother***?" [the teacher always] asked me. Of course, I knew she meant to ask whether I was Jenny's mother—the kid who is different—but all I said was, yes, I'm a mother. People are so stupid sometimes. And so kind other times. Kind people are different from the stupid ones. The stupid ones are stupid most of the time. Same with the kind ones: They are kind most of the time.

But not to worry! TBO has put together an "inclusion taskforce" on how to deal with young adults with special needs. They are inviting everyone—parents, teachers, counselors—except special-needs young adults themselves.

Jonathan is on this. He makes my life so much better in so many ways. Standing up to complaining Jewish women (redundant?) is one of them. Is anything alright?

February 28, 2021: Last day of the month. All the bills are paid. We're ahead of the (financial) game.

Jonathan became a little short of breath during our walk yesterday. He needs to be swimming. Goddamn them for closing the pools & the gyms. If anything happens to Jonathan as a result of the lockdown, I will need to take action […]. [Swimming was my main form of exercise, especially in winter.]

The corruption has been growing for a long time, at least since 1986 ("The Act") and certainly before. Actors got away with taking advantage of the system, so they sought more & more power & money […]. The corruption has already destroyed our daughters' lives (ok, destroyed Flora's life; half-destroyed Jenny's) […].

We watched *Boomtown* last night starring Spencer Tracy, Clark Gable, Claudette Colbert & Hedy Lamarr. It was excellent. Love, family, risk-taking. I never noticed Spencer Tracy as a kid. Now I see what a talented actor he was. *Dr. Jekyll and Mr. Hyde*, *Jim & Pat* (or whatever the name of that film with Katherine Hepburn as a golfing buddy [it was *Pat and Mike*]), and, of course, *Judgment at Nuremberg*. Clark Gable I knew from *Gone with the Wind*, but that's about all. CC & HL were completely unknown to me. What a deprived childhood! Ha, ha. I was busy doing other things. And now I have an enriched adulthood! […].

I love Jonathan so much. His raunchy email today has something to do with Fauci. I'm sure—as always—it's quite good […] & raunchy!!

March 1, 2021: Life seems to be opening up a bit. Murphy is allowing churches to open at 50% capacity. Some restaurants are returning. The

Tyrants—Bill Gates, Anthony Fauci, Governors Cuomo, Murphy, Newsom, Wolf & Whitmer (in MI)—loathe relinquishing their power. But the take-down of Cuomo could be giving at least the politicians pause. His reversal of fortunes is occurring so quickly.

The first-year anniversary of the lockdown will bring contemplation. People have sacrificed a tremendous amount, for what? […].

Yesterday, when I picked up Jenny at Washington House restaurant, I fear I scared some people with my brace. I wanted to say, "No, I'm not a terrorist." But I thought that might make them more upset.

Mistletoe IV today. I'm so grateful to be able to receive the medical treatment that I choose is right for me.

Ugh. I have to deal with the anesthesiologist wanting to charge me another $2,000. If the insurance company can demand its money back, then I will also demand my money back! Ha, ha. Just like the cleaning lady who wanted a sabbatical. And why not? Some people are proposing a guaranteed income. Instead of guaranteeing total income, how about giving every citizen (!) a sabbatical every seven years. Time off to think […] about stuff.

Jonathan has sabbatical in the Fall. I'm doing an online, totally asynchronous course. Ooh, la la. I see trouble […] ☺

March 2, 2021: This morning, I feel a bit tired. As though I had a big workout yesterday & my body needs to recover. No pain, just blocked passageways opening & bad cells being routed out. Some of the cancer cells we might be able to convert back to good cells; others are too far gone & they've gotta go. Unlike many people who do pharmaceutical chemo, I feel better doing natural chemo, not worse. I'd rather do natural chemo than nothing at all. I feel good, really good […].

In other news, the Democrats are eating their own. Cuomo—who killed at least 15,000 by sending them back to nursing homes even when they had Covid—is being excoriated on simple sexual harassment. He's doing the usual *mea culpa*, but—as with almost everyone except Brett Kavanaugh—that is not enough. The progressives want his scalp […].

Jonathan & I bantered about the German term "Herr" this morning. I forget how it started, but I noted that I have hair. Then I remembered the story of a man with the last name of Herr in Germany; he was Herr Herr. His wife with Frau Herr (talk about gender confusion!). And there's Hans Herr, but we always called him Hans Her. So, here we say Herr as her. Huh!

March 3, 2021: […] I kissed my fingers & put them on Jonathan's forehead this morning. I didn't want to wake him, but I needed to touch him.

March 4, 2021: Dr. Johnson was absolutely ecstatic over my scan. Improvements in all areas, he noted. The estrogen blocker itself could not produce results like this. Anastrosole can slow cancer growth, but it typically does not reverse cancer damage. Certainly not at the levels described in the scan. He cautioned we're not out of the woods, but he suggested we're on a good path.

And I feel great. A comment Dr. Levitz made after I acquiesced to taking Ibrance was about a woman who resisted taking the drug but finally agreed. "She said she felt so much better that she wished she had taken it earlier." But I already feel great; I can't feel any better.

Jonathan is with me fully. He was reluctant for a while, as was I for a brief moment. Ibrance is now the standard of care. It keeps the cancer at bay, it suppresses the disease; but eventually nature emerges. With a vengeance. The forces of Nature do not like when you mess with them. That's why using Nature (mistletoe) to address Nature (cancer) is so much safer & effective.

IMO. But what do I know? I'm just some Dumb Broad […].

Jonathan & I will soon be Empty Nesters. Great for everyone. I was afraid for a while that we would get the girls housed & then I would die. If I had followed conventional medicine, I'd probably already be dead. Or worse, half-dead. Now, I feel healthy & well on my way to a vibrant next phase of life. With my BFF.

March 5, 2021: Great day yesterday […]. Jonathan's leg is healing thanks to the cream Lyn gave me! God gave us everything we need to be healthy. It's all right here […].

Jenny is at her overnight [at The Group Home, which] seems to be getting to know her, and they still seem to accept her! The real Jenny is a wonderful person. Lucifer is a person I simply do not know. The look in her eye, the lashing out. She becomes an animal toward me. And that's the key point. Lucifer is directed at me & Jonathan. Her public behavior can be improper—the outbursts at Drew, for example—but those seem to be pretty much gone. Unless I'm around […].

Jonathan & I will have time to ourselves. First time in how many years? First time, actually, ever! We richly deserve fun together.

March 6, 2021: Jenny is a selfish pain in the ass sometimes. Like last night. After a successful overnight at [The Group Home] & a pleasant day, she got upset when Jonathan tried to show me some research about HPV vaccine & fertility (spoiler alert: Merck knew!). She began hitting herself & at some point screaming. After she calmed down, she said she needed to donate blood today in Chatham. This is after the walk we are driving her to.

So, she trashes my work & then wants me to drive her to the mall. At what point, one wonders, will she ever grow up?

I locked the bedroom door & went to sleep. It took so much energy **not** to beat the shit out of her. But I didn't. It just would have made things worse. But it did mean I had to—once again—suck it up.

Jonathan will take her & pick her up from the walk today. I have a ton of work now that I'm back teaching. Also, I have the Monday/Thursday treatments. I feel great, but the treatments are time-consuming.

And the continued paperwork for both Jenny & Flora […].

I would not be able to survive without Jonathan.

March 7, 2021: Flora will be home in less than a month, and Jenny will be moved out in lesser than less than a month (assuming all goes well). Nice!

We do have to get moving—or rather get **others** to move on Flora's placement […]. I'm just so tired of the phone calls & the details & the chasing down of people. But this may be the last push for both girls. At least for a while.

It never ends & it never will […]

We watched *Four Daughters* last night. It was cute, with Claude Rains & Victor's childhood friend John Garfield. 1938. The world was still depressed. Still slogging on & for what? Mismanagement & greed. Like today. Only today is more violent.

No time to correct the errors of the world—I have work to do!

And make sweet love with Jonathan this afternoon […]

March 8, 2021: Finally moving on research. Rejection from *Journal of the Royal Society of Medicine* included no comments. Just "no." This is science? […].

Jonathan & I made sweet love yesterday. I pounced on him right as he was about to come. Ah, heaven!

March 9, 2021: Spring is emerging! And it is beautiful!

[…] as always & forever, I'm grateful for Jonathan. I'm grateful he is on this earth, that I know him & that we share our lives together.

March 10, 2021: Jenny seems calm. Three weeks before move-in (I hope!). She gets upset, but—for the most part—she has a handle on it. Let's pray her equilibrium continues. For everyone's sake, especially hers.

I love waking up next to Jonathan. His smiling face, his warm embrace. Ah, I love Spring […] when the juices start flowing […]

March 11, 2021: Ugh. Although Jenny's move-in date is April 1, she may not actually **move in** on April first. She may not move in at all. There's an approval process that [The Group Home] was very unclear about. Even if she is approved—and Jonathan is convinced she will be—we have to have her support people in place. **What??**

Jenny jumps on my computer & reads my private musing whenever she can. I just noticed that the "2020" folder was recently opened. Not by me. Also, she made her ride wait while she ate dinner. She was messing around on the computer & the phone, arranging something for someone's birthday. That's all very nice, but she needs to focus on what's important. What she needs to do to survive, to get a job, to pay rent. She expects everyone to wait on her with no give & take. Birthday presents for strangers while the rest of us take care of her. Fortunately, the talk of being "underprivileged" has faded. She spends ways too much time on the internet [...].

My Boll & Branch towels & jammies arrived yesterday. They are so soft, so warm.

Just like Jonathan. The warm part, anyway.

March 12, 2021: Much to do over the next couple of weeks. Class prep is time-consuming [...]. Taxes. Helping Jenny get a job [...].

Jonathan is so soothing. He's so good for my soul [...] & my body!

March 13, 2021: We see Flora today. I like when we're a family. It's nice to pretend, even for a moment [...].

I am profoundly sad for both my girls. Their lives are difficult, Jenny's in some ways more difficult than Flora's. Neither is the girl she is supposed to be. But I don't like to dwell. Dwelling is: 1) time-consuming; 2) enervating; 3) cancer-enhancing [...].

Plus, Jenny was a real pill yesterday afternoon & evening. She desperately wanted to donate blood. Doesn't mind how much she puts us out. She lied & said she was going to a church service, but she had made an appointment to donate blood. Last week, when we wouldn't drive her to Chatham to donate blood, she took an Uber ($12 each way). She was turned down, because of her glutathione patch. Then on Monday she took at Uber ($30 each way) to, she claims, "take a walk with friends." She is so dreadful at lying. And so irresponsible. She keeps making the same mistakes—overspending on Uber (and Cameo) and then complaining that she doesn't have enough money. Cameo purchases are getting better, but Uber is getting worse. She cannot be trusted with money.

Jonathan & I peed at the same time—well, we got up at the same time to pee. Our bodily fluids joined & mixed. Ah, glad I could make it. [This was a married couple's inside joke. When we were newlyweds we once arose in the middle of the night and bumped into each other in the bathroom. "Oh, Gayle," I exclaimed, half awake, "glad you could make it."]

March 14, 2021: Iscador—the next major step on my path to healing. Yesterday, I injected about 1/3 of an ampule, and I feel fine. Is my breast-area rash fading or is that my imagination? Time will tell. One red spot became more red, but that could be part of the healing process.

The video playing in my head (á la Scott Adams) takes place 32 years from now. I think back on when that oncologist—I will have forgotten his name—said I had seven to ten years to live. I'll smile & say, "And that was 32 years ago."

The video about being interviewed by a perky 20-something NYU reporter about the time before the common-sense discovery that vaccines could cause harm still plays in my head. [That interview did take place, but the young reporter dismissed her concerns about vaccines.] Getting to that point—where people realize that vaccines can cause harm—is blurry. But I'll be in my dotage, saying, "Yes, people used to think injecting poisons into newborns would make them *healthier*! Can you *imagine?*"

Jenny is on a better keel, though she is running out of some vitamins & didn't tell me. Ugh.

Flora looks good. Calmer for sure.

Dr. Kripsak called. He'll be able to administer the stem cells. Yay! To be honest, I'm not sure how much it's helping, but Jonathan is adamant & I don't see any harm. Flora *is* calmer, & Jenny—though banging her head—is catching herself more often with more control over outbursts.

Travelling through life with Jonathan is a dream, a beautiful, bright dream.

March 15, 2021: Although I feel a little overwhelmed these days, I know I'm so fortunate not to have a real job. Can you *imagine?* Going to an office or even remote activities that someone else dictates each & every day. I shudder.

It would be almost as bad as being married to the wrong person. Though I have no clue what that is like. ☺

PS: Add ungumming Jonathan's computer to my list of awesome things to do today. I love when I can do things for him. He's my BFF.

March 16, 2021: I'd really like to talk with Lyn Redwood about our kids' aggressiveness […].

Yesterday, I cleaned up Jonathan's computer & he was so grateful. I'm so happy when he's happy, especially when I can be part of what makes him happy.

I'm so grateful for so many things. I'm grateful not to have a real job […]. I'm grateful not to have to commute this semester. I'm grateful we can try different therapies with the girls. (I'm *not* grateful they are injured!) Most of all, I'm grateful to have found & married Jonathan.

March 17, 2021: I'm so sick of doctors. Jenny needs a TB test, so we have to deal with conventional medicine. Uck. On the other hand, I'm in the process of setting up appointments for the girls to get stem cell treatments. Not all doctors are so bad […].

Jenny hasn't taken her P5P for the past couple of days & it shows. Edgy, panicky, bitchy. & then she lies about taking her pills—I *did* take them, she proclaims. But she didn't. I had counted the pills, because she was running short, & the number was the same today as two days ago. I tried to gently tell her to sort her pills.

She doesn't change when we advise her gently. Change seems to happen when she's in a heightened state & we're all yelling at each other. Except that change doesn't happen then either. She has so few obligations in life. Sort her pills, put her laundry away, unpack new clothes (her new boots still have tags on them). She expects everyone to wait on her.

But she also wants approval for e.g. cleaning a pot. So, she does want to please.

My neck started bothering me when I was talking with Ruth Beiler last night. Talking was difficult since Jenny was in the room. When I mentioned Mr. Kennedy's name, Jenny reacted negatively. Ruth mentioned abuse in the Amish community. I wish I could have responded, but I didn't know how. I have to let her know that abuse is never ok. That authorities are there to help […].

I so love Jonathan. He was touched that I was so touched when he took such good care of me over the summer. He said he was worried about me, that he could take his mother's passing philosophically [she was 95 when she died], but he would not be able to do that with me [I wasn't]. I will not allow autism to destroy me as it has destroyed our girls.

March 18, 2021: Nice having a meeting with colleagues yesterday. It makes me feel like a grown-up!

And lunch with the girls was fun too. The conversation started with vaccination status. Ugh. "Better than nothing," they said. "Better than getting Covid." No & No. The lies we hear. The lies some of us live by.

Another mistletoe infusion today! I always feel so good when I'm flooded with mistletoe. So strong; so healthy.

Yikes! I forgot to send Jonathan a raunchy meme yesterday. It's as though yesterday didn't really happen.

I tried unsuccessfully to kiss Jonathan this morning silently, so as not to wake him. When I saw he was mildly roused, I explained that I couldn't keep my hands off him. "Just reach out & grab me anytime," he murmured.

March 19, 2021: I picked up Jenny last night, even though Jonathan had planned to do so. It was rainy & crappy; finding the restaurant was easier with

GPS. I like being able to do things for him. Doing nice things for Jonathan is one of my greatest pleasures.

March 20, 2021: It's unbelievable to me that people believe that once they are vaccinated, they can't get sick. I guess they hear that they can get sick, but the illness would be much milder than had they not had the vaccine […]. Plus, if you're under 65, it's never a big deal, unless you had an underlying condition (cancer, anyone?). Still, I'm less afraid of the disease than other people's reactions if I were to get Covid […].

Awk! They've turned us against each other. For what? So they can control our lives. Mediocre people (at best!) finally have power, & they are not giving it up.

Michaela [a friend and personal organizer] said she would help out Jenny. She did ask about the Covid status, though she is fully vaccinated. She wanted to make sure everyone was tested. They are […].

I love Jonathan so much. I didn't have time to make his pudding yesterday—and probably won't today. He's cool about that. He understands. Let me get to work on my lecture so I have time to make the pudding on Sunday!

March 21, 2021: Yesterday was quite a day! Kim called & said Jenny could not come to her party unaccompanied. WTF?!? She's so terrified of Covid […]. Jenny had a huge flare-up, but Jonathan & I went to the demonstration for freedom [in lower Manhattan] anyway. I'm glad we did. Jenny calmed down, so there do not appear to be major repercussions there. We met several very interesting people. A mom who wants a normal life for her kids, a Baruch graduate student who is worried about his future, an artist who is documenting through photographs just how wrong life is going in New York. One of the speakers had us hug our neighbor. What a rebel she is! [With my arm around Gayle, I joked that "Those Sixties radicals were right: protest demonstrations are a great place to pick up hot chicks."]

But that's just it—they want us to hate our neighbor or rather to be terrified of our neighbor. The person living next door could have cooties.

And so many of my friends at Kim's party are falling for it, hook, line & sinker. So sad […].

America is basically a good country. We continue to have issues of race, but let's raise up downtrodden people, not obliterate the middle class that worked so hard to get where it is […].

Jonathan & I make a great team. He really enjoyed being in NYC, eating at a serendipitous restaurant, visiting the Strand Bookstore, which, thankfully, is in full bloom. He looked 20 years younger as we ate outside of the Israeli restaurant. We topped off the day by watching *A Farewell to Arms*. I was hoping they would put a Hollywood Ending on the film (like *Maedchen in Uniform*), but Helen Hayes died in the end. I guess you can't take the "farewell" out of "Farewell to Arms." I keep playing the video in my head, "He told me I had seven to ten years to live [...] thirty-two years ago!" All with Jonathan by my side.

March 22, 2021: Nineteen years. Wow. I miss Dad so much, more than I ever thought I would. He was the only family member who cared about my well-being. He & Mom—in her own way. But Dad really cared. About **all** members of his family. Life is to be enjoyed. We face & deal with issues & then we enjoy life. Period [...]. My family has hurt me so much. Everyone, except Dad. He was always there for me & my family.

Jenny is putting together a tribute for him [...].

The teacher of the Judaism course pointed out we need to rework our brains so that it's ok to socialize again. The statement suggests we've been brainwashed. She doesn't realize that, but she's right. The authorities have brainwashed us—most people anyway—into thinking everyone is an enemy. We need to rethink how we interact with people.

Jonathan went biking by himself yesterday. I was with him in spirit. I'm a little wobbly about going biking. Like the First Time.

March 23, 2021: Jenny created a very touching video for Dad. Family is so important to her. I'm sorry I couldn't give her a better extended family.

Jonathan takes such good care of me [...] in sickness & in health. We both prefer health!

March 24, 2021: We ran into Helene & Paul [neighbors] last night. They were so cute! But then the conversation turned to vaccines—as most conversations do these days. When they asked whether we were yet vaccinated, we said no. When they pushed & asked whether we planned to get vaccinated, I said no & told them why. Jonathan cringed. I do think we need to speak out. We have legitimate questions about the vaccine that should not be ignored.

Jonathan says he admires my spunk. The vaccine issue is one of those areas where I'm spunkier than he. I sense he still loves me. I know I still love him; he's my BFF.

March 25, 2021: I mentioned to Jonathan that now that I'm on Spring Break, we should go to Miami! I crack myself up! Apparently the revelry & rowdiness in Miami is nothing new this year—well, maybe a bit more due to pent-up frustrations from the lock-down—but the media are trashing the activities since Florida is open. Ron DeSantis for President! I say [...].

I look forward to our tour of Kimberton [an adult Camphill community near Beaver Farm]. Reminds me of when I was searching for an academic position. When Jonathan said Baruch had called, I thought, yeah, whatever. Turns out it was the best choice possible. Under all the circumstances.

As long as I can live out the rest of my years with Jonathan in peace, I don't care about the rest of the details. Of course, we want our girls to be safe & happy. That's part of the "in peace" part.

March 26, 2021: Spring is beautiful! The juices are flowing, & I have lots of energy. I also have a small herpes outbreak ☹. Nature can be so cruel. Lysine seems to be helping.

Eleven minutes to coffee.

I'll stave off hunger pangs by reading the raunchy email Jonathan sent me & finding one for him. Excellent use of time, if I do say so myself.

Upon hearing the 7 am alarm, Jonathan started farting reveille. I so love being married to him.

March 28, 2021: [...] We also celebrate Passover via Zoom. I wonder if we were vaccinated whether Suzanne would host an in-person Seder. The idea is totally hypothetical, so forget it.

We watched *Young Cassidy* last night. Jonathan was very pensive afterwards. I was too flighty to partake in his pensiveness, & I regret that now. I should have asked what he was thinking. I'll do that today. Does he think of Catherine when he sees something Irish (even though, yes, I know, she was Welsh? [No. I was not thinking of Catherine, a girlfriend from my remote past who was actually English. *Young Cassidy* (1965) was a fictionalized biopic about the Irish playwright Sean O'Casey. It celebrated his willingness to buck public opinion and tell audiences what they did not want to hear. And it struck me that in 2021 we were trying to tell the world what many did not want to hear: that the autism pandemic was decimating a generation.] I love knowing what he's thinking. His ideas are so fascinating. And—despite all odds against us—we have built a beautiful, caring family.

March 29, 2021: Much to do today. Get *JRSM* article review on paper. The authors are a bunch of snooty "experts" who are telling people, "Don't worry. We'll confirm that the vaccine we approved is safe." Amazing that the general public still put so much faith in these turkeys [...].

We need to get out more, Jonathan & I. Seeing Jonathan's family yesterday for Passover was nice. We're a family, who share stories, memories [...].

Jonathan is stirring. I like to read his raunchy email before he comes down for breakfast. Reading his raunchy email is the highpoint of my day.

March 30, 2021: Slept well. Dreamt Tadeo [our plumber, who has an autistic son] planted a listening device in our house. Soviet-style. Weird. [He would never do that.]

Much work today […]. Review for *Journal of Royal Society of Medicine*. I'm putting way too much time into thinking about that review. But that's how I do things—with my entire heart & soul.

Like the way I love Jonathan—entirely, completely, forever.

March 31, 2021: My Spring Break feels broken. After meeting with The Group Home, Jenny attacked me. I know she's nervous & she's attacking—trying to attack—her autism, but she physically assaults me. Yesterday, it was just pinching, but it's been hitting, punching, pulling hair. Matt [her boyfriend] pointed out correctly that someday she's going to hit the wrong person & regret it.

Being her mother is so difficult. The costs outweigh the benefits […].

And the review for the *JRMS*. The most disturbing aspect of the review is that the more I learn about the covid "vaccine," the more terrified I become. It's not a vaccine in that it does not evoke an immune response. It is a technology that purposely changes RNA or DNA or whatever. Something fundamental to existence. In the short-term, the vaccine appears to be linked to anaphylactic shock & blood clots. No one knows the long-term effects, but people have raised questions about fertility & cancer as well as enhanced immune response when confronted with the wild virus. No wonder the authorities need to coerce people to subject themselves to the medical intervention […].

Yesterday, Jonathan magnified his worth as a human being, if that is possible. He let me vent about Jenny without passing judgement or accusing me of being a bad mother. I could not survive without him.

April 2, 2021: Flora comes home today. Probably for the last time for any stretch of time. I am profoundly sad with what they did to her, but, right now, I need to focus on helping her lead the best life she can. We explore Kimberton this afternoon.

We spoke with several agencies yesterday. Everyone wants Flora! The AVIDD place in Basking Ridge looks good. The residents seem happy. We could see more of Flora. She could probably work somewhere. We could provide the organic food. We'll see.

No parent should be facing these decisions. But, as Jonathan pointed out, at least we *have* choices. Yeah, I guess […].

Jonathan also makes me laugh. He knocked over his computer on Wednesday. Yesterday, we got him a new one & set it up. I'm so happy, when I can do little things for him. He does so much for me. Like yesterday afternoon […]

April 3, 2021: Survival Mode. That's what we're in. It's like Safe Mode, but for humans instead of computers.

Flora is home. Fun food is locked up. Major tantrum about DVD player, but she got past it. NuSera helped.

Yesterday, we visited Kimberton. The souls kind of wander the premises. Flora could get lost. Yes, the fresh air is great & the healthful food is wonderful, but neither the fresh air nor the healthful food of Beaver Farm have helped Flora to blossom. She's still fat & not very communitive or social. Basking Ridge is looking better & better. I could continue to try treatments, but send her back at the end of the day. This could work. We can buy a lot of organic food for $50,000 a year (Kimberton tuition) or $70,000 (Triform).

Too bad about Camphill. I'm grateful we were able to give it a try. Flora did seem to blossom at Beaver Run. She lost some weight, looked happy.

One good aspect of Basking Ridge: low expectations.

And Jenny & Flora could be sisters more often. They do have a camaraderie [...].

Jonathan's raunchy email was two people making out in a laundry room. "Better with a laundryman" was Jonathan's subject line. He's so much fun to be married to. [Jonathan's maternal grandfather owned a commercial laundry.]

April 4, 2021: Jonathan & I watched *Showboat* last night. It was sweet; Jonathan was more touched than I. He loved having me in his arms, while people sang about loving their man. I loved being in his arms while people sang about loving their man. Paul Robeson had a tremendous voice. "Old Man River"—which I like to sing when I have a cold—comes from *Showboat*. I thought it was a classic Negro spiritual [...].

Also, spoke with Sandy Nemeroff yesterday. More precisely, she talked to me. & talked & talked & talked. Interesting, energetic [Orthodox Jewish] vaccine-safety activist.

The idea of Flora living in Basking Ridge is quickly growing on me. Jonathan is correct: The first night she is home, I'm so happy to be a family. But then reality sets in & my nerves fray. If she & Jenny could come for dinner once a week & then go back home, life would be good [...].

Feeling Jonathan so touched by *Showboat* was itself touching. He's amazing.

April 5, 2021: Slept nearly the entire day yesterday. Temperature gyrates, but appears to be 99.9. Could Iscador be creating this fever reaction three days out?

Basically, I missed the Passover Seder. So sad. There are worse things, but I wish I had felt better. Jonathan led a wonderful Seder. Flora sipped some wine (!) & Jenny read beautifully.

I don't think I have Covid, since taste & smell seem fine. I'm listless, though, & no appetite. I'm certainly not going to get checked into & then put in a database […].

I love Jonathan so much.

April 6, 2021: I'm feeling better. Yesterday, my temperature went as high as 101.5, if the thermometer is to be believed. My sense of smell is fine: Jonathan farted this morning & PEE EWE! I'm assuming it's the Iscador doing what it is supposed to do […]. If the downward trend in my temperature continues, I'm fine […].

It's not helping that the girls are both (each?) being a pain. Jenny doesn't watch Flora when we ask her to […]. She's so irresponsible, yet when we point that out, she goes into a rage. Flora is just being the pain she always it—eating too much, going her own way. As long as I don't have Covid, we only have two more weeks of this hell […].

April 7, 2021: I'm feeling better, though my appetite is still in the tank […] & I'll finally make an appointment with the Rabbi for the first Thursday after Flora is gone. I'm dragging my feet on this. Mom said I can bullshit my way through anything; I'm not sure I can bullshit my way through this one. The Progressives are *so* pious & sanctimonious. People of a certain political persuasion are treated differently from those with different political ideas. Or not even political "ideas," more manifestos.

Flora was up very late this morning. At 3:15 am I caught her almost eating an entire box of cereal. Then she wanted bread. I had lots of energy at 3:15 am—the kind of energy you have after sleeping for three days—but when it was time to wake up this morning (6:30 am), I didn't want to. Flora wrote a lot of [unintelligible] stuff on yellow papers. I wish I understood. [We joked that Flora could become a federal bureaucrat, filling out meaningless reams of paper.]

I love Jonathan so much. Nothing new there; just love.

April 8, 2021: Yesterday, when Flora & I asked what we're looking forward to tomorrow, Flora said, "Going to Montville." She absorbs so much! Also, she cleans so beautifully. She's so much like me!

I love Jonathan, madly!

April 9, 2021: Jenny is a parasite who expects her hosts—Jonathan & me—to take care of her every need. When we aren't around, whoever is can be *in locus hostus* […].

Now she wants us—neh, ***demands us***—to take her to Randolph to drop off baby wipes for a charity. So giving to others; so demanding of us. She said she told me the baby wipes were for charity when she bought them. I had to stop & think for a minute; she didn't tell me the charity was in Randolph. I thought it was at the church in Morristown. Donating items to a church in

Morristown makes sense; donating to a charity in [far more remote] Randolph does not.

When we refused to take her, she became violent. I locked myself in the bedroom so not to be attacked. She hit Jonathan & kicked Flora. Jonathan called the police. They are absolutely terrific at defusing the situation.

On a lighter note, my cancer seems to be moving. A red spot has now turned to a blister, which strikes me as being a good thing. My temperature went to 101.5F at one point on Monday. Yes, I felt like crap for a couple of days, but if the cancer clears up, it's worth it. Today, I take another dose of Iscador. Let's see what happens.

We saw a group home yesterday in Montville. It was nice, but the residents seemed a little low-key for Flora.

Today, it's stem cells & then Basking Ridge.

How could I survive all this without Jonathan? I couldn't.

April 10, 2021: Flora's very allergic reaction yesterday to the stem cells was scary. She started to itch, her ears turned beet red, she started to wretch. Dr. Kripsak—I get such a kick out of saying his name—said he never saw anything like this with stem cells. He said the stem cells were probably too concentrated; they aren't supposed to push the cells […] Flora recovered with Zertec & is absolutely fine now. But for about five minutes, *she didn't want to eat.* Something was wrong. But she came around relatively quickly […].

Could Flora have an autoimmune condition? Maybe we can test for that […].

The colder I am to Jenny, the nicer she is to me. Ice Queen, here we come. & it feels so right […].

The hotter I am to Jonathan, the nicer he is to me. & it feels so right.

April 11, 2021: Jenny continues to be a conniving wench. My being an Ice Queen toward just feels right. "You like Flora more than you like me!" she protests. "Flora doesn't hit me," I reply.

Why on earth should I continue to bang my head against a brick wall; I'm not autistic. And yet the abusive relationship Jenny & I have—Jenny abuses me—continues. When she graduated, I didn't care. She had hit & scratched & kicked me so often, I was numb by the time she earned her diploma. Ditto her book. I tried & tried & tried. There's no reservoir of understanding, of caring. She's blamed me one too many times. No longer will I enable her to treat people—including me—so shabbily.

Yes, yes; I realize it's her condition. But she's not even trying. She blames her condition for her shoddy behavior. I will go along no longer.

Flora is somewhat more verbal! & more eye contact. Stem cells seem to work a bit.

Jonathan & Flora went biking yesterday. He's such a great dad. & husband. & lay.

April 12, 2021: Jenny continues to be a pain in the ass. I wish she would just leave me alone. Yesterday, I lent her my keys; she forgot to return them & they ended up in Flora's Coach bag. "This is why you can't have your own keys, Jenny," I pointed out. So, she gets mad at me. Then, when she didn't clean up the mess she made dishing up Flora's ice cream, she got mad at me. That's ok, Jenny; don't help. I'm better off without your help.

I've played along for too long, encouraging her "helpfulness" & overlooking the messes. "She's trying," I kept telling myself. She's trying, for sure, but she's not succeeding. When I try to help her to succeed, she gets mad at me, starts screaming, "I can't do anything right!" & tells her friends (and mine when she was able to access my phone) what a terrible mother I am.

ENOUGH!

Flora was still up at 4:30 this morning. Amazing that she is able to get back into the Camphill routine relatively easily. I hope she can find worthwhile employment that occupies much of her day.

I love Jonathan. I know converting would make him happy. Maybe I can convert on my terms.

April 13, 2021: Jenny has been reading my Musings on my Chromebook. Perhaps that's why she's so angry. She knows my true feelings. She has a choice—either believe me or believe the garbage on the internet.

She's looking over my shoulder right now.

Flora seems to be making very positive changes. When she gets upset—again, typically when Jenny gets upset—her reactions are not nearly as intense and they don't last as long. Last night was somewhat of an exception, but Jenny's tirade was also very intense & very prolonged.

And Flora is more with it. Gradually, but steadily.

The allergic reaction to the stem cells—could something have been in the solution that made her so sick? Fortunately, whatever it was was temporary.

OK, I'm going to stop writing. Jenny is peering over my shoulder.

I love Jonathan. I could not survive the living hell without him.

April 14, 2021: Jenny went on a bender last night. That's the only way to describe it. It's like living with an alcoholic, never knowing when they are going to explode.

We were watching Tucker Carlson, who did a great piece on whether Covid vaccines were safe & effective. He raised questions, that's all. Just like Jonathan

& I are doing. We're definitely not alone. [Carlson and Sharyl Attkisson were practically the only television personalities who questioned the safety and effectiveness of vaccines. After he was dismissed from Fox News in April 2023 he became an apologist for Vladimir Putin and offered an uncritical platform to a Holocaust denier, and then I would have nothing more to do with him.]. Jenny was starting to get twitchy. She chewed on her blouse & the TV remote. Then she started banging her head on the glass. I wanted to throttle her, but I resisted the urge & hit the couch with my fist & said, "Stop!" She lunged at me with the hateful, out-of-control look in her eye & started choking me & hitting between my shoulder blades. When Jonathan tried to intervene, she started kicking him. Like a wild animal. Jonathan eventually called the police, who eventually calmed her.

God, Jenny, why? Why are you reading those awful websites that you know upset you & then why do you take it out on us? Why? Dad & I are part of the solution. You seem intent on ruining your life & it's getting worse. There is no universe in which this behavior is acceptable.

Of course, in the heat of battle, I forget about Passiflower & NuSera.

Also, Jenny could avoid the garbage websites. At least until we take Flora back to Camphill.

Speaking of Flora—who, understandably, got very upset last night—we put in train her moving to Basking Ridge. I'm at peace with that decision. While I had envisioned her staying within the Camphill community, Basking Ridge is close & we can be a family (of sorts!). Have dinner once a week […] and then send both girls home. There's beauty in that arrangement.

Speaking of beauty, Jonathan & I have one of the most beautiful, caring, giving relationships in the world. Love in the Age of Autism.

April 15, 2021: Jenny is doing better. It's so difficult for me to be warm to her. Yes, I treat Flora differently. Flora doesn't beat me up. Or attack me verbally.

Flora was upset, because internet didn't work […] on her cell phone! She is exploring more. Also, her DVD player isn't working, but she found other things to do last night (until 4 am). Things are changing. Hope springs eternal […].

Every day—but these days in particular—I'm so glad to be married to my soulmate.

April 16, 2021: Two more nights of Flora's soul wandering through the house after we go to bed. She does seem a bit more with it after stem cell & Dr. Johnson's remedies. It will be fun having her close by […] but not in the house.

Jenny remains on a more even keel. Yeah! […]

Jonathan is my knight in shining armor. Yesterday, I felt like crap after my xgeva shot. He stepped in, no hesitation. And he never seems to tire of helping me. He seems, in fact, to enjoy it.

April 17, 2021: Flora responds well to PMS homeopathic remedy. She had a hissy fit yesterday in Lyn's office, but calmed almost immediately after the remedy [...].

Jonathan & I will soon be empty nesters. He's already getting quite horny. I'll actually believe the girls' being settled when I see it [...]

April 18, 2021: Flora's last returning-to-Camphill supper at the Famished Frog (where else?) went nicely. We were in the bar at a round table. Noise level was perfect, & Flora could come & go to the bathroom whenever she pleased. She decided she wanted an ice cream treat at home instead of dessert at the FF. Yeah! I think she would do great on a low-keto diet. But that planning is for later.

Right now, I need to get some things ready for her trip back [...]. Since I can't get to the bathroom as our bedroom door is locked, I'll put together my response to the Judaism topic—social justice.

[...] I just posted a rather explosive response concerning social justice that no one will read. Still, writing it was cathartic.

April 19, 2021: We took Flora back to Camphill yesterday. I'm decompressing. Appetite was shot last night. Not quite sure why.

I could take each girl at a time, but not both together. While we were focused on Flora, Jenny signed up for two more "free trials" without asking. Also, a new email account in the name of Jessica Rothenberg (get it? JR.).

And I can't find the recharging cord I always place on my cabinet handle so I can recharge my phone while I'm on the computer. Take & break. Jenny is so good at that.

Anyway, just a few more weeks of Jenny [...].

I had a romantic dream about Jonathan last night. Something about all the time we'll have together. I said, "I have some ideas," and winked at Jonathan. Calling Dr. Freud!

April 23, 2021: Katie Weisman is gone. Unbelievable.

Ed Yazbak is gone. Sad, but not tragic. He lived a very full life with a wonderful family he built [...]. [Katie Weisman used chelation to treat her three autistic sons and agitated on behalf of the vaccine-injured. She died of cancer at age 55. Dr. Edward Yazbak, who had vocally defended Dr. Andrew Wakefield's theory that the MMR vaccine could cause autism, died at age 89.]

Spoke with Rabbi Satz yesterday. This conversion process won't be so bad (he didn't ask my ideas about social justice). He & I are going to study the book of Ruth together.

Boaz showed great compassion toward Ruth the way Jonathan shows great compassion toward me.

April 24, 2021: Finding a place for Flora in New Jersey for right now makes sense. We'll see how it goes. Bridgette knows the keto diet! *And* she's into organic food. This arrangement could work for a while […]. [Bridgette was the manager of a group home in Boonton, about 20 minutes from our home, where we ultimately placed Flora in September.]

I love Jonathan so much. My herpes outbreak is still here ☹ It was bad this time.

April 25, 2021: A very pleasant evening with Angela & Mark. They are such a cute couple! I'm so happy for Angela. She deserves all the happiness she can find. It's so nice getting to know Mark; he's a solid mensch […].

One more week of Jenny—as long as I don't kill her (or vice versa) before then. Angela mentioned she had to call the cops on *Michael*. Woah. And how Graham [her ex-husband] never peeled Amy off of Angela when Amy attacked. What a *shit* […].

Jonathan continues to be great during everything. My herpes outbreak is quite severe, & Jonathan is very understanding. I look forward to being fully healthy & expressing my love with him.

April 26, 2021: For a brief moment yesterday, I was able to think clearly while preparing for class. Flora's living arrangements are taking care of themselves as are Jenny's. I could focus on my work.

Then I stumbled upon Jenny's $95 payment to talk with some "movie star" for two minutes. Ninety-five dollars. For two minutes. How can she be so smart & creative with writing & so stupid & lame with money?? I laid down the law. No advances this week. If she doesn't have enough to buy something at Writers Group, she can't go; no lunches; nothing extra that costs money. Period. She had $95 for all the extras she enjoys. She blew it.

Jonathan was *not happy* with Jenny & he let her know it. Part of his anger, I suspect, is that he sees how Jenny's poor decision-making takes such a toll on me. No one on earth loves me in all the dimensions that Jonathan does. And I him.

April 27, 2021: Another day of health yesterday followed by a great night's sleep! Oh, bliss!

We bought Jenny's furniture—to be delivered on May 2—as well as her desk […]

After our day of shopping, we stopped off at Ikea for some fød.[That's how it was spelled in a Simpsons episode.] My chocolate almond bar was delicious; the Swedes do chocolate quite well. It was a nice outing.

Jenny kept it together until we got home. Her falling apart was mild compared to the past.

I need to find or request an SSI letter for Jenny. It never ends.

And the anesthesiologists sent me a bill in mid-April that Jenny didn't give me. I'm ticked at Jenny; I'm even *more* ticked at the anesthesiologists.

Shopping—and eating fød with Jonathan—is *so much fun!* He's so decisive & doesn't settle. Just like when he was looking for a wife […]

April 28, 2021: Jenny went on another bender yesterday morning. Punched another hole in the wall. This time in the hallway. That has *got* to hurt. NuSera seemed to help calm her. Today, she needs pads. An explanation—*not* an excuse […].

I so love that the last person I see at night is Jonathan & the first person I see in the morning is […] Jonathan! My sympathy goes out to Queen Elizabeth these days; no longer able to snuggle up to her Prince. I have more riches than the Queen of England!

April 29, 2021: Jenny's move-in date postponed until May 15. She took the news better than Jonathan & I. She may sleep over, but needs to wait for supports to be in place before living there […].

Jonathan continues to be my Prince Charming. Can't wait to read his raunchy email of the day!

April 30, 2021: Very tired yesterday. I think a combination of the end of the semester, mistletoe treatments & Jenny along with Spring (pollen is quite high) makes me spacy.

Right knee hurts a little […].

Appetite is still weak. Energy good in the morning, then peters out […].

I so want my health back […].

Jonathan & I might make love this afternoon. Ah, bliss!

May 1, 2021: [Gayle ordered organic pillows for Jenny.] Four times (at least!) as expensive, but we have to do everything we can to help her succeed.

Like be organized with her medical cards. She started hitting herself yesterday when she realized she screwed up again. Maybe she should stop screwing up. Just take my simple advice.

It's so painful to see her hitting herself. But I'd rather her than me. In the future, though, I'll recommend the pillow […].

But I'll attend to more immediate work.

And play. Jonathan & I have plans for this afternoon. Ooh, la la!

May 2, 2021: We watched *That Hamilton Woman* with Vivien Leigh & Laurence Olivier. Oh, enchanting! But also makes me realize how little I know about Napoleon […].

I so love being married to Jonathan.

May 3, 2021: Jenny's furniture arrived! She seems so at peace at The Group Home. And the people seem to adore her! Lovely!

She & I watched John Denver last night. Such innocent times […]

Jonathan is now having breakfast & I want to join him. I so love being with him. Today is his last day of classes until *January 2022!* Oh, bliss […] for us!

May 4, 2021: May the Fourth be with you!

Slept well. Amazing what a good night's sleep can do!

Jenny has an overnight tonight at The Group Home. Good for her! & us!

I could write more freely if I knew Jenny wasn't reading my musings […].

I so love Jonathan!

May 5, 2021: My God! It *is* the little things that make or break life. Jenny slept over at The Group Home last night. We could talk about any topic at dinner. I had control of the remote. No one started harping about "How soon are you going to be finished watching TV?" […]. We need to get her to The Group Home as quickly as possible—for everyone's sake […].

I made a mistake yesterday, & I'll apologize to Jenny. She was about to go in the back door of her house when I said, "Go to the front." She was right; I was wrong.

Jonathan & I are going to be able to hang out together. Just the two of us. Time together that we've never really had. I hope he still likes me; I think he will ☺

May 6, 2021: Melanie publicly humiliated Jenny by telling her she needed to read the passages before coming to the Writers Group […]. I wish Melanie had alerted me that Jenny needed to read the passages earlier so we could have worked with Jenny […]. ["Melanie" is the fictitious name of the leader of Jenny's weekly Writers Group.]

Jonathan continues to be my rock […] and my hard place.

May 7, 2021: Right leg hurt a bit at joints—especially knee & hip. Before the injection, I noticed a few red bumps near incision in neck. Right ear lobe is tender. Oh, my God! My right ear lobe!! What could it mean? Actually, right side of neck is a wee bit tender. It could mean something. It could mean nothing. It could mean something that goes away on its own […].

I look so forward to spending time with Jonathan. Really, the little things are so important […] and his big thing.

May 8, 2021: What an unbelievable selfish bitch is Jenny Rose. Everything is about her, her, her. Nothing has changed since she was a toddler. Life would be good, until she had a tantrum. There was no getting through to her then, and there is no getting through to her now.

I get it—she's caught between two worlds. Her autism is not nearly as severe as Flora's, yet Jenny is far from "typical." But she wants all the rights of the typical world without any of the responsibilities. She's a perpetual teenager, only she's growing worse, not better.

She has a choice. Either she takes on the responsibilities of being part of the typical world—reading the passages before Writers Group, just to give an unbelievably simple example—or she is shut out of that world. I'm surprised her friends put up with her as much as they do [...].

The tantrums need to stop, or she will live in an institution. There is no universe in which her behavior is ok. She is ruining my health by her intermittent yet violent attacks, both physical and verbal. Currently, I have a rash on my neck & behind my right ear that could be hives, but reminds me suspiciously of the rash that occurred in my breast area that turned out to be cancer.

Either way, I'm in pain. The rash hurts—a stinging—I get periodic twinges of a pain on the right side of my head. That's where the bone mets are most dense on my skull (I think).

Yesterday, I was trying to be sympathetic about Melanie uninviting Jenny to Melanie's party tonight. But then Jenny attacked while Jonathan was helping me put together a blurb for the DeLong Prize in Book History [an academic prize honoring Gayle's father and mother]. Females, in her twisted mind, do the writing; males do the numbers. "Real men" and "real women." She ran outside, scaring the twins next door. There is no universe in which such behavior is ok. When Mark Berger [husband of Dara Berger] called, she grabbed my phone. We're associating with the "wrong people."

Jonathan & I have done everything we can to help prepare her for the world. She's picked up on the rights, but not the responsibilities. Or even mild corrections [...].

I want to have nothing to do with Jenny.

I need to focus on Jonathan, who is worthy of everything I can possibly give him.

May 9, 2021: So sick. Hives. In great pain.

Jonathan helped out.

May 10, 2021: Severe pain. Rash over right side of neck. Dr. Johnson said he's never seen this kind of reaction to mistletoe [...].

Jonathan just went out to get Benadryl. When I ask him to jump, all he asks is how high. ☺

May 11, 2021: SHINGLES! I have fricken *shingles!* And, yes, they hurt like hell. Burning twinges. One side of my body. Around (in?) the ear.

Jenny seems concerned. In her own way. "You can't have shingles," she told me. "That's an *old person's* disease!" Very sweet.

Jonathan is a wonderful caregiver. I look forward to taking care of him.

May 13, 2021: Finally, the last day of class. What an awful semester.

Shingles are subsiding! [...] Lyn recommended some homeopathic remedies as well as antivirals [...]. As with treating our girls, I am the hub of many medical spokes.

May 14, 2021: Not only am I going to live [...] I *want* to live! Feeling better, though tired & welts are still quite large (but crusting). Could I have had covid & now shingles? Could covid clear out cancer? Is there a God?

Odd dream—couldn't get to a group leaving for New York. Needed to use bathroom & then retrieve pocketbook from apartment. Nice people in apartment—including a special-needs young lady. Missed bus. (My brilliant career?) Found happiness, fulfillment elsewhere (went back to have lunch with people in apartment).

May 15, 2021: Jenny moves to [The Group Home] today. She's ready, and she'll do just fine.

Of course, there are details to manage—which clothes to take & extras (toothbrush, toiletries, etc.). I'm still too sick to accompany her move, but maybe it's that better that way. She'll figure out stuff.

Coffee. That's important. We have to figure out how she can get her morning caffeine.

The shingles are crusting over. They are *so gross!* It's amazing that the body would do this to itself.

It's also amazing at how the body heals itself [...] given half a chance [...].

Things are working out. It's good to know that Jonathan & Jenny can figure out things without my being there. Not that I'm planning to go anywhere; in fact, I'll probably become healthier when the girls are settled. It just relieves some pressure [...].

Hesed—going beyond that which is required by law & duty. That is Jonathan.

May 16, 2021: Health is returning, slowly, but surely. I'm beginning to think straight again. Ah, bliss!

Jenny got off yesterday. We haven't received any phone calls. ☺

Jonathan & I watched *The Taking of Pelham One Two Three* last night with Walter Matthau. Excellent film that showed the grit of New York City in the 1970s. A major difference between NYC in the 1970s & today is that in the 1970s, people were not calling to defund the police. I do sense that the Chinese—along with the elites (Gates, Zuckerberg, Bezos, Soros, Google, Apple, Clintons, Obamas) want us all to be servants to their grand schemes. Shut up & obey! Grand scheme of what, exactly? World domination, I suppose. Whatever that is. Typically, things do not end well for tyrants. The question is only how long will it take? How many more lives—like the lives of our daughters—will be wrecked?

So, I'll just keep doing what I do. Research on vaccine safety. Now that Jenny is out of the house, I'll be able to pursue my projects in peace.

Everything I do, I do for her & Flora. I suppose my life started out in pursuit of fame & glory as a top-notch researcher in banking. Publish in top journals; receive multi-thousand dollar consulting gigs. Haha. How empty.

Jonathan showed me the way. By the time I met him, he knew what was important in life. Love, caring, the next generation. Jenny is carrying on that tradition—contacting family members on their birthdays, staying in touch with Mom. And we will find worthwhile employment for Flora. We will be trailblazers in helping people find meaningful lives, even in New Jersey.

May 17, 2021: I do believe I'm getting stronger every day. (Chicago? 1973?)

The house is deliciously quiet. Jenny seems to be settling in nicely. Already looking outside herself. Ah, bliss!

She noticed that my shingles appeared to be healing nicely. The comment struck me as different, but I couldn't quite figure out why. Jonathan noted that Jenny said something *positive* about my appearance. Yes, that's different. She also hopes my letter arrives on time.

I'm taking some time off from cancer treatments. I haven't taken pancreatic enzymes in a week; the last time I took mistletoe was Thursday a week ago. Maybe I'll go a few more days, get tested at Dr. Levitz' office. See where we stand […].

Jonathan is up & we're going to have breakfast together. How sweet it is to be loved by you (James Taylor, c. 1970).

May 18, 2021: The silence is so sweet.

Jenny seems to be settling in nicely […].

I so love Jonathan. Hanging out with him (inter alia) is my favorite thing to do.

May 19, 2021: I am feeling stronger every day, but I'm still quite wiped out. I'm sick & tired of being sick & tired.

But I plug along [...]. Scabs from shingles are falling off like leaves. As soon as my rash is gone, I want to get my nails done at a professional salon. Funny, that.

Jonathan continues to be my everything. It is delicious spending time with just him.

May 20, 2021: I'm healing more slowly now, but still healing. I can't wait for the shingles to be ***all gone!*** [...]

Today, I see Dr. Levitz, which I always dread. He's so nice, and I always feel I'm letting him down for not taking Ibrance. But I just can't. Yes, I know he has years of education that I do not, but he also has years of brainwashing that I don't. Reviews from people who took the drug continue to be mixed. Even according to Pfizer (whose name I curse), the drug is to extend life with no cancer growth by 7.8 months. At $15,000 per month for the drug (!), you could buy a nice sized house in Cleveland instead of taking the drug. Assuming you'd ever want to live in Cleveland. And side effects do exist, according to the people who have taken the drug (or their loved ones after the people die). It shoots the immune system to hell. White blood cell counts tank. The only universe in which that is ok news is a universe that ignores blood analysis. But I thought blood analysis was the whole point of oncology hematology. And Dr. Levitz is trying to hold the—in his mind—inevitable cancer growth at bay. Building a dam, instead of reducing the forces that are causing the tidal wave [...].

My covid antibody test results should be in soon. They said turnaround time is 24 hours. Sometimes, they lie.

Jonathan never lies. Not to me anyway. And I not to him. We both have lust in our hearts [...] for each other ☺

May 21, 2021: Beautiful day for a protest! The sun is out; it's not too hot. Vaccine mandates, you don't stand a chance!

Dr. Levitz did it again. Pushed Ibrance. But now I realize—after my appointment, of course—that none of his pills address the underlying cause of ***my*** cancer. The constant stress of raising two children with autism—two very different types of autism—has overwhelmed my immune system. His pills don't—and can't—address that. Jonathan had a great analogy—it's like trying to keep a beach ball underwater. At some point, the beach ball will explode to the surface. That's what Ibrance seeks to do: keep the beach ball submerged a while longer. But deflating the beach ball while it's underwater would be a much healthier way to approach cancer. The question arises as to whether I should take Ibrance "for a while." I think the downsides—tanking the WBC counts; the risk of lung inflammation, especially in the age of covid; the unknown unknowns—render the drug for me useless.

The regimen that Dr. Isaacs prescribed should have worked. The reason it didn't is that I was still fighting a constant battle with autism.

Now that the girls are more or less settled, I can heal […].

Jonathan continues to be my saving grace. He showed me how to find raunchy—**really** raunchy—images on Brave. My setting was wrong. One little flick of the switch, and *voila!*

May 22, 2021: I wonder if Dr. Levitz ever thinks about where cancer comes from. It's obviously very individual. Plus, he doesn't have the tools to deal with underlying sources. So, he probably doesn't. Maybe I should **politely** ask sometime. I will certainly make more explicit why *I* have cancer. It's what I was trying to say during our most recent appointment […].

Yesterday was a lovely day for a protest [at Rutgers University]. A nice-sized crowd against mandates for college students. Several news outlets.

I so love going through life with Jonathan.

May 23, 2021: Jonathan & I watched an early Lucille Ball film, *Beauty for the Asking*. I liked it, more as a period piece, though it did have a plot. Jonathan was bored. He gets to choose next week. Even if it is Groucho Marx.

We're able to cuddle again. Oh, bliss!

May 24, 2021: Pleasant evening at overpriced Italian restaurant. Jenny mentioned she feels comfortable in her own skin. That was wonderful to hear […]

[…] until we realized how irresponsible she's been. I told her three times to check her emails from ESS [an employment service]. There was a glitch in one of the forms. She hadn't done that. Then, we find that the issue of their not having Jenny's fingerprints has been outstanding since the end of March.

So, it's easy to feel comfortable in your own skin when no one is making you do anything that's uncomfortable.

*** I had to stop writing abruptly. Jenny got up & of course always wants to know what I'm writing.

[…] Sadly, unless we bring her to a state of agitation, she does not seem to understand the importance of some issues.

We now have a deal that she reads every email that arrives. If it is from a site she doesn't care about, she searches for & deletes all emails from that site. For every site she totally deletes, she earns $3. Oh, God, I hope this works […].

Jonathan stays so calm whenever Jenny & I rip at each other. I'm so glad. I hope Jenny is, too.

May 25, 2021: Ugh. Sore throat. Congestion. Body aches. I'll get tested for Covid. If I have Covid, I'll stay home. Even if I don't have Covid, I'll stay home. I feel like crap, & I don't want to give anyone else what I have […].

Jonathan, without hesitation, said to let him know where he can take me to get tested. I feel so bad for him. With me, it's one thing after another. We *will* have sex again, we ***WILL!***

May 26, 2021: Kishore [her former department chair, who also had cancer] passed away on Monday. How sad. Ever since his radiation treatment for his throat, he struggled with pneumonia. So, that's what he died of; not cancer. What a farce. He died from cancer treatments. Bastards.

Facebook censors accurate information. It demotes comments derogatory about the Covid shot. So, I'm making the best decision I can based on the information I have, but the available information is incomplete & biased. Wonder what else they are hiding. Is Zuckerberg so hung up about being part of the establishment, the society he felt closed out of at Harvard, that he bows to their every demand? Fauci obviously did not like Zuckerberg's very astute question about messing with people's DNA, & then Zuckerberg changed his tune.

Jonathan & I drove to Chester yesterday so I could get a Covid test that I'm almost sure is covered by insurance. As usual, we had so much fun on the road trip & then making snide comments about *The View* (what a pathetic excuse for a television show). I love romping through life with Jonathan! I'd like to romp a bit more […] And I will as soon as I am better!

May 27, 2021: Jonathan & I are having a blast reading the *New York Post*. I'm so glad we subscribe […].

Jonathan continues to be my rock […] and hard place (someday *soon* I hope).

May 28, 2021: Kishore's funeral today. So odd. He's no longer here. Jonathan asked whether they are going to scatter his ashes into the Raritan River. We'll see.

May 29, 2021: Kishore's funeral yesterday. Very touching. Such a family man. And we were ***all*** his family. Neeta's father [Neeta was a niece] pointed out that Kishore was not interested in a homogenous "melting pot," but rather in bridging two cultures Some from each. So true; we see it in the Indian names of his grandchildren. Some traditions live on, others replaced. (I doubt, for example, that his girls' marriages were arranged […].)

Who will speak well of me at my funeral—which I hope is a long way off (I still have that tape running in my head about Dr. Levitz saying I had seven to ten years to live. "And that was ***thirty-two*** years ago!") Jenny, of course!

She was the first from the audience to jump up yesterday. Also [...] Victor's & Ruth's; she was too young for Dad's [...].

I wish I could do more to show Jonathan how much I love him. I will, but right now I'm healing. His ***chesed*** is beyond measure. But ***chesed*** usually is.

May 30, 2021: Jonathan & I watched *36 Hours* last night with James Garner, Rod Taylor & Eva Marie Saint. It was intriguing! Mind games [...].

I'm feeling somewhat better. Typically, I feel better in the morning, but start to drag as the day wears on. Let's see what happens today. I so want to be better. I want to get back to work. I want to get back to love.

Love. Jonathan. The words are synonymous.

May 31, 2021: Memorial Day. Both of Jenny's grandfathers fought to keep our country free. Now look at U.S. Her life is so difficult due to government-mandated policies. She'll be able to deal with them—but why? [...]

Jonathan, Jenny & I watched *1917* last night. Very powerful. Jonathan said he wouldn't fight for our country—not with what our country has done to our girls. I agree. The elite don't care. The soldiers in *They Shall Not Grow Old* were merely cannon fodder.

My love for Jonathan sustains me. It's my reason for being. Love for Jonathan & the girls.

June 2, 2021: Pleasant walks with Jonathan yesterday. Last night, we ran into several neighbors. We wonder what they'll think when we display our "We love & respect our police" sign. Jonathan likes "love & respect" better than "support." I hadn't thought about it, but when I did I realized that "support" does sound like a jock strap.

I'm healing slowly. Too slowly for my taste. But at least I'm able to get back to research. The results aren't quite as clean as the first time, but the main result remains—women who receive the HPV vaccine are less likely to have ever been pregnant. This is before Covid.

The new "unwashed" (the unvaccinated) are to be segregated. All the Trump-supporting white men who refuse vaccination. Except that the main groups not to vaccinate are African American (gee, I wonder why; Tuskegee, anyone?) and Hispanic. Asians are the most likely to get vaccinated. Traditionally, their cultures are very trusting (communist rule in China notwithstanding). Whites are close behind with vaccination.

I look forward to healing more & faster so that I can take care of Jonathan. I'm sure he's getting frustrated.

June 3, 2021: Victor would have been, what?, 102 today. Jenny knows. She wanted one of his shirts to wear today. L'dor v'dor [Hebrew: From generation to generation]. She gets that from Jonathan's side of the family; certainly not mine.

Recovery is taking longer than I want, but I do seem to be getting better. I'm able to function. I'd like to gain in function. Haha. Get it? "Gain in function" research is getting Fauci's dick in a wheel (deservedly). That bastard has done more harm to more people—under the guise of "health"—almost any dictator or tyrant. He *is* a tyrant. Yet in the current political environment, I doubt we will get justice. I hope I'm wrong [...].

It's raining again today. Jonathan & I will nestle together in our ark. I love nestling with Jonathan. It's one of my favorite things to do.

June 4, 2021: Had ¾ of a good day yesterday. Did research in the morning—results strong for married women—got my nails done (!) a pedicure. It was so decadent. Very nice. [...]. Then came home and **crashed**. Struggled through dinner—no appetite. Took shower at 8 & felt better.

I want to be better for a *full day* [...].

Intake for Flora went ¾ well. AVIDD *not* happy that Flora is not vaccinated. Quarantine. The overreaction to Covid is beyond belief. Terrify *everyone* & then they obey [...].

June 5, 2021: Melanie is being particularly cruel to Jenny. Melanie wrote Jenny an extremely nasty email, detailing everything that Melanie perceived was wrong with Jenny. After Jenny said to us that everything went so well on Wednesday—Melanie was not there, Jenny presented a chapter in her new book, received helpful feedback, provided insightful comments on the works of others—the problem became clear to Jonathan. Melanie cannot allow this to happen. Jenny, already a successful published author, is writing a second book as well as participating in a meaningful way. Melanie is an extremely unstable, jealous young lady. Why on earth should she write to the parent of a participant? Why on earth did I put up with it? Melanie is abusive & I assisted. For that, I am deeply sorry. Jenny has outgrown this group (at least with Melanie at the helm); it's time to move on [...].

Jonathan prepared dinner last night &—sensing I wasn't feeling well—cleaned up. I am not worthy. I remember when we were first married, I had been stupidly pissy about something—I forget what—so I bought some flowers for Jonathan as an apology. "I am not worthy," he said. Woah, I thought; I didn't marry that other guy from Princeton.

June 6, 2021: Last night, I had a nightmare. Jonathan & I watched *Night Must Fall* about a sociopath & the people he ensnares in his orbit by his charm. I dreamt several of us—Jonathan, me, three other people—were in an apartment. We knew a sociopath was trying to get me. We barricaded the door, boiled coffee to throw on him & baked a cheese soufflé also to use in an attack. We walked away from the front door of the apartment; when I returned, the barricades had been removed & the door was wide open. I think I tried to scream (in real life) "He's here!" but the words didn't come out. The dream was so vivid!

Jonathan didn't much like *Night Must Fall*, but he watched it to keep me happy. I thought it had some interesting plot twists, in particular how the Rosalind Russell character was taken in by the sociopath's charms. Overall, though, Jonathan was right (as usual). The plot twists were difficult to believe & the story really had no redeeming insights [...] except to give me nightmares! Next week, Jonathan gets to watch anything he wants.

June 7, 2021: Delightful garden party yesterday at The Group Home. I'm still not feeling 100%, but I enjoyed myself. [The residents'] parents are special—reasonable, understanding, caring. They have their priorities straight—their families—without needing to totally control their children [...].

Jenny has friends at The Group Home. Katelin seems to genuinely enjoy Jenny's company & Jeremy likes being with her as well. At first, I thought Jenny might be the Great Disruptor in a perhaps negative way by wanting to bring R-rated movies into the home. But her yoga & other activities can provide positive disruption. Yin & yang.

I so look forward to having sex again. So does Jonathan (he likes me!). Soon the time will be right.

June 9, 2021: I'm still in survival mode. I can get done what needs to get done. For example, yesterday I got Jenny to the polling station at 5:30 am. [She had a job as a poll worker.] She was correctly dressed (oops, forgot underwear & a bra [...] details!) with hair brushed. But then I came home & semi-crashed.... Jenny had left her lunch in the car (☹) so I dragged myself over to where she was. Forced myself to eat a slice of bread with pb for lunch. Saw Dr. Gatto for the last time (unless I have pain)—pity that, he's the only conventional doctor I like. I should have told him that. Then came home & crashed. Slept in bed; dragged myself to enema & shower. "Dinner" of ice cream at 7:30 pm.

Slept ok [...]. But I'm still so drained. It's draining still taking care of Jenny. We need to change her duvet, because the one she has has a hole in it & the stuffing keeps dribbling out. Her purse zipper doesn't work anymore. "I'm sorry, Mom!" she proclaimed as though if only she had my approval for the broken zipper, then everything would be ok. Never mind that her purse could spill at any moment. & how did it break to begin with? She destroys purses. Take & break.

& there's the preparation for Flora [...]. Flora might need to get a TB/hep B/lead test. Ugh.

The girls will be more & more out of our hair, but we're not there yet. One of the reasons I think shingles emerged when they did is that The Group Home kept postponing Jenny's move-in date. "It's never going to happen," I kept thinking to myself.

Plus, my poor body has just had enough. Enough of autism. Enough of conventional medicine. Enough attacks from all sides, including (especially?) Jenny. In a book I'm reading about God's love for my conversion, I read that children are to assist their ailing parents. Really? I'm not seeing it. Maybe next time Jenny attacks me, I'll remind her that being a good Jew means honoring your mother & father.

I want more from life than mere survival. I want to make mad passionate love with Jonathan. Maybe I should "just do it" even though I don't feel completely ready.

June 10, 2021: Saw Lyn yesterday & I'm feeling much better. Why do I even see conventional doctors? Lyn's remedies address the underlying causes as well address symptoms of my (all too many!) ailments.

Lyn was so excited about my dream where the sociopath trying to kill me left the apartment. The more I think about it, though, I'm not sure the sociopath was cancer. I think it was Dr. Levitz. Not that Dr. Levitz is a sociopath—far from it! He's one of the nicest, most sincere doctors I've met. But his drugs are trying to kill me & the people behind the drugs—the researchers & the salespeople—*are* sociopaths. They have no regard for human life. Only making money & covering up mistakes & side effects.

I wonder if I can transform my dream to ushering out cancer? Why not? It's a pleasant thought. And the door is open [...].

We have to figure out a way for Jenny to remember to take her remedies during the week. Envelopes marked with the day of the week & a phone call from me? [...]

Jonathan & I did it yesterday! By *it* I mean *sex!* I've shrunk, so it was slightly painful. More of my super lube next time. Ah, bliss.

June 12, 2021: Jonathan got up very early yesterday morning—earlier than I! So, I dragged myself downstairs—I so love being with him—but my morning was discombobulated. Hence, no musing.

Not much to report any way. Mild leg pain is back. It sucks growing old. With cancer treatments. One person described women with metastatic breast cancer as "walking chemical miracles." What the F*CK! I **REFUSE** to be a walking chemical *anything*. "Better living through chemistry" as Jonathan noted.

Reading all the adverse effects of the chemicals these ladies were taking & the new chemicals to replace the ones that stopped working or caused too many side effects made me want to stop all unnatural cancer treatments. The only unnatural treatments I'm taking are anastrozole & xgeva. I wonder how much good they are doing versus how much harm. I'm such an economist.

Today, Jonathan & I are going to a demonstration against mandating Covid shots for students. I'm so glad someone organized this rally. I'm not an organizer, but I certainly believe in the cause. These kids should *not* be taking the shot. They have a greater chance of getting killed by lightening than by Covid; they don't spread the disease as we had feared; and the side effects such as heart inflammation are beginning to become apparent.

Jonathan pointed out that one of the best natural treatments is cock therapy. How true!

June 13, 2021: Rally yesterday was small, but meaningful. Totally new people, similar causes (no mandatory vaccines, starting with Covid), fabulous energy. The tyrants have really overplayed their hands. We're mad as hell, & we're not going to take it anymore […].

Jonathan & I watched *Ship of Fools* last night. People going out of their ways to make their lives & the lives of others miserable. (Ship travelling from Mexico to Germany in 1933.) The only one with any sense was the Jewish salesman, who uttered, "Germany has almost a million Jews; what are they going to do, kill us all?"

My health is still volatile. I enjoyed the rally yesterday, but came home & crashed. Dinnertime is the worst. Tired, no appetite. I want to be all better *right now!* Jonathan—or was it me?—pointed out that my body was crashing after decades of caring for others. "I don't know how you did it," Jonathan observed. Because of you, Jonathan. I would not have been able to survive without you. With you, I can (obviously!) survive anything […].

Lately, I'm purchasing organic clothes. They feel quite nice.

Jonathan continues to be my everything. It is a blast spending time with *just him*. Even traffic jams are fun with him. Yes, I *am* in love!

June 14, 2021: Flag Day! Yes, it's a grand old flag. Jonathan is cautiously optimistic that the tide is turning, that the tyrants are on the run. America is one of the few places where we can rise up & succeed […].

Jenny was here yesterday & truly concerned about my well-being. She even opened the door for me […]! What a nice young lady she is becoming.

Jonathan is so patient & understanding. He's certain I'll get better & I am! Thanks in large part to him.

June 15, 2021: I want my body back [...] completely [...] totally [...] & for the entire day! Mornings tend to be good. I feel ok now. But as the day wears on, I tire easily. Most days I crash at some point. Sunday, I couldn't pass a couch or a bed or a chair without wanting to collapse in it. So I guess today is already better than Sunday. Still, I don't trust my body. Are you going to keep going? Are you going to crash? What can I do to help?

"Taking it easy" is still not yet possible. Jenny's smoke alarm still isn't fixed as well as her air conditioning. The Group Home is mandating orientation. Flora needs tests [...].

My sex drive is in the basement. I love my husband more than anything—& I want to show him—but my body just hurts. It's probably the anastrozole.

Jonathan continues to be a peach. Last night, I was able to eat some dinner. He's so caring, so nurturing. I love him so much.

June 16, 2021: If my cancer is estrogen-fueled, but stress allows what little estrogen I have to do its dirty deeds, then we still need to get rid of the stress, right?

And getting rid of the stress we are. Life is so much better for Jenny & me now that she's on her own. Of course, I always get nervous when [The Group Home director] needs to talk with us (like now). For two decades I've had to field "Your daughter did this; your daughter did that." What's surprising is that I didn't develop cancer earlier.

Urile has a vaginal moisturizing cream that I will order. I want to keep Jonathan happy. He's my most precious find on this earth.

June 17, 2021: [We had to deal with an array of agencies which required confusing forms, did not call at prearranged times, and demanded repeated background checks, fingerprinting, and TB tests.]

Jenny came over last night & quickly resolved the form for ESS. She also fessed up to crashing a [wedding] party at a neighbor's house. That's probably what [the director] wants to talk with us about. Not the worst thing in the world. In fact, Jonathan's smirking, "That's my girl!" [The newlyweds did not mind at all, so this was a victimless crime.] As she explained the situation, Jonathan pointed out something & Jenny said he was going all Immanuel Kant on her. I didn't get the allusion, but Jonathan was *very* impressed. [An allusion to the philosophical principle of the Categorical Imperative: what if everyone crashed parties? I told Jennifer, "Look, you're a writer. If writers followed all the rules, they'd have nothing to write about."]

June 21, 2021: Temperature gyrating between 97.1 & 101.8. Energy level as well on a roller coaster.

Drinking tea with heavy cream. It is absolutely delicious. Tapioca is a food that currently appeals to me.

Jenny & Jeremy went to the movies yesterday. It's so nice. For both of them. This week & early next week will be tough. After that […] who knows?

So glad Jonathan is by my side […].

June 23, 2021: Rough night. Headache. Leg pain. Ice packs all night. Water helped. One hour plus of HBOT this morning alleviated headache ☺ Still draggy from interrupted sleep.

So, I'll take it easy today. Reply to reviewers & send off HPVs in HPV vaccine recipients paper. Another hand grenade. We'll win eventually. You can't suppress Nature forever. I just hope there are enough healthy members of the human race remaining to carry on.

Saw Dr. Weiss yesterday. He found no infections. I like his old-time doctoring manner of poking & listening to see/hear/feel if there are issues. He said he could give me an antibiotic, but why? He could also order a lung scan, but sees (hears) no reason. I walked out of his office without any prescriptions, because I don't need any. I need rest & self-focus after twenty years of autism.

Jonathan's been through 20 years also. Fortunately, he's strong right now, very strong. My vaginal cream is coming in the overnight package from Uriel. Let's see what comes up tomorrow!

June 24, 2021: I have little strength. Everything is a chore. Tea with cream tastes good—up to a point. Otherwise, no appetite.

I do hope this is Flora related & that once she is settled, I'll feel better. Otherwise […] I just don't know.

Anticipation is (almost) always worse than the actual event (in this case, Flora coming home).

I love Jonathan on a spiritual level. Bodily, I'm just too frail & tired. This is known as Living Hell.

June 26, 2021: Dad's birthday. He would have been 99, except that the goddamn medical establishment killed him. Removing the anger from my heart might help me to heal, but I'm not there yet. The medical establishment killed my dad, probably my grandmother, totally screwed up Flora & made Jenny's life much more difficult that it should be.

I'm so sick. We picked up Flora yesterday. Are the two connected? You decide.

Diarrhea. ZERO appetite. I do wonder how I keep going. Tapioca does taste good. Yes!

I've decided to suspend pancreatic enzymes while I do mistletoe. Pancreatic enzymes did not prevent the metastasis of the cancer. Therefore, I want to try mistletoe. I can't do both.

So many burdens on Jonathan, but he takes it in stride. I love him so.

June 27, 2021: I'm a mess. No energy. Lots of iron in my blood—not getting to where it is supposed to go. No wonder no energy. I wonder if/how we can address this. Also, diarrhea.

I'm floating between the well & the sick. I'm not totally on my back, but I can't remain vertical for very long.

Unless I have to. Like yesterday, when Jenny dislocated her shoulder.

So, I'm able to function. But for how much longer? Yesterday, I ate some tapioca & raspberries for breakfast; a slice of bread with a slice of ham for lunch; & buttered toast (one slice) for dinner.

If this phase doesn't kill me, it will make me stronger! […]

Jonathan is my everything.

June 28, 2021: Another episode with Jenny at dinner. She was so proud of Flora for not eating any popcorn. I lamented the fact that she tempted Flora with popcorn & Jenny flew into a rage.

I sense her mission in life has been to destroy me. My happiness, my health, my research. She wants it all destroyed […].

Jonathan is worried. I'm sorry he's worried, but he has reason to be.

June 29, 2021: [Problems continued to escalate at Jennifer's group home, including a failure to provide 24/7 coverage.] Need to find new place for Jenny. She'll figure stuff out. She'll find the local library, the pool, the yoga classes.

It's so odd—just Jonathan & I. A wonderful oddness!

July 6, 2021: Was in the hospital since Friday night. Probably colitis, though no one gave me an official diagnosis. Appetite came roaring back yesterday. When I eat foods good for colitis, I feel better; when I eat foods bad for colitis, I feel awful. Probably not related to cancer, though many of my cancer markers are haywire. And I have two lumps, one under each armpit. Lymph nodes? […]

I'd like to do some cleaning every day. I'll start with my closet—my clothes. I don't want to leave a huge mess for Jonathan.

Jonathan is optimistic that we dodged another bullet. But so many bullets. April exhaustion; May shingles; June colitis. Gotta keep going.

Jonathan is my everything.

July 8, 2021: It is fantastic waking up in my own bed next to my best friend. Let me unpack that: It is fantastic a) to wake up; 2) in my own bed; 3) next to my best friend.

Gratefully, the hospital stay was short—three nights. They never really told me what I had, though they indicated it might be something called "colitis" […].

Scans not yet back. Tumor markers are sky high, so I'm expecting the worst. Results probably won't be quite as bad as expectations.

See Dr. Levitz today […].

Jonathan is truly an angel. And a hero. My angel hero.

July 9, 2021: Cancer has spread to lungs & liver. Just little spots. 7 mm. But there we are. Time to up the game. Ibrance ☹ as well as GcMAF ☺ Both Jonathan & Fabrizio reminded me about GcMAF. Fabrizio says the world needs me. More importantly, I know Jonathan needs me […].[GcMAF is a protein which some alternative physicians use to combat cancer, though this therapy is controversial and has not been approved by the FDA.]

Jonathan is my everything. If I were to exit now, it would be so unfair to him. We've worked so hard as parents for 25 years. Now, finally, we get a break. Time for heal, for both of us.

July 10, 2021: Did I mention Josh G. from Israel had a heart attack two and half months after getting a Covid shot? Due to a blood clot. No family history of heart attacks, no risk factors. Just imagine—with my family history of blood clots—if I were to submit to the shot. No, don't imagine, because it is not going to happen.

Saw Lyn yesterday. Jenny had a series of tantrums in the car, including hitting me several times. When I walked into Lyn's office, I must have looked like the shell-shocked creature that I was. Lyn gave Jenny a new once-a-week (yeah!) remedy. Jenny was uber apologetic afterwards, but the roller coaster is almost worse than if she would be in a crazy mood all the time. Almost. At least with the roller coaster, we get glimpses of the real Jenny. I suppose. Or maybe she's really the selfish bitch she presents as Lucifer & her Jennifer personality is simply a façade. Nah, the real Jenny is incredibly sweet & thoughtful. She got a sympathy card for Helen [her support person at the Group Home] when Helen's sister-in-law died. Helen was very touched.

Lyn—and also Dr. Isaacs, who called while Jenny & I were at lunch— interpreted my scans as tiny indications that we need to up the game. Nothing life-threatening. Maybe even exaggerations.

My questions to Dr. Isaacs—are these results exaggerations? Indications of future issues? What am I doing wrong? Can pancreatic enzymes still help? […]

Jonathan continues to be my everything. I tried to find a raunchy email to send him yesterday, but couldn't. He understands. His raunchy emails are just so spot on.

July 11, 2021: To heal, I need to stay away from Jenny. Our relationship is toxic. I will have as little to do with her as possible. For my sake. For the sake of my health & healing.

What I can't understand is her attitude. She knows she's a burden—she says it all the time. Yet she does nothing to address why she is a burden. Figure out a place to always place your phone so you don't lose it. Not rocket science. And don't attack me for making suggestions.

Jonathan & I watched *The Wild One* with Marlon Brando last night. He found it a great period piece; I found it a bit annoying, but delighted to share a movie with my BFF […].

I thought of some raunchy ideas to search for to send to Jonathan (sex & motorcycles). He always sends me the best—and by "best" I mean raunchi-est—emails. The ones I send him are so lame, but he seems to appreciate them.

July 13, 2021: Spoke with Dr. Isaacs. She's not too worried. Yes, I should begin Ibrance due to tumor markers & everything else that seems to be going wrong. But the spots on my liver could have been from colitis infection & spots on lung are too small to "count." Anything less than 10 mm typically is not of concern. The largest spot I had was 7 mm. Oh, & the "fissures" in the lung could have been from the fluids they gave me in the hospital. Water collects in the feet (& how!) & lungs. Levitz did this on purpose. He wanted to scare me into taking Ibrance. OK. I'll take it for a while. But I'm not happy.

Dr. Johnson said mistletoe can aggravate colitis. However, we agreed to retry mistletoe. It almost seems as though the colitis was a one-off attack. Could it be my body is collapsing after 22 years of autism? Autism squared. I'll have to suspend mistletoe for two weeks when I start Ibrance. & I'm still searching for GcMAF […].

Jonathan took Jenny to the orthopedist yesterday. I need to have as little to do with her as possible, & Jonathan understands. He doesn't call me a bad mother—far from it!—& he steps up when needed. How did I get so lucky?

July 14, 2021: I am mending every day. My feet are still swollen, but I'm hobbling around just fine. The weight is all going to my tummy—I really do feel pregnant.

Jonathan's right—I really do feel snookered by Dr. Levitz. Do the scan in the hospital when my body is already a mess. It will be bound to show some-thing. Dr. Isaacs thinks I should try Ibrance due to the high tumor markers. OK, I'll try it. But first, I'll do some mistletoe & I'll hold off beginning Ibrance until I have a couple of mistletoe sessions under my belt […] "Gee, the Ibrance just didn't arrive."

My appetite is still strong, though not quite as roaring as when it first returned. My body is amazing, given half a chance. And now is the time to heal. The girls are out of the house & more or less settled.

We are looking for a group home for Jenny that is better organized [...] (***that*** won't be difficult), but not as restrictive as Flora's [...].

Saw Miriam & Michelle [autism moms and friends] yesterday for lunch. It was so nice seeing them, sharing things that only girlfriends can share. Like when I told Michelle I thought it was over for me. I couldn't tell that to Jonathan; he was scared enough as it was. But I did think this past episode meant the end was near for me. I was sad for Jonathan. We finally had the girls out of the house & I was going to up & leave. I didn't want to do that, but diarrhea was so explosive & so bloody & my energy & appetite were so low, I thought it was over. I'm so glad I was wrong. I also realized—once again!—what's important. Jonathan, the girls, friends. Not articles, teacher ratings or crabby students. Good students are important in my life, but the crabby ones are probably leading miserable lives that I can't help shape.

Jonathan & I continue to send raunchy emails. Sex is just around the corner [...]

July 15, 2021: I am seen; I am heard; I am loved. Not by God—what has Hashem ever done for me?—but by friends & especially my BFF, Jonathan. ***That's*** what matters in life [...].

Jonathan & I will have sex soon. My nether regions are healing from a herpes outbreak & my decrepit bag of bones is healing. I love expressing my love for him.

July 16, 2021: Saw Mary Holland yesterday. We're going to have fun on our road trip to Lancaster County. Jonathan—as am I—is a little shy to ride over to Lancaster (from Philadelphia) with RFK, Jr. But Mary offered & I'm sure she was sincere. I can help prepare them for the event with my great Amish Insights [...]

My herpes have cleared up, so I think I'm ready for sex. I know Jonathan is. I don't want to make promises I can't keep—so I won't send a raunchy email indicating as much—but if I'm still ok by this afternoon then today is the day.

July 17, 2021: Normalcy is returning to the greater world—at least the United States—as well as my own life as we all continue to mend. When I got my haircut yesterday, Nino was no longer wearing or requiring a mask. And he was one of the most skittish—understandably, because a case of Covid could have shut his business for good [...].

I'm not just my cancer & blood results. In fact—except for the red patch in my breast area—I still don't feel as though I have some horrific disease. I have a bunch of cells that aren't behaving correctly, so I need to whip them into shape.

Sex today with Jonathan? Let's give it the college try!

July 18, 2021: Alison McNeil once pointed out that we autism moms are like the cog in a wheel of medical professionals. They form the spokes, we are in the middle, deciding what makes sense for our children. I'm using the same philosophy with treating my ailments. No one doctor knows everything. Gotta say, when I saw Dr. Levitz's assistant who immediately suggested Imodium upon hearing that I had diarrhea, I lost some respect for the practice. It's this, so take that. Deal with the symptom, no need to be concerned about the underlying cause. Except in this case the underlying cause was colitis & Imodium did nothing. I get it that they want people to feel better & that they have limited time with each patient, but I totally disagree with the here's A so do B mentality. I'm not a machine (or a "walking chemical miracle" for that matter). I'm a human being with stresses & past illnesses & heredity (think blood) & a diet & (some) exercise. I also take pancreatic enzymes & mistletoe & homeopathy. I am unique.

Jonathan & I watched *Requiem for a Heavyweight* with Anthony Quinn, Mickey Rooney & Jackie Gleason. Heavy, very heavy. Camera angles, chiaroscuro, violence off camera (but still devastating), music. They really don't make movies like that anymore [...].

We made love yesterday. Very nice. Penetration still hurts—I guess I've shrunk—but intimacy is delightful. NO LOCKED DOORS!

July 19, 2021: Kids came over yesterday. No change in Flora—Jonathan is bummed about that. Jenny & I didn't fight. She picked her nose during the movie as well as gnawed on her shirt. I only pointed out the nose-picking. "Sorry, Mom," she replied, as though I make the rules she breaks. She still doesn't understand that I'm trying to correct her behavior so she can thrive in the outside world [...].

Flora put the "Happiness is Being Married to Your Best Friend" pillow on the bed [...] where it belongs. She's right. The pillow is also right.

July 20, 2021: The girls are getting settled. That helps immensely with my healing [...].

I'm spending money as though I have it [...] which I do! Organic sheets **&** duvet. Jonathan balked at the $700 price tag. Then we both laughed. Not having to shell out 8 grand a month for Flora [her tuition at Beaver Farm] ***does*** put money in our pockets. I'll reach a shopping saturation point at some point, like I did with buying organic clothes. But it sure is going to be nice having sheets that are organic & ***that match*** [...].

Jonathan continues to be my everything. This morning, he asked how I was doing. "Great & getting better," I told him. When I returned the question, he replied, "Great that you're doing better!"

July 21, 2021: Life is so peaceful now that the girls are out of the house. No land mines; no hand grenades; […] no Taylor Swift songs saying I'm an abusive mother; no wondering what Flora is up to.

I'm looking forward to Family Days on the Farm. It's really happening. I hope the weather is good & the people receptive. The latter is a foregone conclusion. Let's pray for the former.

Ruth had the Community pray for my health. I'm really touched by that. Hey, it worked!

Ibrance will arrive the end of the month. Being part of the "copay assistance program" means I don't even pay the copay. Nothing. I pay nothing. To be poisoned. Well, at least I don't have to pay for it. Reminds me of when I said to Phyllis Mast, who played the flute in the marching band, how cool it was that she got to go to football games without having to pay. She didn't like football and replied, "Getting into hell is also free." Of course, **someone** pays for it […] in monetary terms, that is. **I'll** pay for it with lowered white blood cells & the host of other side effects. But Dr. Levitz is happy. I'm not, but he is.

Pfizer makes Ibrance. What Pfizer has done to my kids constitutes crimes against humanity, but I'm now entrusting them with my survival. What's wrong with this picture?

I'm up to 104 pounds! I do feel heaps better than the beginning of the month. **HEAPS!** *[…]*

Jonathan is glad I'm pursuing GcMAF. Finding a practitioner is difficult. There is a woman in NYC. I'll see her in September, unless someone else emerges.

Being with Jonathan is so peaceful, so blissful. How did I get so lucky?

July 22, 2021: The world was too much with me yesterday. Stress about the GcMAF decision […]. Stress about the Amish handouts. Stress about [errors in] Jenny's ESS [pay]check [for her occasional work as a per diem classroom assistant].

At every turn, Jonathan helped me out. Especially with the ESS check. I mentioned on our walk that I was nervous. When I actually sat down to write the email, I freaked out. "I don't know what to do!" I exclaimed in a panicky voice. "Uh, do you want me to help?" Jonathan offered. "Oh, please. YES!" After we (he) composed the email to ESS, he pointed out that all I had to do was ask. So, I practiced last night in bed, "I'm feeling overwhelmed. Can you help me out?" It's so easy […].

And I ordered GcMAF. The strongest available shipped as quickly as possible. Jonathan repeatedly said I'm worth it.

We are worth it, Jonathan. Earlier this month, when I thought the cancer had attacked my colon & that it was all over, I thought how unfair to you. The girls are finally gone, we have time to ourselves & then I exit. I'd be gone, so I wouldn't notice; but you would be alone & that would be so unfair. Part of the feeling that it was all over for me came from Dr. Levitz's prophecy that I would feel great until I didn't anymore. I figured my body was shutting down & quickly.

But, alas; the world doesn't get rid of me that easily. I'm so glad, for my sake & Jonathan's sake.

July 23, 2021: Just think of what [Flora] could have accomplished if her brain had not been scrambled?

We'll keep trying to unscramble her brain, but the most important thing now is for her to enjoy life. New Jersey is paying $100K for her to be housed. That doesn't include the day program. [The total annual cost is $235,000.]

Crimes against humanity: Pfizer, Merck, GlaxoSmithKline, Astrozeneca. And now I'm supposed to trust Pfizer to keep *me* alive. I will take Ibrance for the shortest amount of time possible. If it works & my numbers go down, I'll stop; if it doesn't work & my numbers stay high, I'll stop. I do not trust those bastards.

Babylon Bee had a headline, "Debate between well-respected medical doctor & Dr. Fauci." I think a more appropriate headline would be, "Debate between well-respected medical doctor & Bureaucrat Fauci."

It's so wonderful coming home to Jonathan. I had a mistletoe infusion yesterday & then came home to Jonathan. Ah, bliss!

July 24, 2021: Almost totally pleasant day yesterday at Flora's Farewell Celebration. The weather was delightful. Flora was calm most of the time—didn't fight us about food. Jenny was pleasant—except for two "panic attacks." She was so, so sorry afterwards. It doesn't matter. I warned her that if she misbehaves, I will not drive her to see Lyn on August 20th [...]. Regardless of how short the "panic attacks" are, they are dangerous. I cannot, for safety reasons, drive alone with Jenny.

She has one more chance—our trip to see Dr. Johnson. Let's see if she can control these outbursts. If she can't, all the more reason to avoid driving with her alone [...].

Discussed Ibrance with nurse yesterday. Blood clots a big issue [...]. Other side effects include vomiting, diarrhea, loss of appetite. Remember the first time you tried smoking? Your body was trying to tell you something [...]

It was wonderful to retire to our home, just Jonathan & me, after being with the girls. I love our empty nest.

July 25, 2021: Jenny is taking my criticism in stride. She knows I won't drive her to see Lyn unless I see that she can behave. And guess what? She's behaving! It's one thing to see your mistakes, which she's getting good at. The next step is to address & prevent those mistakes. I'll try not to overdo it, but it sure is nice to point out her weak areas—like hanging up towels properly— without her going ballistic.

Jonathan & I watched *The Petrified Forest* last night. Leslie Howard was *so* romantic. No wonder Ruth had the hots for him. Humphrey Bogart was *so* young, but already had his characteristic swagger […].

Jonathan is stirring, so I want to read his raunchy email before he appears in the study. I love thanking him for his dirty mind early in the morning. It sets the tone for the entire day. Of course, I'll look for something for him.

July 26, 2021: The girls were here for dinner last night. What a disaster! Jenny got upset when I tried to assist her in sorting her pills—an activity with which she has had issues in the past. She started adding the pills helter skelter. When I suggested she go down the list in order to make sure she gets all the pills, she threw a fit. Flora then became upset. A joyous evening then ensued […] NOT.

Jonathan was particularly tired from his bike ride in the heat & humidity. He's concerned that all dinners are going to go this way. We might just have to set a few ground rules.

But Jenny can be such a pain in the ass sometimes. At this point, I will *not* drive with her to Lyn's. It's too dangerous if she cannot control herself.

Jonathan & I had a drink last night for the first time in a long time. Campari. We had our "safe space"; how pleasant!

I love sharing time with just Jonathan. I wish the rest of the world would go away.

July 27, 2021: GcMAF arrived unexpectedly yesterday! So far, I've used the cream once (last night) & the spray once (this morning). I feel fine. In fact, I feel great. Adjusting to something unexpected took some time […].

It's so much fun playing house with Jonathan. Our enchanted house.

July 28, 2021: Jenny did pick up her own medicine yesterday! I was pleasantly surprised she was able to take the initiative to do that […].

Playing house with Jonathan is such a blast.

July 29, 2021: One thing I really like about alternative medicine is how much in charge I am. Since alternative doctors freely admit they don't know how people are going to react to, say, mistletoe, they have the freedom to say,

"Let's try this & see what happens." Conventional doctors—yes, Dr. Levitz, I'm talking to you—say "This is going to happen & this & this." Also, taking Ibrance is so different from taking GcMAF. With GcMAF, the manufacturer says if there are any side effects, then suspend the treatment for a day or two. *You decide*. With Ibrance, I am to report any side effects to the doctor who will decide for me.

I wonder how soon my CA 27.29 numbers should fall after starting Ibrance. They are already beginning to fall (now that the colitis is subsiding?) […].

Jonathan is adorable. So kind, so sweet. So great in the sack.

July 30, 2021: We go to Lancaster County today. I do hope everything works out well. That Bobby finds the trip useful.

Driving through the horrible rainstorm yesterday all I wanted to do was be home. Home is where you want to be. [When she was very young, this was Jennifer's definition of "home".] I so love being with Jonathan. He's my home.

August 1, 2021: Jenny is 25 today. What a life she is leading. She's getting there.

Very pleasant day in Lancaster County yesterday. Everything worked out fine. We could not have asked for better weather—sunshine, breeze, not too hot. The crowd was large & respectful. [Gayle keenly noticed that the young Amish men were magnificent physical specimens, thanks to vigorous farm labor and an organic diet.] Bobby helped people with their questions & concerns. He explains issues so well.

Jonathan is right, though. I would not want to be the jet-setter he is. Jonathan & I are both homebodies. That's who we are. Bobby thrives on this kind of work—fundraising & publicizing Children's Health Defense. Mary & Laura manage the implementation of the strategy. Amazing how this rag-tag group of passionate parents has risen the #2 source of "misinformation" in fewer than ten years. Mercola is #1. "Huge disappointment" Bobby said when we asked why he wasn't #1. [The "Disinformation Dozen" was a blacklist of 12 vaccine skeptics. Dr. Joseph Mercola was ranked first, followed by Robert F. Kennedy, Jr.]

One thing I learned—the CDC counts as "vaccinated" only those people who are two weeks out from their second shot (for Moderna & Pfizer) or from their first shot (J&J). Many cases & deaths occur between or shortly after shots. Even if a person has received the shots, if the disease or death occurs within the two-week time frame, the CDC considers them "unvaccinated." What a bunch of pricks. Anything to terrify people.

More lockdowns starting August 8. Ugh. I mean, my life doesn't get rearranged too dramatically, but Jenny might have more difficulty getting a job

& Flora a day program. The small businesses—the ones that survived—will again be under attack. The Dark Side just doesn't know when to stop. Jonathan is optimistic (!) that that will be their downfall. The vaccinated people, when exposed to the virus or a variant, indeed seem to be more affected.

I so love showing off Jonathan. A man of few (fortunately, not as few as his father), but choice & interesting words. Plus, he's great in the sack. Who could ask for more??

August 2, 2021: Yesterday, I was draggy all day. Then I had to see the kids. I felt worse—mainly backache (muscle cramps?) & a touch of nausea. Dinner I was able to eat, but only a salad. I felt bad, because it was Jenny's birthday. I apologized for ruining her birthday, but she said I didn't.

Jenny also got her pills together on her own. Steadily, methodically. She even found more Neuroprotek in the side cabinet & put away the supplements. She's growing.

Flora kept asking to go to the bathroom, when the food would arrive & in general did not show any growth in behavior. She was good when Jenny got ice cream & she didn't. The promise was that she would get ice cream at home, which she did.

How do you unscramble an egg?

I don't know. But I do know I need to focus on my own healing right now […].

Jonathan—as usual—took excellent care of me yesterday, making sure the girls didn't bother me too much. He's a wonder.

August 4, 2021: It's so much fun just hanging out with Jonathan. We both richly deserve this special time together.

August 6, 2021: The world has gone mad. Protests in Berlin look like Hong Kong. Police patrols in Australia look like East Germany before the Wall fell. The Gestapo will soon be asking for our papers before allowing us to eat in NYC restaurants & children must hide their faces "in the name of health." This is insanity. We're going to take all the same measures with the Delta variant that we took originally […] and didn't work. Masking, social distancing (an oxymoron), vaccines. God, if you do exist, Planet Earth could use Your guidance right now.

Mark Steyn pointed out that the farther East you go, the more Western you become, i.e. Hungary & Poland are more Western than France & Germany.

From the profound to the profane: Jenny's room was an utter mess when I went in yesterday while Flora was going to the bathroom. Junk everywhere, no pillowcase (how do you not have a pillowcase on your pillow?), Jasmine's payment envelope on the floor, along with the stamps Jenny stole from us (ok, "took

without asking") [Jasmine was one of Jenny's support staff] [...]. Jonathan &
I need to go to Jenny's apartment, lay down the law that her room needs to be
orderly before she does **anything** [...]. Jenny will not be able to live on her own
until she acquires basic cleanliness skills [...].

Hard ridge around my cancer rash is receding. Thank you, GcMAF! I
wish I could try GcMAF for three months before doing Ibrance. But everything is set in motion, & at least I have the next two Thursdays off from mistletoe so maybe Lyn & Mary Coyle & I can get together. If any NYC restaurant
will have those of us who are unwashed.

Jonathan gallantly stuffed my duvet onto the top shelf of my closet. He indicated he wanted to stuff another thing somewhere. I so wish my body would
cooperate, but right now it's pained when he stuffs.

August 7, 2021: It's early—a little past 6:30. Nice time of the morning.
Everything is quiet, except a few birds going about their morning routines.
Hustling the kids out of the nest. Off to catch worms.

The world has gone mad. Suzanne & Mark will not attend [Cousin]
Hannah's Bat Mitzvah, because there might be unvaccinated people there.
Say, what?? The fear, the misinformation, the compliance [...].

Tomorrow, I begin Ibrance. I don't want to, but everything is in train, especially time off from mistletoe. I'll give it a month. Any negative side effects & I
will halt the "treatment." Liz Johnson says if I don't want to take the treatment,
it isn't going to work anyway. We'll see what happens. Maybe it will suppress
the cancer long enough for the mistletoe & GcMAF to kick in. I'll call the
Ibrance hotline today to find out whether Ibrance is an immunosuppressant. If
so, GcMAF won't work. Also, if it's an immunosuppressant, why would I take
it with Covid swirling around? [...]

Jonathan & I have a date to make love today. I hope my body cooperates. Our Bulgarian neighbor who speaks no English was so sad the other day.
She walked with us a while. She indicated [wordlessly] how beautiful it is that
Jonathan & I are two; she is only one. So sad. Made me realize—once again!—
how fortunate I am to have Jonathan.

August 8, 2021: Jenny's room was almost presentable yesterday morning! I wonder what motivated her? [...] I still become physically ill when I am
near her. The chewing, the defensiveness. I try to be warm & loving, but it is
so difficult when I can't get through to her without being cold & hard-hearted.
Plus she hits me, especially when I am most vulnerable (e.g. in double brace,
driving).

My body seems to be coming around. Rash is flatter; ridge not as pro-
nounced. I'd hate to screw up this progress with Ibrance. I called to ask whether

Ibrance was an immunosuppressant, but Accredo has not yet gotten back to me. GcMAF won't work if I'm taking an immunosuppressant. Plus, we have a pandemic raging through the streets. Do I really want to suppress my immune system when viruses are everywhere?

We watched *Shoot the Piano Player* last night, a French film. When we were choosing movies, I was just about to say that I'd like to watch any film except *StPP* last night, because I just didn't want to have to follow the subtitles. But Jonathan very much wanted to watch the film & we did. It was cute, but one of those French films that I didn't really understand. Philosophic, heavy, no resolution […] except death […].

Jonathan & I made love yesterday. Everything in working order! Penetration for the first time in a long, long time. (My lady parts have shrunk, making penetration painful up until now.) Ah, bliss!

August 9, 2021: I have until tomorrow to decide whether to start Ibrance. My inclination is to buy some time to let GcMAF kick in. Do I really want to start a drug that lowers my immunity in the middle of a pandemic? Right now, I'm leaning toward waiting a few months to start Ibrance. Three maybe […].

Kids were over yesterday. I was sick; I'm always sick around them. The aggravation, the stress returns. Jenny lost her phone again. Said Uber drive stole it from her. Also, took Uber to ice cream social. Spent $15 (or $17) for an ice cream cone […].

Jonathan suggested we abandon our Sunday dinners. Theoretically, they should be a joyous occasion—see the kids once a week, talk about the week. All Flora could talk about was Brendan Criscone & glue. Jenny started screaming, so Flora started crying & throwing napkins. I held back on what I really wanted to say to Jenny—How could you be so stupid as to lose your phone *again??* And lying to us about carpooling. I don't like you. I don't like your lies. I don't like that you learn so slowly. Did you sort your pills correctly? I'll check, *because you left them here*.

Jonathan is the only person I can trust. He's always there for me. Really cares. And I really care about him.

August 10, 2021: No Ibrance. At least not now. Is it really wise to start a drug that lowers the immune system *during a pandemic?!* The earnest, young pharmacist (EYP) asked whether I was vaccinated. When I replied no, he regurgitated the party line that the vaccine is safe & lowers the probability of contracting Covid. It's so sad that the energy these earnest, young people are expending on the party line can't be employed toward useful purposes. Like actually saving lives.

Since the EYP informed me that Ibrance lowers immunity & GcMAF doesn't work if one is taking drugs that lower immunity, yet another (the main?) reason not to take Ibrance. Of course, I can't tell that to Dr. Levitz et al. I have to play the pandemic card. Jonathan is totally behind GcMAF. He helps me so much in making decisions & feeling at peace with the choices [...].

Jonathan & I are having so much fun together. We care about each other's happiness (something he says he's still getting used to). Get used to it!

August 11, 2021: Jenny's behavior is so odd. If she would only think before she acts. "If I tell my parents I'm about to do this, what would they say?" Not that we have to agree with everything she does, but she needs to ask herself "If they would object, why?" She wastes so much time doing odd things—obsessing about an ice cream social; getting an Uber instead of telling us she needs a ride—that her book suffers.

Of course, B----- is a piece of work, not allowing unvaccinated people in her car. *Stop watching CNN!! [...]*

Jonathan is the only person on earth with whom I feel completely comfortable. How did I get so lucky?

August 12, 2021: Jonathan was so cute this morning without his underwear. Guys are lucky that way.

August 13, 2021: Twenty-six years! Wow. Best 26 years of my life. In 20 years, we will have been married 46 years [...].

Jonathan looked at me with such desire yesterday. "Do you want to have sex?" he almost pleaded. I was just about to tape the class. After my moment of hesitation, he said, "Oh, it doesn't have to be right now." But he wanted right then. Maybe I should have. But I was torn—torn between work where students don't care much & a husband who cares totally. Choices. Opportunity costs. Sunk costs. Next time, I'll do it. Sex, that is, not tape.

August 14, 2021: Enchanting day yesterday in the city. Walked around. Went to Everlane. Bought a great pair of jeans. Ordered a too-expensive pocketbook for Jenny that I may confiscate (& give her my purse, which would be perfect for her). I've never owned a $200 purse before [...] I wonder what it feels like.

Perhaps like owning a $50 purse, only made out of real leather.

Several people told us how cute we were, which we are. "I want to be like you when I grow up!" crowed one young lady. "We never did grow up!" I returned. When Jonathan got on his knee to re-propose, the ladies across the way stopped their conversation about anxiety & their anti-depressant drugs & stared. "Our wedding anniversary," I explained. "Oh, wonderful! How many years?" And so it went. An Asian young lady in the street said we looked so cute. We were just holding hands! We weren't even smooching! I guess New Yorkers are not as jaded as we think.

Or maybe they are. If just holding handing elicits positive comments, what kind of lives of quiet desperation do New Yorkers live? I sense they want some of our magic to rub off on them—& that's ok; we have plenty of magic to share— but we're just **holding hands!** The most natural of human interactions.

The restaurant was very nice. Too bad it was its last night in NYC; it's moving back to Italy. Next year […] Italy! […].

Being back in NYC with Jonathan—for the day!—was delightful. We became young again.

August 15, 2021: Jonathan & I made love yesterday. Ah, bliss!

August 16, 2021: The girls came over for dinner last night. As usual, it was hell. Flora & I went shopping for glue—what else?—& she ate something off the street. I blew up. Jenny lost her wallet with her insurance cards. At least it was just that, but, my God, can't she keep anything organized? I'll bet it's still in her purse somewhere.

Of course, I couldn't find the Metro Card on Friday when we wanted to come home. Yet, I remained calm & eventually found it. OK, Jonathan found it. But I remained calm.

Yes, I'm exhausted from Jenny losing things & my being the person who has to replace the items. Phones, insurance cards. If I were calmer & if she hadn't lost so much in the past & if she wouldn't hit me, replacing the items would not be a big deal. But she resents my suggestions.

By the time dinner came around, I had no appetite […].

What Pfizer has done to my children constitutes Crimes against Humanity. Now, I'm supposed to entrust them with my health.

Jonathan is pushing for me to put in for a vacation from the girls. We deserve it, he notes. He's better to me than I am to myself.

August 17, 2021: I'm hungry. After I write this musing (& read Jonathan's raunchy email!), I'm going to have breakfast. Typically, I wait & join Jonathan for breakfast, because I so love spending time with him. But this morning, I'm too hungry to wait. At least part of the reason I'm hungry is that I'm not in much pain […].

Going to Dr. Levitz's office today. Dreading the idea. I have to once again explain why I am not poisoning myself with pharmaceuticals that do not improve my chances of survival. Ugh….

August 18, 2021: Ugh. Saw Dr. Levitz yesterday. He's pushing Ibrance. He's a drug pusher. "I don't want you to feel I'm selling you anything," he said, as he tried to sell me Ibrance. I asked about the study that said the survival rate of women who took Ibrance was no different from the women who did not take Ibrance. He pointed out the study was from 2019, that it must have been updated. He looked for the update, but could not find it; he seemed genuinely perplexed. Hey, maybe the information Pfizer is giving you is a lie or at least exaggerated.

Anyway, I want to give GcMAF a 3-month chance. I didn't tell Dr. Levitz that; he wouldn't understand about GcMAF […].

Jonathan wants me around. I like being around Jonathan.

August 19, 2021: Leg pain interfered with a good night's sleep. Stupid letrozole. Stupid Dr. Levitz. You said you had many tools to help & you're frustrated, because I won't avail myself of them. How about the tools that boost my immune system; let's start there. What tools do you have to improve my health? None. I thought so.

Jenny opened my musings yesterday when she was on my computer when I expressly told her to clean out her emails. She is not to be trusted. It's odd; she opened some only for a minute or less. How could she possibly have read them?

Trip to see Dr. Johnson yesterday. Jenny read at Flora, who insisted on listening to—what else?—Coffeehouse. Jonathan & I could barely talk. Flora was very good at the [diner] buffet […].

Gene O'Brien wants to talk about Jenny's position in Watchung. [O'Brien was her employment counselor, who thought she could get a per diem job at a Watchung school.] I pray she doesn't need vaccination. We may have to start driving her there, which, of course, would disrupt my morning routine until we could find assistance. Cross those bridges if/when we get to them.

Jonathan is my perfect partner. Period.

August 20, 2021: Jenny has a job! I know she'll do well. She just needs to stay on top of the notices from work. She almost didn't reply to the offer.

Flora & I were on the phone for almost half an hour yesterday. Just chatting. She called me […].

It's so great being married to Jonathan. Greatest thing in my life.

August 21, 2021: We're getting the outside of the house fixed up! New roof; new siding. No more stuff growing everywhere.

So much fun playing house with Jonathan. Maybe we'll grow up someday. Hahahahahaha. I crack myself up.

August 23, 2021: Jonathan & I made love yesterday. Ah, bliss! We're both getting stronger.

August 24, 2021: Tomorrow, classes begin & Jonathan & I go into NYC to protest vaccine mandates for city employees. What a day it will be! […]

The world is going to hell in a handbasket. Vaccine mandates, gender studies, Afghanistan. No more logic, no more democracy […].

Jonathan—who was a bit uncertain about going to tomorrow's protest—yesterday announced that, yes, we should definitely go. We must do everything we can to stop the madness. A peasant revolt, while the elite enjoy a maskless, crowded event to raise money for the Democrats. Enough!

Being married to Jonathan is my greatest joy.

August 25, 2021: I wonder what great & wonderful things will happen today! […] Dad's mantra. ***That*** is the way to live […].

Rabbi Satz […] telling people to wear masks & get vaccinated when he has no earthly clue about individual circumstances. Telling people to "have the conversation" with your unvaccinated cousin. What conversation? He doesn't elaborate.

Jonathan supports me in my decision not to become a member of Temple B'nai Or […].

Protest against mandates today. The weather will be hot, but at least not raining.

I love going through life with Jonathan. Protests, rabbis & all!

August 26, 2021: I wonder what great & wonderful things will happen today! […] Thank you, Dad […].

Jonathan & I attended a protest in NYC yesterday against vaccine mandates for union members. We didn't know a soul. Bodily autonomy is attracting all sorts of strange bedfellows—gays, Republicans, pipe fitter unions […].

Jonathan wore his "Sorry, this guy is taken by a smokin' hot ECONOMIST!" tee shirt yesterday. At least ten people made positive comments. Who says New Yorkers are jaded? I so love being his economist!

August 27, 2021: I so missed having dinner with Jonathan last night. Sometimes we talk a lot; sometimes not much at all. But we are together […].

The worst part about not feeling well last night was not having the wherewithal to get Jonathan his ice cream. I so love him & I want to do the little things for him. By bedtime, I was able to straighten his sheets. I don't know if he even notices [I did]; I do it because I care.

August 28, 2021: Afghanistan is a complete & utter disaster. Who saw anything like this coming? Putting a doddering old fool in the White House & expecting nothing bad will happen […].

Feel good with mistletoe & GcMAF. & supplements & diet & enemas. Still need to reduce stress.

Jonathan helps me reduce stress. He's an angel […] when he's not a devil!

August 29, 2021: Getting Jenny ready for her new job. How exciting!

The world is literally going to hell in a handbasket. It seems people are realizing it now. Maybe it had to come to this. The corruption had to get so intense, had to affect so many individuals, before people saw what was going on. Many still don't. Those that watch CNN. Even CNN is trashing Biden over Afghanistan. Meagan McCain as well, even though she helped get him elected.

Now we know who shot Ashli Babbitt. He came forward. The officer strikes me as total mediocrity, if that.

Jonathan & I watched *Waterloo Bridge* last night. So Victorian! Vivien Leigh & Robert Taylor were excellent. I'm glad we're not Victorians.

August 30, 2021: Jenny's first day of work. Last night was awful. She drained me of any energy I had, which wasn't much. We transferred her purse. Picking out clothes was so exhausting to me that I had to leave the room. I put out some of Flora's nice blouses & skorts.

So helpless she is.

After I collapsed into bed & was asleep, she barged into our room & screamed that Jonathan was watching everything she was doing or something like that. He had told her to go to bed, because she needed to get up early. Then she started hitting herself.

That's when my legs started to hurt.

She treats us like dirt & expects that we wait on her hand & foot.

When she banged her bed against the wall & we asked her to stop, she replied that all we can think about is ourselves.

This morning there was some head banging in the powder room.

I wonder whether she realizes we have our own lives—lives separate from taking care of her every need.

I'm exhausted. She drains me; being in the same room drains me.

August 31, 2021: If it weren't for Jonathan, I would not have survived yesterday.

September 1, 2021: Jenny lost her first job yesterday [...]. Apparently, it was The Sneeze. When she sneezed at lunch & they asked her whether she had the Covid vaccine & she informed them of her unvaccinated status, everything changed. People who were formerly nice & warm & friendly suddenly became mean & cold & obnoxious.

The Elite really hate us. They are dividing us. They want it that way. Or they don't care. Whatever it takes to control us. Fear is good. Those of us they can't scare, they isolate. It's a brilliant diabolical plan.

Fortunately, Takenya—the manager at ESS—is excellent at what she does. She agreed the fit wasn't good—apparently the school told her that Jenny was sneezing & coughing & running a fever (they forgot to mention that the "fever" was a temperature of 99.1!).

Mary Holland said tyrants can't last. But when? When do we get rid of them & get our freedoms back? How? […]

Jonathan keeps me going.

September 2, 2021: I have hunger pangs! Small, but real […]. Last night, I ate ice cream—real, honest to God, store-bought with sugar ice cream! It tasted very nice […].

We need to talk with [the Group Home director] about Jenny's not being vaccinated. We can offer to use the home test once a week. [He] will insist upon masks. I'll show him the science. He won't care. We need to put up a bigger stink. [He] doesn't like hassles […].

So glad I'm going through this crazy world with Jonathan. Otherwise— quite literally—I would not be able to survive.

September 3, 2021: Where to begin? Jenny is on the verge of getting kicked out of [the Group Home] for not being vaccinated. People have gone mad. There's nothing we can do. So, we explore other options. Got a message about Jespy House yesterday. Divine intervention?

The conversation with [the Group Home director] was cordial. Jenny sets the kitchen on fire & that needs to stop. OK. She's out late at night. That needs to stop. Totally agree! But […] Jenny needs to wear a mask because she is unvaccinated. I should have pushed back—not that it would have mattered. If the other resident is vaccinated & thereby protected, why does it matter whether Jenny is vaccinated? Second question: The CDC now says even vaccinated people can transmit Covid. Should then not all residents be required to wear masks?

Questions you think about later […]

The email from [the director] was not so cordial. It was a threat, an ultimatum. Covering his ass so that he has a paper trail when he boots Jenny […].

Speaking of Divine Intervention, we could use some right now. DI, if You do exist, HELP! The world You created is being run by tyrants who are determined to destroy Your creation.

A few sane voices exist—RFK Jr.—but they are being threatened.

Let me know what I can do to help save Your creation. I won't worship the false gods of pharma. I will speak out more, calmly & with facts. I will remain in awe of the Tree of Life & Knowledge, but I will not try to eat its fruit.

I am getting stronger. Yesterday, I started drinking beef blood & my appetite seemed stronger. This morning, I'm drinking straight coffee (not keto coffee with butter & coconut oil) in hopes that I have a strong appetite for breakfast. I think I do […].

Jonathan said he's so glad to have me. Imagine that, **he's** glad to have **me!** I would have collapsed years ago without him.

September 4, 2021: It's too bad Jenny couldn't rise to the occasion. She's getting kicked out of [the Group Home] for not being vaccinated, but we see the lack of impulse control & the inability to handle money. Those are the real issues & the [Group Home] is not able to address them […].

Jenny is going to feel less anxious if she is more organized. She won't lose things so much. She won't be going to the bank so often to get money back. She can concentrate on her writing […].

I'm speaking out more, telling people why I'm not vaccinating. Cordial & clearly, but forcefully […]. The vaccines are unsafe & ineffective. The disease is nothing to young people; older people need to do a cost-benefit analysis. I did & decided the vaccine has more potential costs than known benefits.

It's so much fun playing house with Jonathan. We have a new roof! It's so nice. No green stuff growing between the shingles. The house will look great with new siding.

September 5, 2021: So glad the girls aren't coming for dinner. I couldn't handle them today […].

Jonathan & I watched *Les Girls* with Gene Kelly. It was cute. He is cute. We are cute.

September 6, 2021: Moving slowly. Hannah's Bat Mitzvah Celebration today. Suzanne & Mark won't be there, because "there might be people who aren't vaccinated." I can only shake my head. Just when I was getting the hang of this family thing, the family has to dissolve. Thanks to Bill Gates, the Clintons, George Soros, Jeff Bezos, Mark Zuckerberg, Jack Dorsey.

I had a dream last night I was interviewing for a new position—an academic position, I believe. I had an ethical stain on my record—unclear what—& my CV (which the interviewers did not have) was very thin. Kind of like now. Except for the ethical stain pain. Maybe the greater society thinks I have an ethical stain—that I'm being selfish for not vaccinating. The greater society is brainwashed by CNN, mouthpiece to the above-mentioned tyrants. I was planning to discuss my *Review of Industrial Organization* paper on vaccine safety before & after delitigation [that is, before and after the 1986 National Childhood Vaccine Injury Act shielded vaccine manufacturers from virtually all lawsuits arising from vaccine-related injuries or deaths]. But the elevators stopped working at the firm (at this point, it felt more like a firm than an academic institution). Something like a boat. I did manage to find some of the people with whom I was to interview & they contacted their higher-ups who were also to be part of the interview. We waited, watching some kind of propaganda film about the firm. It was almost as though the lower ranking people were preventing me from talking with their higher-ups. I then realized I hadn't done my homework on the products the firm creates & why I wanted to work at the firm.

I slept most of yesterday, punctuated with […] making love with Jonathan. At least I'm able to partake in life's greatest pleasures.

Jonathan & I enjoyed ourselves (see above). We still have it!

September 7, 2021: Yesterday, I felt awful. It's such shame, too, because it was Hannah's Bat Mitzvah. I had no energy. No appetite. Slight fever, chills. I just didn't feel like socializing. The music prevented most conversations, anyway.

When I got home—I was able to drive us back safely—I collapsed. Temperature was 102.3, but went down to 101.8 by the time I went to bed. This morning, it's 99.8. I'm feeling somewhat better. Was able to eat jelly toast for breakfast, after having no dinner last night […].

Jonathan is so sweet. I imagine that his mom was not the world's best caretaker, but he is! I'm just sorry he has to be.

September 8, 2021: I so love being married to Jonathan. Besides everything else, he makes sure I eat. If I were living alone, I'd starve to death. Jonathan said he's glad I'm not living alone, for many reasons.

September 9, 2021: Semi-rough night. Right leg pain. Jonathan's snarky sounds; he stopped when I asked him to. I felt bad. He's such a wonderful husband; I hate to criticize. But I couldn't rest & his funny sounds weren't helping […].

We Unvaccinated are second-class citizens. We, the unwashed, the irresponsible, the selfish. [My hair stylist] put on a mask when he remembered I wasn't vaccinated. He said it was to protect me. Please. Suzanne & Mark probably won't get together with us for Thanksgiving in person; we're unsanitary, dirty […].

I do so love being married to Jonathan. I wish life weren't so difficult for us, but there's no one I'd rather go through hell with. It used to be micro-hell (autism) & now it's macro-hell (Covid). Hell is hell, only now we're sharing it with more people.

September 10, 2021: Biden mandating that employers require vaccines (or tests). Why go out of his way to get half of America to hate him? Why this huge push? From so many sources—government, schools, media, social media. There's something nefarious going on & I'm no longer convinced it's just money. Do the injections change us somehow? Do they track us? Make us more obedient? All I know is that *I* am not getting one.

Yesterday was a great day. Morning a little slow—very tired—but lunch-time delightful with my girlfriends. Even if I couldn't remember a single thing we said when Jonathan asked what we talked about […].

Jonathan takes such good care of me. He's so precious.

September 11, 2021: Twenty years ago. Look what the Taliban have achieved. The United States is pathetic. Joe Biden is pathetic.

I need to get back to research so I don't micro-analyze every bodily function.

Speaking of bodily functions, Jonathan & I are going to have sex today. Yeah!

September 12, 2021: Twenty years ago, I felt such unity with all Americans. We were all in this together. What a fool I was. We were never in this together. The Clintons had already divided America; George H. W. Bush smirked during his "The State of the Union is strong" speech. We've been becoming more divided ever since. Who would sign up for the military now? By the way, why are we glorifying only the firefighters? Certainly, they deserve the glory, but weren't there one or two police officers on the scene? […].

Jonathan & I watched *To Kill a Mockingbird* last night. I had seen it before but forgot everything except the scene where Scout was a ham for Halloween. It's so much fun sharing movie night—and everything!—with Jonathan.

September 13, 2021: Pleasant day at the beach—or as pleasant as a day at the beach surrounded by vaccine-injured people allows. [It was a special event for autism families.] Nice breeze. Friendly people. Flora enjoyed herself, but then started perseverating about the missing piece on her purse […].

Popped into HBOT after returning home, exhausted. Whose cheerful little face should appear but Jenny. Ugh. I thought. No. Go away.

She wanted to print out something for Larry's birthday. I asked her how she was going to get home & she said Jonathan offered, which he had not. She just comes waltzing in, expects us to chauffeur her everywhere. When I asked her—several times—whether she had sorted her pills, she lied & said she had. There were no telltale signs of her having sorted her pills—she always has telltale signs.

She detected I was annoyed. "Be honest, why are you annoyed?" When I told her, she flew into a rage. "Most parents care about their children" etc.

Jonathan drove her back to [the Group Home] as she pounded the dash-board & hit herself.

There's nothing more I can do. I need to focus on my health […].

Jonathan stays so cool. It's a good thing. He says his mom was also insane.

September 14, 2021: Jenny came by yesterday […]. She managed to attack me when I was down. Fortunately, it was just verbally.

Jonathan & I had dinner on the couch. It was nice. I could rest my head between bites. He's such a gentle soul.

September 15, 2021: Whew! Second day in a row that I'm feeling good upon rising. Yesterday was a good day. Jonathan noticed more color in my face right away. I had energy & even a modicum of zest.

Hemoglobin down only slightly (7.95). The physician's assistant suggested a blood transfusion, which I declined for the time being. I sensed yesterday I had turned a corner […].

It's so nice to have energy.

Jonathan sticks with me through sickness & in health. Literally. Ditto.

September 16, 2021: Jenny is back here because she had a violent outburst at [the Group Home. The director] keeps moving the goal posts. He wants her out.

The first half of the evening, Jenny seemed to be scared straight. She seemed to understand the consequences of her actions. However, while we were watching Tucker Carlson, she became agitated. He did a great segment on Nikki Minaj & how she's standing up to the vaccine bullies. Jenny kept getting more & more agitated. When she asked whether I would pay her for staying calm & allowing me to use the remote, I said no. She EXPLODED. The tantrum lasted from about 9 pm to midnight. Headbanging, screaming.

She read some of my musings. I need to change my password.

We may have to commit her. But where? We'll hang there today—Jewish Family Services is closed due to Yom Kippur—& talk with Danielle Weiss [our support coordinator] tomorrow.

This is hell. This is absolute hell. There's no one I'd rather go through hell with than Jonathan.

September 19, 2021: Finally able to write a musing. Friday, I was flat on my back, in pain. Yesterday, I was flat on my back, but fortunately, the pain had more or less subsided. Having Jenny back living with us in not helping […].

AVIDD [the agency that provided a group home for Flora] can be a pain in the neck sometimes with the paperwork, but that's the deal. They need every t crossed & i dotted. And we all have the best interests of the resident. The procedures provide protection […].

Jonathan sticks with me through thick & thin, in sickness & in health & every stage in between. How did I get so lucky?

September 20, 2021: Jenny is so flakey & flighty & irresponsible. I hope Jespy House comes through. Soon.

Jonathan & I made love yesterday. It was very nice. The Uriel cream helps immensely.

September 22, 2021: Having Jenny here is a pain. Two explosions yesterday. One right before leaving for work. Couldn't find purse. Kissed me good-bye & then bopped me on the head […].

Jenny interrupted my writing by peering over my shoulder. Seems as though her second day at work [as a per diem teacher's aide] went well.

Disappointing news from Dr. Isaacs. She's not pushing my returning to pancreatic enzymes because, at this point, it probably wouldn't help much. I was taken aback. She's rescued people with stage 4 pancreatic cancer, but then I realized—I wasn't supposed to go to stage 4 on her protocol. But I did. To her great credit, she didn't drop me as a patient when her protocol stopped working. Almost all other doctors would […].

I love Jonathan so much. What more can I say?

September 23, 2021: My birthday! Funny what metastatic breast cancer will do to you—***happy*** to be another year older.

Much work today, getting ready for class next week. Also, appointment with Dr. Levitz, who will push Ibrance. Maybe soon. Not yet […].

Cords scattered everywhere as Jenny looks for recharger (I think). She has a specialized cord for recharging […].

Works seems to be going nicely for her. I'm glad. I'm exhausted from supporting her, but I'm glad. Jonathan transports her. He's protecting me.

He loves me so much and I him.

September 24, 2021: Yesterday I started Ibrance, & dammit, I am feeling better. I had a good night's sleep; woke up refreshed.

The cancer appears to have gone to my bone marrow, which explains the anemia.

Jenny behaving nicely. No explosions yesterday […]. She has this unfounded fear of talking with me. Yes, I give her a lecture if she does something stupid, but I find out about her doing stupid things any way. If I don't give her a lecture—and in the past I've tried to ignore stupid behavior—no one else tells her, but they treat her differently […] and not in a good way.

Jonathan is my rock. He's upset about the new medical news, but taking it in stride. One day at a time. We're kissing even ***more*** now, if that's possible.

September 25, 2021: Very nice birthday dinner last night. Flora didn't ask about Brendan Criscione until well after an hour. There's still no conversation. Pfizer, I will never forgive you.

However, dear Pfizer, you have created Ibrance, which is helping me. I slept well last night, woke up refreshed. I don't know how long the drug will help & I don't know the side effects—you lie about side effects—but I will take Ibrance until the cancer is under control. I have the energy now to discuss Ibrance & Pfizer in chat rooms. Yes, Ibrance is really helping me. However, I don't trust Pfizer, because Pfizer poisoned my child with Prevnar. Pfizer, if you really want to redeem yourself, find a way for me to have a conversation with my child. In the meantime, f*ck you.

Things seem to be moving with getting Jenny better housing […]. Jenny is being nicer. I'll enjoy it while I can. She still doesn't understand the danger from candles, but doesn't explode when I make suggestions. In fact, she hasn't exploded in at least a day, maybe two.

I'm glad I'm sticking around for Jonathan.

September 26, 2021: Jenny is a monster. A manipulative, calculating animal out to destroy her life & our lives. But why?

Wrote to a stranger that I had been attacked on the set of *The Act 1986*. Kim Rossi let me know about it. Jenny is so sick. She keeps calling Jonathan a "simp," which means "Suckers Idolizing Mediocre Pussy."

I forgot to take Ibrance yesterday. Didn't feel as energetic as previous two days. It will be interesting to see what happens today.

I need to write paragraph on how burdens shifting to Jonathan will affect his health.

I love Jonathan so much.

September 27, 2021: Feeling better with Ibrance. I suppose women feel better with Ibrance for a while until the cancer overwhelms the drug. But what if a woman addresses the cancer while on Ibrance? For example, with GcMAF or mistletoe? And, of course, diet & stress-reduction. I guess we're about to find out.

Jenny has a gig today. Assistant teacher in Madison. Starting at 11:10 am. Nice […].

Jonathan is doing more of the paperwork. He senses when I need help & steps in immediately. The world's greatest BFF.

[On this date Gayle and I wrote to the Division of Developmental Disabilities appealing for emergency housing for Jennifer. Jenny made the same request in her own letter, which reveals that, when she was lucid, she fully understood her out-of-control episodes and felt real remorse. "I can no longer handle living at home," she wrote. "Recently, the fights I have been having with my mother have gotten so hostile that every day we're at each other's throats […]. For example, yesterday, I posted online that she was sexually assaulted (which wasn't true) to spite her after a particularly brutal fight […]. I can't keep going on like this. If I want to be a mature adult, I'll have to learn to take responsibility for my own actions [...]. When I'm in a state like this, it's difficult for me to calm down or be reasoned with—if anything, telling me to 'calm down' only makes matters much worse."]

September 28, 2021: Jenny is involuntarily in the hospital. Her rages have become more frequent & more violent. She can't control herself. The peace in the home is palpable. I hate to say that, but it's true. Jenny is very sick & it's time for drugs. Probably past time. As few as possible. As natural as possible. But her paranoia ("my parents are making fun of me") coupled with her physical aggression against me & her screaming—in public now—show she is totally out of control.

Jonathan & I are both deeply saddened by the family we could have had. We both tried so hard. We have each other.

September 29, 2021: Day 2 of Jenny being held in the ER psych ward. She became a little agitated when I reminded her why she was there, but otherwise, she is her sweet self. She wants out & who can blame her? [...]

Jonathan & I are surviving this together. Today is his day with Jenny. Being around her is no longer draining but being in the hospital is [...].

September 30, 2021: Jenny moved back in with us [...]. Jenny is being incredibly sweet & cooperative as well as innovative. When the remote didn't work last night, she attempted to fix it by turning around the batteries. That takes some logic, even though it was incorrect. I'm not sure why the remote didn't work for her—perhaps the batteries had popped out—but I got it work & she allowed me to use it during the programs. Without a fuss [...]. Solitary confinement—with no cell phone or computer—has had a salutary effect. Let's hope it lasts [...].

Going through hell with Jonathan is not the worst thing in the world. I look forward to a little more heaven again.

October 1, 2021: Jenny had another rage last night when I received a text from Dara Berger. DB is huge trigger for Jenny. Screaming, kicking, hitting herself, chewing [...] the usual. "Some parents care about their children's self esteem" & "So-&-so's parents love her more than you love me." What a piece of work. Jenny started sobbing after her outburst. Jonathan consoled her; I went to bed.

Baruch is trying to force all students to get vaccinated. What's up? [...]

Yesterday, we moved Jenny out of [the Group Home]. The whole experience was a disaster. Jeremy was upset. He said he didn't want Jenny to leave. Jenny, quite maturely, said, "You can't always get what you want." We said the two of them could still get together [...].

Going through hell with Jonathan. No one I'd rather go through hell with. When does heaven appear?

October 2, 2021: Jenny called [the Group Home director] on Thursday night during her fit. Of all the people on Earth, she chooses the one who cares least about her. That really hurts. & it shows what a bad judge of character she is. She knows he's a shit, yet she reaches out to him. Almost as though she wanted to sabotage her recovery. So sick […].

Yesterday was a Jenny day […]. Dr. W prescribed lithium. We'll see.

I hope Jonathan & I can make love today. As long as Jenny doesn't have a rage & I'm able to stay on an even keel, I see sex in the near future.

October 3, 2021: Jenny is still here. Yesterday, she had two explosions—one mild, one medium. I don't even remember the cause. Typically, there isn't really one. OK, I guess there are triggers. Dara Berger, "Dad is a words person, I'm a number person," nurses are fighting vaccine mandates. Jonathan pointed out that my work has nothing to do with Jenny's outbursts. Had I been a housewife, Jenny would have been a radical feminist.

I'm tired of walking on eggshells. Dr. Weiss said one theory is to expose Jenny to the triggers over time. Jonathan & I do that naturally, I suppose, when we read & discuss news articles […].

We watched a documentary about Buster Keaton last night. I wasn't all that thrilled with the idea, but Jonathan wanted to watch it. I'm so glad we did! It was marvelous & Jonathan really enjoyed it. I can only be happy when he's happy.

October 4, 2021: Jonathan & I made love yesterday. It was so, so sweet. I'm dry & need to figure out how to make it hurt less. He's so BIG!

October 5, 2021: Yesterday, I did feel a little dizzy right before leaving for Sylvia Shire's funeral.

She was an amazing woman, Sylvia [a cousin of Jonathan's on his mother's side]. Strong family & community values. Her children—at least one daughter—admired her as well as her platoon of grandchildren.

I have these visions while reading Joe Dispenza. We're going on a trip, the girls & I, to meet Jonathan. I open the satchel to pack & rays of sunlight come pouring out. There's light & sun & breeze & salt air. It's enchanting. A good feeling. A healing feeling.

Jonathan & I are both sad about the dissolving of our families. My family fell apart after Dad died; his as a result of Covid (though extended family fell apart before then). Greed, fear, intrusion by the Dark Side (if you have family, who needs government?). We have each other.

October 6, 2021: Appetite is back. Food tastes so good. Especially Linda's sugar-free baked goods. She is an angel.

Jenny had zero explosions Monday or Tuesday. I don't think anything on Sunday either […]. Maybe it's been low lithium all along. Wouldn't that be a pisser?

Life's journey with Jonathan is enchanting. Period. No, exclamation point!

October 7, 2021: I restart mistletoe injections today. Jonathan pointed out that my rapid response to Ibrance is probably a function of GcMAF able to kick in. His hypothesis is that Ibrance reduces the growth of the cancer enough so that GcMAF can attack the cancer. All I know is that Ibrance is supposed to suppress my appetite, which it has NOT, and that I'm feeling better […].

Jenny had one explosion yesterday. Jonathan told her to clean up her desk area. She had spent all morning cleaning her room, so she was tired of cleaning. Still, her reaction—screaming, hitting herself, banging her head—were totally inappropriate. The explosion, while intense, was relatively short-lived. About a half an hour. I sense she's getting better. The lithium seems to help […].

I so love Jonathan. We had a nice, quiet dinner—Jenny went to game night at a bar. I love our quiet time together.

October 8, 2021: We weren't sure whether Jenny was needed at Madison Junior School today. She called this morning & found out she was not needed. She did a great job with the phone call […].

Jonathan & I made mad passionate love yesterday afternoon. It's hurting less & less. He's very gentle, even though he is so BIG.

October 9, 2021: I continue to feel good. Energy, appetite, desire to work […] & play. According to the chats on "Health Unlocked" (what a name, eh?), Ibrance wears off after a while—stops working. Maybe by that time GcMAF will kick in, assuming Ibrance—which lowers to some extent my immune system—allows the GcMAF to do its thing. And the mistletoe.

Anyway, I'll enjoy this time while I can […].

We see Flora today. We're taking her out for lunch in Boonton. I'm looking forward to that.

Jonathan was lost in thought during our walk yesterday. I just let him work & didn't prattle on the way I normally do. I so want him to be happy.

October 10, 2021: Several days now without Jenny exploding. She came close a couple of times—last night when I wasn't sure whether "stupendous" was a) a word & b) a good description of the music in the film *Exodus*. Yes & yes.

Jenny spent $40 on shot-gunmess.com. No concept of money or understanding of "free offers" […]. Ugh. When will she become responsible?

Pleasant lunch with Flora. Latin American restaurant where language was a barrier. Nail place overcharged for Flora's "manicure." So, we don't go back. Market capitalism—in its true form—is great.

Do I still want to convert? Good question. The response to coronavirus is really showing people's reactions to fear. Instead of asking questions & debating issues, people fearfully follow government edicts. Even Jews. Especially Jews? I'm just so surprised & disheartened. Disillusioned perhaps. Disillusioned definitely. The data from Israel show how ineffective the vaccine is & the data from VAERS show how dangerous it can be.

I need to speak up more. Not as a crazy person, but as a person who has reviewed the data & observed anomalies.

Jonathan is descending the stairs. I have not yet read his raunchy email. He just promised me I'll be a little surprised. Huh? Gotta go find out what he meant by that […]

October 11, 2021: Today, we go to Jespy House. I hope it's a good fit. Jenny really needs guidance that I can't provide—because I'm living my own life (trying to, anyway) & she reacts so negatively when I try to provide advice. Her room looks like a tornado hit it, really. Ditto her desk area. Why things on the floor? It's so much easier not to make a mess in the beginning […]. When will she become responsible?

I've always been more than responsible, so I don't know how to assist in her growth. I simply do not understand her […].

Looking so forward to research again. Teaching-research-home balance. Ha! That's a joke.

I love travelling through life with Jonathan.

October 12, 2021: I'd like to continue with mistletoe. I'm not sure how effective GcMAF is since Ibrance suppresses the immune system & I want to do more than Ibrance. We'll suppress the cancer, kill the "escapee" cancer cells with GcMAF &/or mistletoe & live a good life to 104.

Jenny had a great interview with JESPY House yesterday. The only glitch might be vaccination, though Frank [the Intake Coordinator] didn't seem put out when he learned we belonged to the unwashed. (The unpolluted, in my mind, but that's a different thought thread.) […].

Jonathan helped me fill out Jenny's JESPY form. No one I'd rather go through hell with.

October 13, 2021: I so resent Jenny's being here. I know the resentment is making me sick, but for God's sake, she requires so much work—the forms, the doctor appointments, the chauffeuring. You can do that when kids are little, but I'm trying to have my own life. I do fear that we get Jenny settled &

then I die. That would be so unfair to Jonathan, so brutally unfair to such a wonderful human being.

No, I have to hang in there. Once Jenny is gone, I can focus more on my healing. She won't be here forever; she can't be. It just feels that way, sometimes.

Her tantrums are fewer, but I still never know when she is going to explode. She got upset when she couldn't find the blender, which she had put in the refrigerator. Oh, please. She said I yelled at her.

I so love Jonathan.

October 14, 2021: Child abuse—I'm being abused by my child. She hates me. She obviously wants me to die. Her tantrums create so much stress that I am one step closer to death. There are only two people on this earth who can attack me the way she did without my calling the police—she & Flora. If I had a husband who abused me the way Jenny abuses me, I would obtain a restraining order […]. She is literally killing me. Why does she hate me so much?

With my intense diarrhea, I'm not quite sure what to do. I sense it is the mistletoe, but it could be the Ibrance. I'll be suspending Ibrance for a week. Should I continue with the mistletoe to see if the diarrhea goes away sans Ibrance? Or do I cut back (or suspend) mistletoe? The diarrhea does make me miserable—*almost* as miserable as being Jenny's mom.

There's no one I'd rather go through hell with than Jonathan.

October 15, 2021: Jenny didn't hit me, even though I mentioned Dara Berger's name! Dr. Weiss is upping the lithium. Let's hope—for everyone's sake—it works […].

I so love "Mr. King" (Jonathan). We saw a movie a long time ago about King George III. His wife referred to him as "Mr. King" & he referred to her as "Mrs. King" [as Gayle and I did in bed].

October 16, 2021: Jenny went on another bender last night. It is like living with an alcoholic. One moment, so sweet & caring; the next, raging, screaming & punching. Jenny self-medicates with alcohol & is usually quite pleasant when tipsy such as Thursday. But yesterday, dear God, edgy all day, but kept it together. Then at night, explosion. Screaming, lying that "Dad violated me," banging her bed against the wall (even after we moved it; quite a feat), hitting herself.

We've lived with this behavior for so long we sometimes forget that *it is not normal*. If JESPY House can't straighten her out, she will have to be committed.

I have to finish the application, which is difficult because I'm exhausted. I'm tired of all the forms & the doctors & the pills. Her room is a pigsty, her supplements are not sorted, her clothes torn from her chewing.

We received a shocking email from Bridgette yesterday reporting that Flora's behavior is very disruptive. I guess I shouldn't be shocked about anything anymore—all the calls from schools & colleges & workplaces for each girl. Just as my stomach lining repairs itself, I would get another one of "those" phone calls & I wouldn't be able to eat again […].

I was also searching for some emails to piece together Jenny's hospitalizations. Man oh man, I wrote hundreds of emails to various doctors & healthcare providers. The amount of time & energy I've spent on getting the girls well is ***not normal***. Yes, I could have been a contender, but autism denied me my fate. Worse—***much*** worse—it denied my girls their fates. They will never be the women they were supposed to be […].

Jonathan & I are considering going to a protest against vaccine mandates (or something like that) in NYC today. That was one thing that set off Jenny yesterday. I really want to go for at least two reasons—to get away from Jenny & to let her know she can't bully us into changing our plans. Also, we'd be fighting for what's right; that too. Jonathan is bit more ambivalent than I. Let's see how he feels this morning.

How could two such wonderful people as Jonathan & I have created such a monster? As Jonathan pointed out, ***we*** didn't create the monster. The pharmaceutical companies did along with Big Tech & politicians. How can I possibly have cancer when I am married to my best friend & love conquers all including the stress of autism?

October 17, 2021: Jonathan & I had a delightful day in NYC protesting vaccine mandates. The crowd was large & diverse—in the blue middle of a blue state! Bobby Kennedy spoke & then a slate of people telling us to feel the "love." We decided to feel the warmth of baked goods & had a wonderful snack at a nearby coffee shop. We sat outside, because we didn't have a vaccine passport & we (I) didn't want to get the shop in trouble. Two police officers were there, also feeling the warmth of the baked goods, & I thanked them for all they do. It felt good. I later saw them along the route we walked to Hudson Yards. I thought how sad it might be—for all of us—if they needed to arrest us. They didn't need to, as we were peaceful & no one attacked us […].

Jenny was up & down yesterday. Head banging […]. Then bed rattling & two screams in the middle of night. Then sleep. What an awful guest she is!

It's so much fun going through life with Jonathan. Even riding the PATH train is easier & more fun with him. **Especially** riding the PATH is more fun with him.

October 18, 2021: Jonathan asked me a very simple question, which, as often happens, I could not answer. How does GcMAF work? Let me explore right now. "GcMAF is short for Glycoprotein Macrophage Activating Factor." Apparently, a healthy body makes GcMAF on its own. One of the functions of GcMAF is to activate macrophages, "which eradicate viruses, tumors, antigens and other unwanted cells from the body."

Jenny hasn't had work in a while. Odd. The incident manager has not yet called us back, even after we left two messages. I hope Jenny isn't being automatically eliminated from possibilities [...].

Jonathan is up now, so I'll go enjoy breakfast with him. We made sweet, sweet love yesterday. It's getting easier, though I'm still very dry. Old age sucks, but bearable (& bareable) with Jonathan.

October 19, 2021: I just started reading *It's OK That You're Not OK* or something like that. I don't want to dwell on my anger & sadness, but I guess I have to recognize it.

My hair is thinning. Stupid cancer treatments. But I am feeling better. Diarrhea is subsiding [...].

Jenny was away during the day yesterday. Why isn't she getting jobs? It's odd. Odd jobs.

Sometimes her chatter is so annoying. It's close to the topic, but not quite. Plus the interruptions. Ugh!

Jonathan keeps me sane. Then drives me insane, in the nicest possible ways!

October 20, 2021: Have two parents ever tried harder to have a happy family & failed so miserably? The ballet lessons, the girl scouts, the outings (to watch the leaves turn!), the doctors' visits, the supplements, the therapies. Flora seems to be unhappy in her new home & Jenny, my god, Jenny, such an ingrate. Matt called late last night. Jonathan suggested Jenny take the call in case it was something important about their date today. Jenny was "in the middle of something" on the computer, but was able to take enough of a break to take a swipe at Jonathan. Then she lunged at me; she didn't make contact, but it was still scary.

She will be out of the house by the end of the year. Either JESPY House or another housing arrangement or an institution. Of course, I hope for JESPY or something similar, but her violence is so ingrained that it may be too late. That's how she handles frustration—attacking. Fortunately, it seems that it's only been toward Jonathan & me. But what happens when we're not around for a while? Will the violence calm down or will she find other targets? Others will always put demands on her […].

I'm sharing the burdens more with Jonathan now. That's bound to affect his health. We so very much need each other.

October 21, 2021: Alex Berenson gave me a great research idea. He claims all-cause death is higher among countries that are highly vaccinated. The overall death rate has increased in countries such as the United Kingdom & Israel, especially among people (men?) aged 30 to 50. Heart conditions in particular are causing death. We could determine a) whether this is true & b) whether the Covid vaccine is somehow implicated. The dependent variable would be the death rate for a particular area; independent variables would include vaccination rate along with control. Perhaps over the past two years […].

Spoke with Dr. Isaacs yesterday. She's not giving up on me; she just felt having me take pancreatic enzymes when I was already so tired would be too much. That made me happy.

Jenny is still up & down, understandably. Who wants to live at home when she's 25 & has tasted the sweet nectar of freedom? Still, she needs guidance wherever she goes.

Lunch with Kim yesterday very nice. She suggested Jenny might have concussions from her headbanging. The son of a friend of hers developed anxiety after a concussion playing sports […]. Hey, you never know […].

Jonathan & I have a hot lunch date today at Chestnut Ridge […]. It's so much fun travelling through life with him.

October 22, 2021: Workmen are here. We're getting a new outside! We'll wait for Jenny to leave before we fix the inside.

Pleasant lunch with Mary [Holland] & Heidi [Kidd, now also an officer at Children's Health Defense]. Women do prattle on about unimportant topics. Still, I like going out with my girlfriends. I'm also glad Jonathan was along; when a man is present, women are somewhat less prattling […].

Jonathan is up & I want to enjoy breakfast with him. He's so much fun. First, I will read the raunchy email he sent me.

October 24, 2021: *Man from Laramie* with James Stewart—very good! […].

Having her here is such a pain. From now on, I will use "she" & "her"—I suppose those are the pronouns she prefers—instead of her name. That way, she can't search on her name & I can vent without her snooping.

& vent I need to do. She's such a selfish bitch. Everything is about her. Yesterday, I wasn't feeling well & I was a little slow in changing the radio station in the car. She exploded & hit me. Not everything is about her, but then it becomes about her.

Flora is still Flora. No hope. All we've done [...] to no avail.

Jonathan is still Jonathan. Blessed be he.

October 25, 2021: She wants me dead; my daughter wants me to die. That's the only explanation for her keeping the stress level at fever pitch. She knows the stress is killing me—she sees me fading. The worse I get—sleeping all day, cutting short a walk—the nastier she becomes. She thinks if her mother dies that she'll be the "right" kind of victim; that people will feel sorry for her. She's so sick [...].

I so love Jonathan. Life with her here is hell. He & I find our oasis. Like yesterday afternoon [...]

October 26, 2021: She had an explosion yesterday when she couldn't find her insurance cards. Instead of staying calm, she exploded. Eventually, she found them in a side pocket of her purse. I pointed out that had she stayed calm, she might have found the cards earlier.

She demanded a kiss good-bye. I don't want her touching me. I'm afraid of her when she's in one of those moods.

Jonathan protects me [...].

I so love Jonathan.

October 27, 2021: She changed my password. She f*ckin' changed the password I need to get into my computer. And I'm *not* supposed to resent her? Well, I do. I resent her living here; I resent having to drive her everywhere; I resent her complete & utter lack of appreciation [...].

Jonathan is eating breakfast & I so love eating with him.

October 29, 2021: Sometimes the woman who lives with us says things that are spot on [...] & sometimes she just interrupts. Most times she interrupts & I lose my train of thought. It's the worn-out "jokes" that get to me the most, but I could also do without the marginal comments that do not contribute to the conversation. I don't think she & I ever had a conversation. Everything is about her & it's quite boring.

October 30, 2021: Lunch with Miriam & Michelle yesterday. Miriam's sister-in-law won't come for Thanksgiving, because her 5- & 9-year-olds are not vaccinated. It must be awful to live with such fear.

November 3, 2021: Election yesterday. Moderate Republican Youngkin won in Virginia. Too close to call in New Jersey. Wow. Restores my faith in the American people. Democrats have gotten between us mama & papa bears & our cubs. We in the enlightened autism community have seen it for years. Now the rest of the parents see it as well—critical race theory (which VA Dems deny is being taught), lockdowns, masks. Vaccines for kids—and the ensuing injuries—will push people over the edge. You can't deny what people see with their own eyes. It's too late for Flora, but we can save others […].

Watching the elections with Jonathan I was calm. I'm almost always calm around Jonathan […].

November 4, 2021: [Steve] Sweeney [President of the New Jersey Senate, who in 2019 had led the effort to abolish religious exemptions for vaccinating schoolchildren] seems to be on his way out! What a shocker. Restores my faith in the American—even the NJ!—public! Elections matter […].

Still uncomfortable watching television with the woman who lives in our house. She either won't sit still during commercials or sits & chews on her shirt. I know she's upset because she lost her phone—again!—but that's all the more reason to get organized. My suggestions go unheeded or worse—she hits me […].

Jonathan is such a wonderful soulmate. We're both pleased about the election results. […] It's fun sharing good news with my soulmate.

November 5, 2021: […] The woman who lives in our house has been good lately. Let's hope the new house comes through & is what we think it is.

Jonathan was like a little puppy dog this morning in bed, kissing me all over. He's an adorable puppy dog!

November 6, 2021: We're still feeling the aftershock of the election. Murphy is shaken. Americans are even greater than I thought. We know what we see & we can't be brainwashed. And you never, *ever* come between a mama & papa bear & their cubs. ***That's*** what makes America great.

I'll draft a letter to Ed Durr [the truck driver who scored an upset victory over Steve Sweeney] & include a check for $153 for his re-election campaign. I'll also contact the political wing of the NJ vaccine safety movement. I sense Mr. Durr will be receptive. We're just parents wanting to do right by our kids […].

Cancer rash is bigger; along the sternum. Bumpy. Bad stuff coming out?

Other than that, energy is level is glorious. Sometimes I feel like an Alzheimer's patient—wouldn't it be awful to have such a dreaded disease named after you?—who knows the lucid (in my case energetic) moments are probably fleeting. Still, I refuse to live in fear & I will enjoy the delicious moments I have.

Jonathan & I stopped drinking about a week ago since my liver enzymes are high. I don't miss drinking.

November 7, 2021: My daughter is slowly killing me. Her erratic explosions; the eggshells upon which we walk ***in our own home***; her insane insistence on being the "right kind of victim"; her demands that we cater to her every wish, with no regard for how she taxes our lives. The holes in the walls are evidence of her animal behavior as well as all the chewed items around the house. I can no longer tolerate this & my body is fading.

Yesterday, we discovered that she overdrew her account (again). She spent $40 looking for a $60 phone, when we have a replacement phone at the ready. When we pointed out the stupidity of her actions, she did what she always does—attacked us, especially me. Then, of course, she ranted while I was on the phone [...] discussing my HPV & fertility paper [...].

She's a tyrant & a monster. Perhaps she thinks she'll be the "right kind of victim" if her mother dies. She's certainly doing everything in her power to find out. No respect; no appreciation; no ability to learn from mistakes.

I see these students at Baruch who had far less going for them & they overcome so much. I'm so glad I work [...].

First, I'll read Jonathan's raunchy email. He keeps me sane [...] & drives me insane (in a good way) [...]

November 8, 2021: That woman continues to be a monster & a tyrant & a bully. She used my computer last night & managed to chew on several of the items on my desk, including a small flashlight. I got it to work, but her policy of "take & break" is so selfish.

There's going to be a webinar about a girl who was violent—especially against her mother—but the father addressed her viruses & the girl is good now. The girl took Valtrex along with other supplements. Not sure why I'm going to waste my time & energy, but I have to try this one last thing.

Getting back to research is grand. Too bad that woman is sapping so much of my energy. I'll ignore her as best I can.

That man is **not** sapping energy. He makes me feel warm & loved & needed.

November 9, 2021: We watched *Top Secret!* as a semi-family on Saturday. It was quite nice. The woman who lives in our house sat still during the entire movie, unlike when we watch the news & she jumps up during commercials to dash to her computer & then dash back. It's annoying.

Jonathan is **not** annoying. Quite the opposite. What is the opposite of annoying? Enjoying? Warm & fuzzy & enjoyable to be around. Yes, that's Jonathan.

November 10, 2021: Saw Lyn yesterday. She wonders how Jonathan & I can keep giving & giving & giving to JJR [Jennifer Jeanna Rose]. No gratitude, no sense of responsibility for her actions, **not even trying** to improve. She's up now; gotta run (or else she'll read over my shoulder & get upset)!

I love Jonathan.

November 13, 2021: Jonathan has [a minor surgical] procedure this morning. You always worry a little when someone you love goes to the hospital […].

JJR is useless at putting away dishes. Stacks them too high & not in the correct places. If I say anything, she blows up. Life around her is not fun […].

Jonathan & I made love yesterday; he may be out of commission for a while. It's hurting less. I love him so.

November 14, 2021: I'm in a toxic relationship I very much want to get out of […] with my daughter. She's so cruel—both verbal & physical abuse. And yet here we are.

I can't give any more. There are glimpses of gratitude, but they are so fleeting as to be almost invisible.

How did Jonathan & I raise such a self-centered, unfeeling, unthinking brat?

I so love Jonathan. He's healing & I wanted to make his healing process easier. But JJR goes out her way to needle me & does such stupid things—e.g. opening my mail, throwing out catalogues I'm interested in—that I have to react. I'm sorry, Jonathan.

November 15, 2021: Yesterday, I was in so much pain that I got nothing accomplished. ***Nothing***. Days like that are awful. Right shoulder blade mainly.

JJR is such a drag. A drain. A parasite. She tried to choke me on Saturday. Thanks a lot.

The only decent relationship I have is with Jonathan. Of course, if I'm only going to have one decent relationship, having it with my spouse is the best!

November 18, 2021: JJR is visiting Jespy House. A great weight is lifted.

Except now my body is falling apart—ulcer? (Drinking 1,000 Guilder tea seems to help.) Bladder infection or is that tingle the beginning of a herpes outbreak? Back hurts. Cancer rash area hurts. I really need to trade in this old bag of bones!

It's fun playing house with Jonathan.

November 19, 2021: JJR is back. Stress up. Jespy said they'll let us know in a week or two. That all sounds positive, especially since JJR seemed to have a good visit. She's good at impressing people in the special needs community. The issues arise when she tries to interface with typical people […]. The general population doesn't understand.

Jonathan continues to be my everything.

November 20, 2021: According to my most recent blood analysis, I should be dead. But I'm not dead (last time I checked). And I feel poorly only occasionally (after a mistletoe infusion, after JJR tries to choke me). **WHAT** is going on? CA 25.27 has exploded to over 32,000; liver enzymes are more than triple what they should (& I even gave up drinking!), ferritin—whatever that measures—is tenfold normal levels.

I'll talk with doctors sooner rather than later [...].

Jonathan put my mind at ease last night when I told him about my blood levels. I should be feeling awful if the numbers reflect anything. So much for numbers. Love prevails.

November 21, 2021: Feeling better. Was able to work yesterday on HPV & fertility paper. Slept a lot. Getting over shock of blood results. Honestly, what the **hell?** I thought my tumor markers were supposed to go **down** after subjecting myself to Ibrance [...].

We watched *Niagara* with Marilyn Monroe & Joseph Cotton yesterday. It was fun watching it with Jonathan.

Everything is fun with Jonathan. Well, maybe not **fun** (e.g. autism), but better, definitely better.

November 22, 2021: JJR has been good lately. Stress levels have fallen. Prospect of Jespy House helping immensely.

November 23, 2021: JJR tried to kill me last night. We were watching [television] when the phone rang. Suzanne was concerned that my condition has worsened because Jenny posted I have stage 4 breast cancer. So, the phone call was a result of Jenny's action. Anyway, when she didn't return to watch the show, we continued without her. She exploded. Threw a brush at my head. Had I not caught it, it would have smacked into my skull. My weak, cancer-ridden skull. Then she wanted to "hug her dolly" & proceeded to squeeze me. Jonathan got up to call the police & she started kicking him.

How could Jonathan & I have created such a loathsome human being? She's a parasite; a leech. So selfish.

She calmed enough to watch the rest of the show as well as *Gutfeld!* "Good night, Mom. I love you," she then said. "You have a funny way of showing it," I pointed out, which prompted another outburst.

I thought we had finally gotten through to her. That my illness is very serious & I need peace & quiet. I guess she offers peace & quiet as long as it doesn't interfere with her computer activity.

It's either Jespy House—if they'll have her—or an institution. She cannot remain here.

What would I do without Jonathan?

November 24, 2021: JJR goes to verge of outburst, but pulls back. Still unsettling. She wrote what an ogre I am, without mentioning why I might be so negative—constant phone calls from schools, her attacks on me, trying every conceivable treatment with minimal results. Yes, I have collapsed.

Jonathan is helping me to recovery from my collapsed state. Where would I be without him??

November 25, 2021: JJR went into NYC yesterday without telling, yet expecting us to wait up & pick her up from the train station. I wonder how she affords all this. Not my problem.

November 26, 2021: JJR almost exploded while I was getting brownies [for Thanksgiving dinner]. I mean really close to exploding. She didn't, but the threat is always there. Flora fine until we all went to bed. Then she raided the kitchen. She can't stay here overnight. We can't lock up everything.

Jonathan an absolute doll. Very concerned about my stress. I was thinking about the moment I fell in love with him. We were waiting for Jackie Mason to come on stage & Jonathan described an event as a "bacchanal" just like in a little-known Don McLean song. I thought, "Woah. This guy is smart & fun & he seems to like me." He smelled good, too. Fresh & clean. …

November 28, 2021: Excruciating leg pain on Friday night into Saturday. Wailing helped relieve the pain to a very small degree. JJR got up & started wailing, too. She seemed sincere. Difficult to take her seriously, when she's been so mean to me. Time will tell whether her concern is sincere & long-lasting or just a fleeting moment.

Legs felt better yesterday during the day so I was able to sleep, since I missed a night's slumber.

Discovered a bump on the left side of my upper forehead that is not symmetric. Probably a brain tumor. Better to think the worst.

I have to go eat since I ate very little yesterday.

Jonathan wants me to waken him when I'm in pain. I guess he could have massaged my legs.

November 29, 2021: What a disrupted life I have. Both Jonathan & I. Very disrupted lives.

Lunch with Flora yesterday was annoying. I think we over-Flo'ed this weekend. No more sleepovers, that's for sure.

How did Jonathan & I create two such creatures? He's right *we* didn't create them. We created two beautiful children. The government turned them into the creatures they are. Thanks, corrupt government. FU.

Glad to be going through this disrupted life with Jonathan. There's no one else on earth with whom I could survive.

November 30, 2021: I'm in a lot of pain. Now it's my liver. Every time I breathe deeply, it hurts; when I cough or sneeze, it hurts.

Having JJR here sure as hell doesn't help. She said we should have had her get over her mental illness before college. So, it was our—read my—fault. The thing is, we did address her illnesses before, during & after college. We're still addressing her illnesses. It would help if she would take some responsibility for her actions […]. JJR seems to have no capacity for self-reflection, or at least not how her behavior affects other people.

She accuses me of being negative. Yes, I'm negative now. I wasn't negative when we started this journey. Each doctor we visited, each treatment we followed to the "t" was going to rescue my girls. I was so hopeful. But JJR's outbursts continued through the treatments, sometimes getting worse, sometimes getting better; but they continued. They continue to this day […].

Jonathan manages to stay upbeat. I'm glad he can because I can't. I need my energy to heal.

December 2, 2021: Yesterday, went early for mistletoe infusion.

Right side very painful, especially at night. Sore throat. Anemia, big time. *I want a new body!*

JJR not bothering me since she sees how sick I am. She's still concerned about who is going to drive her places. I so hope Jespy House comes though. Soon […].

Jonathan is the world's best caretaker. Suggested Advil, which helped for two evenings in a row. So selfless. In so many ways.

PARTING

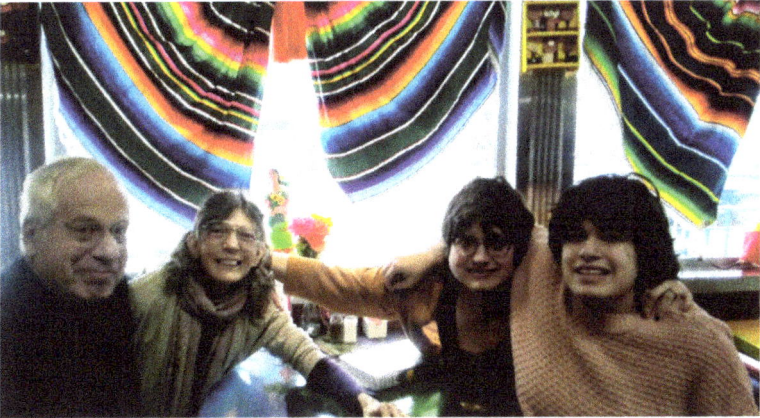

Our last family photo, November 28, 2021.

Shortly after Gayle's final diary entry, Jespy House did come through, at least provisionally. Jennifer was accepted into a community for special-needs young adults that provided housing, life skills training, psychological and medical services, job placement and coaching, and cultural activities—precisely the supports that she had always needed. But she would have to wait another year for an apartment, and meanwhile Gayle's health continued to deteriorate. She developed fluid in the lungs, which could have been caused by her cancer or by Ibrance. Dr. Levitz immediately stopped the Ibrance and checked her into Morristown Medical Center. His plan was to remove the fluid around her lung and start chemotherapy. Realizing this was her last line of defense, Gayle agreed.

It was too late. When I visited her in hospital on Christmas Day, a doctor pulled me aside and told me that the cancer was spreading throughout her body, and she was much too weak for chemotherapy. It was the bleakest of midwinters, when another Covid wave was shutting everything down, and that only magnified the indescribable loneliness that overwhelmed me. In my darkest moments of despair, I prayed, something I normally never do. I didn't seriously think that God (if He existed) would suspend the laws of medical science as a personal favor to me. But now I understand why people pray: when your back is to the wall, and you're confronting the unendurable, and you have nowhere else to turn.

Until very late in the game, we had proceeded on the assumption that Gayle would beat the odds, like her father at Pearl Harbor. After all, pessimism has no therapeutic value, and optimism greatly enhances the quality of life. Her father always said, "Never worry about the bullets you dodged." But for all of us, there will eventually be one bullet we can't dodge. Nevertheless, if, when I first met Gayle, I had known in advance what our life together would be—all the joys and all the sorrows—I would have still pursued and married her without a moment's hesitation. Whenever I think of her I think, "How did I get so lucky?"

Gayle gradually lost her grip on reality, imagining that she was hospitalized for a nervous breakdown—understandable, given what she had been through. But even when she could barely speak, she could still kiss. (Boy, could she ever!) And when, in the hospital's hospice ward, I asked if she wanted anything, she coolly said, "I want to fuck your brains out." The most life-affirming part of Gayle was still there.

Then Governor Murphy all but ended visiting hours at hospitals. When Jennifer and I were turned away at the front entrance, I exploded at the hospital worker who was just following orders. ("Gee, Dad, just like Liam Neeson!") On December 31 Gayle was moved to home hospice, where friends could freely pay a final visit. Jennifer had finally expressed sincere remorse over how she had treated her mother, and they were reconciled before the end. From that point on Jenny's violent hysterical episodes ceased completely.

Gayle lost her battle shortly after midnight on January 5, in the bed we had shared for 27 years. Though cancer had been a fact of our lives for seven-and-a-half years, we had never acquired a burial plot. We had talked about finding a bucolic spot where the girls could conveniently visit us, but never seriously looked for one. We were entirely focused on living, and I think we were right to do so, even if I had to scramble at the last minute to arrange a cremation. Gayle never thought much about an afterlife, and she may have been attracted to Judaism because it emphasized making the most of this life. L'chaim was her favorite toast. The Talmud says that we will ultimately have to answer to God for every permitted pleasure we did not enjoy in our lifetimes. I have no doubt that Gayle aced that test.

It is difficult to believe that someone as radiantly alive as Gayle will not enjoy some kind of immortality, through her work and through her children. Her diary is the monument she designed for herself: it tells us much more than any gravestone, and it is far more durable. As Winston Churchill once said, "Books last forever."

DECEMBER 25, 2022: A POSTSCRIPT
BY JENNIFER ROSE

Two things are often said by people with astute observations—that people tend to feel depressed around Christmastime, and that the worst situations tend to bring out the best in people. Last Christmas was a reflection of both viewpoints.

Things weren't easy, living with my mother struggling with cancer. We would often, but not always, butt heads, especially concerning things we didn't agree with. It drove her nuts, as it did me. There are times when I did and said things so unspeakable I couldn't believe I did so, and would do anything to take those times back. Eventually, we got into a fight over something as trivial as Christmas cards, and that was the last straw for her health.

When I realized I wouldn't be seeing my mother over Christmas due to the significant stress, I was almost heartbroken. I felt as though my own world was falling apart—support from others notwithstanding—and that there was nothing I could do.

Until I realized, I could do something for her.

I couldn't walk over to the hospital due to visiting hours, but I could reach out to others for support. So, the first thing I did when I got on my computer was log on to Twitter (as it was called then) and start posting about my mother and her health, reaching out to everyone I could. And what do you know, Tara Strong herself—one of if not the world's most famous voice actress—retweeted me. Short of actually curing my mom, it was the nicest thing she could do.

Of course, while I appreciated what Tara did for me, I couldn't help but feel guilty that this didn't come under better circumstances. After all, I didn't mind to get the attention of someone who's been an integral part of my childhood—I just didn't want Mom to die for it to happen. Talk about a double-edged sword!

Eventually, when Dad left to go see Mom at the hospital, he told me, "You wrote a lovely tribute for your grandfather for the 10th anniversary of his death. Perhaps you'd like to write something for your mother?"

"Of course," I told Dad. However, it proved to be a little easier said than done. After all, what was I going to say about her? We had so many stories together, but so few that could be put into words.

There was, however, one story that stood out.

You see, in 2019 I was slated to go to Israel for a Birthright trip during the Christmas season, but got kicked out for various reasons (poor mental health, not filling out the form on time, etc.) After getting kicked out on the 10th anniversary of my bat mitzvah, I was so heartbroken, I cried all day. At which point, Mom said, "Isn't there another trip?" Dad Googled and found one specially for handicapped young people, and in January I went on one of the last Birthright trips before they were shut down by the pandemic.

After telling Mom my story on the phone, Dad said, "Jenny, that was beautiful! Your mother was so touched!" She may have been too sick to say anything, but I could tell that deep down she knew, truly knew, that I loved her.

It's often said that miracles happen to poor kids on Christmas, and in a sense, it did. Did Mom get better? Sadly, no—her cancer was deemed terminal literally the next day. Did a miracle happen that Christmas? Yes, she finally knew, truly knew, that regardless of the way I acted, deep down I truly loved her. Many people don't even get to tell their loved ones they much care before they die, and Mom and I were lucky enough to have the opportunity.

Mom, if you're reading this, I hope you're having a wonderful Christmas, wherever you are, and just know we all love and miss you. Merry Christmas, and God bless us all.

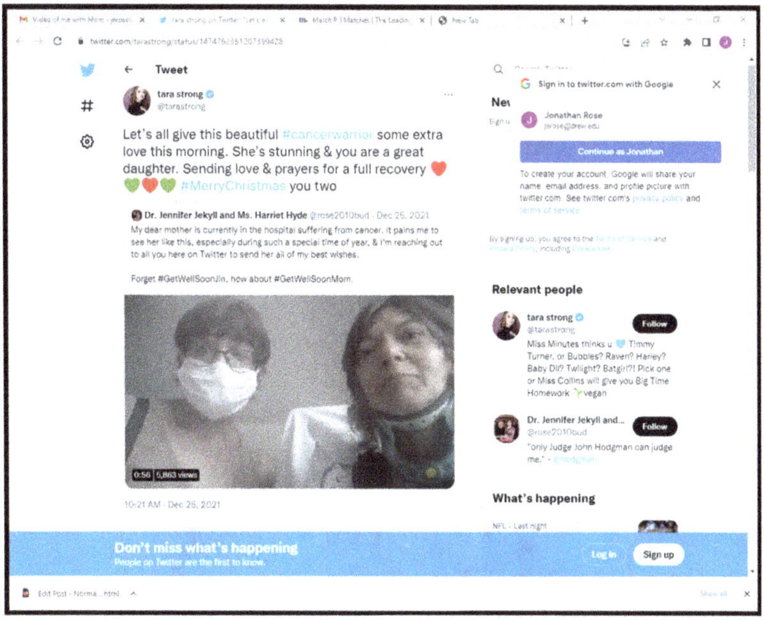
Tweet
tara strong
@tarastrong
Let's all give this beautiful #cancerwarrior some extra love this morning. She's stunning & you are a great daughter. Sending love & prayers for a full recovery #MerryChristmas you two
Dr. Jennifer Jekyll and Ms. Harriet Hyde @rose2010bud · Dec 25, 2021
My dear mother is currently in the hospital suffering from cancer. It pains me to see her like this, especially during such a special time of year, & I'm reaching out to all you here on Twitter to send her all of my best wishes.
Forget #GetWellSoonJin, how about #GetWellSoonMom.
0:56 5,863 views
10:21 AM · Dec 26, 2021
Sign in to twitter.com with Google
Jonathan Rose
Continue as Jonathan
To create your account, Google will share your name, email address, and profile picture with twitter.com. See twitter.com's privacy policy and terms of service.
Relevant people
tara strong
@tarastrong
Follow
Miss Minutes thinks u Timmy Turner, or Bubbles? Raven? Harley? Baby Dil? Twilight? Batgirl?! Pick one or Miss Collins will give you Big Time Homework vegan
Dr. Jennifer Jekyll and...
@rose2010bud
Follow
"only Judge John Hodgman can judge me."
What's happening
NFL · Last night
Don't miss what's happening
People on Twitter are the first to know.
Log in
Sign up